OXFORD MEDICAL PUBLICATIONS

Cardiac Electrophysiology and Catheter Ablation

D1707457

Oxford Specialist Handbooks published and forthcoming

General Oxford Specialist Handbooks

A Resuscitation Room Guide
Addiction Medicine
Hypertension
Perioperative Medicine, Second Edition
Post-Operative Complications, Second Edition
Pulmonary Hypertension
Renal Transplantation

Oxford Specialist Handbooks in Anaesthesia

Cardiac Anaesthesia
Day Case Surgery
General Thoracic Anaesthesia
Neuroanaesthesia
Obstetric Anaesthesia
Paediatric Anaesthesia
Regional Anaesthesia, Stimulation and Ultrasound Techniques

Oxford Specialist Handbooks in Cardiology

Adult Congenital Heart Disease
Cardiac Catheterization and Coronary Intervention
Cardiac Electrophysiology
Cardiovascular Magnetic Resonance
Echocardiography
Fetal Cardiology
Heart Failure
Nuclear Cardiology
Pacemakers and ICDs
Valvular Heart Disease

Oxford Specialist Handbooks in Critical Care

Advanced Respiratory Critical Care

Oxford Specialist Handbooks in End of Life Care

End of Life Care in Dementia
End of Life Care in Nephrology
End of Life in the Intensive Care Unit

Oxford Specialist Handbooks in Neurology

Epilepsy
Parkinson's Disease and Other Movement Disorders
Stroke Medicine

Oxford Specialist Handbooks in Paediatrics

Paediatric Dermatology
Paediatric Endocrinology and Diabetes
Paediatric Gastroenterology, Hepatology, and Nutrition
Paediatric Haematology and Oncology
Paediatric Intensive Care
Paediatric Nephrology
Paediatric Neurology
Paediatric Palliative Care
Paediatric Radiology
Paediatric Respiratory Medicine

Oxford Specialist Handbooks in Psychiatry

Child and Adolescent Psychiatry
Old Age Psychiatry

Oxford Specialist Handbooks in Radiology

Interventional Radiology
Musculoskeletal Imaging
Pulmonary Imaging

Oxford Specialist Handbooks in Surgery

Cardiothoracic Surgery
Colorectal Surgery
Hand Surgery
Liver and Pancreatobiliary Surgery
Operative Surgery, Second Edition
Oral Maxillofacial Surgery
Otolaryngology and Head and Neck Surgery
Paediatric Surgery
Plastic and Reconstructive Surgery
Surgical Oncology
Urological Surgery
Vascular Surgery

Oxford Specialist Handbooks in Cardiology

Cardiac Electrophysiology and Catheter Ablation

Yaver Bashir

Consultant Cardiologist, Department of Cardiology, John Radcliffe Hospital, Oxford, UK

Timothy R. Betts

Consultant Cardiologist and Electrophysiologist, Department of Cardiology, John Radcliffe Hospital, Oxford, UK

Kim Rajappan

Consultant Cardiologist and Electrophysiologist, Department of Cardiology, John Radcliffe Hospital, Oxford, UK

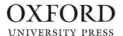

OXFORD
UNIVERSITY PRESS

OXFORD
UNIVERSITY PRESS

Great Clarendon Street, Oxford OX2 6DP

Oxford University Press is a department of the University of Oxford.
It furthers the University's objective of excellence in research, scholarship,
and education by publishing worldwide in

Oxford New York

Auckland Cape Town Dar es Salaam Hong Kong Karachi
Kuala Lumpur Madrid Melbourne Mexico City Nairobi
New Delhi Shanghai Taipei Toronto

With offices in

Argentina Austria Brazil Chile Czech Republic France Greece
Guatemala Hungary Italy Japan Poland Portugal Singapore
South Korea Switzerland Thailand Turkey Ukraine Vietnam

Oxford is a registered trade mark of Oxford University Press
in the UK and in certain other countries

Published in the United States
by Oxford University Press Inc., New York

British Library Cataloguing in Publication Data
Data available

Library of Congress Cataloging in Publication Data
Data available

Typeset by Glyph International, Bangalore, India
Printed in China
on acid-free paper through
Asia Pacific Offset

ISBN 978–0–19–955018–0

10 9 8 7 6 5 4 3 2 1

Preface

Cardiac electrophysiology is an expanding field with rapidly evolving technologies. The role of interventional electrophysiology in the management of patients with arrhythmias is increasing, particularly for atrial fibrillation. We intend this book to not only be used to provide specialist level knowledge for a broad range of medical, technical and industry personnel now involved in the specialty, but also as a resource for anyone with an interest in learning more about cardiac electrophysiology and catheter ablation.

The aim of this pocket-sized handbook is to both simplify and clarify the basic electrophysiological principles of many arrhythmias in a highly illustrated way, as well as providing practical advice on performing catheter ablation in patients with a variety of arrhythmias. Despite its small size it comprehensively covers supraventricular and ventricular arrhythmias, ablation technologies and techniques. The step-by-step approach provided is designed to facilitate the use of the book for real-life scenarios in the catheter laboratory and to demystify this traditionally inaccessible field for the wider cardiology community. Schematics, fluoroscopy, electrograms recordings, and illustrations are used to explain simple and complex electrophysiological concepts and procedures. Hints and 'top tips', gained from the authors' extensive experience, are provided to help put theory into practice.

Where necessary we hope that readers will be stimulated to look for more detail in larger, traditional textbooks or journals, but this book will serve as the day-to-day resource to which they can turn in those moments in the electrophysiology laboratory or clinic when there is a need for just a little guidance . . .

Dr Yaver Bashir
Dr Timothy R. Betts
Dr Kim Rajappan

Contents

Detailed contents

Contributors

Joe de Bono
Specialist Registrar in Cardiology,
John Radcliffe Hospital,
Oxford, UK

John Paisey
Consultant Cardiologist and
Electrophysiologist,
The Royal Bournemouth Hospital,
Bournemouth, UK

David Tomlinson
Consultant Cardiologist and
Electrophysiologist,
Derriford Hospital,
Plymouth, UK

Kelvin Wong
Senior EP Fellow,
John Radcliffe Hospital,
Oxford, UK

Arthur Yue
Consultant Cardiologist and
Electrophysiologist,
Southampton University Hospital,
Southampton, UK

Symbols and abbreviations

~	approximately
↓	decreased
↑	increased
→	leading to
±	plus/minus
🕮	cross reference
ACS	acute coronary syndrome
ACT	activated clotting time
AD	after-depolarization
AERP	atrial effective refractory period
AF	atrial fibrillation
AFl	atrial flutter
AH	atrial-His
AP	antero-posterior
AP	accessory pathway
APB	atrial premature beat
ARVC	arrhythmogenic right ventricular cardiomyopathy
ASD	atrial septal defect
ASIS	anterior superior iliac spine
ATP	anti-tachycardia pacing
AV	atrio-ventricular
AVN ERP	atrio-ventricular node effective refractory period
AVNRT	atrio-ventricular nodal re-entrant tachycardia
AVRT	atrio-ventricular re-entrant tachycardia
BBB	bundle branch block
BCT	broad complex tachycardia
BP	blood pressure
BRK	Brockenbrough (needle)
CABG	coronary artery bypass grafts
CFAE	complex fractionated atrial electrograms
CHB	complete heart block
CL	cycle length
CNS	central nervous system
CRT	cardiac resynchronization therapy
CS	coronary sinus

CT	computerized tomography
CT	crista terminalis
CVA	cerebrovascular accident
CXR	chest X-ray
DAD	delayed after-depolarization
DC	direct current
DCM	dilated cardiomyopathy
DCS	distal coronary sinus
DP	double potential
DSM	dynamic substrate mapping
DVT	deep vein thrombosis
EAD	early after-depolarization
ECG	electrocardiogram
EF	ejection fraction
EGM	electrogram
EP	electrophysiological
EPS	electrophysiological study
ERP	effective refractory period
EV	eustachian valve
FAT	focal atrial tachycardia
FBI	fast, broad, irregular
FFP	fresh frozen plasma
FO	fossa ovale
FP	fast pathway
FPERP	fast pathway effective refractory period
GA	general anaesthetic
HA	His-atrial
HCM	hypertrophic cardiomyopathy
HIFU	high frequency ultrasound
HOCM	hypertrophic obstructive cardiomyopathy
HRA	high right atrium
HRS	Heart Rhythm Society
HV	His-ventricular
IAP	incremental atrial pacing
IAS	inter atrial septum
ICD	implantable cardioverter defibrillator
ICE	intracardiac echocardiography
INR	international normalized ratio
IST	inappropriate sinus tachycardia
IV	intravenous

IVC	inferior vena cava
IVC-TA	inferior vena cava-tricuspid annulus
IVS	inter ventricular septum
JET	junctional ectopic tachycardia
LA	left atrium
LAA	left atrial appendage
LACA	left atrial circumferential ablation
LAO	left anterior oblique
LAT	local activation time
LBBB	left bundle branch block
LL	left lateral
LIPV	left inferior pulmonary vein
LMW	low molecular weight
LPV	left pulmonary venous ostia
LRA	low right atrium
LSPV	left superior pulmonary vein
LUPV	left upper pulmonary vein
LV	left ventricle
LVEF	left ventricular ejection fraction
MEA	multi-electrode array
MI	myocardial infarction
MR	magnetic resonance
MRAT	macroreentrant atrial tachycardia
MRI	magnetic resonance imaging
MV	mitral valve
MVA	mitral valve annulus
NSVT	non-sustained ventricular tachycardia
NYHA	New York Heart Association
PA	postero-anterior
PCI	percutaneous coronary intervention
PCL	pacing cycle length
PCS	proximal coronary sinus
PDF	portable document format
PES	programmed electrical stimulation
PFO	patent foramen ovale
PJRT	permanent junctional reciprocating tachycardia
PMVT	polymorphic ventricular tachycardia
POTS	postural orthostatic tachycardia syndrome
PP	Purkinje potential
PPI	post-pacing interval

PPV	positive predictive value
PSVT	paroxysmal supraventricular tachycardia
PV	pulmonary vein
PVAC	pulmonary vein ablation catheter
RA	right atrium
RAO	right anterior oblique
RBB	right bundle branch
RBBB	right bundle branch block
RCA	right coronary artery
RCT	randomized controlled trial
RF	radiofrequency
RIPV	right inferior pulmonary vein
RL	right lateral
RRP	relative refractory period
RSPV	right superior pulmonary vein
RV	right ventricle
RVA	right ventricular apex
RVOT	right ventricular outflow tract
SA	sino-atrial
SACT	sino-atrial conduction time
SAN	sino-atrial node
SCD	sudden cardiac death
SLRAT	small loop re-entrant atrial tachycardia
SLRT	small loop re-entry
SNRT	sinus node recovery time
SNRT	sinus node re-entrant tachycardia
SP	slow pathway
SPERP	slow pathway effective refractory period
SVC	superior vena cava
SVT	supraventricular tachycardia
TCL	tachycardia cycle length
TIA	transient ischaemic attack
TOE	transoesophageal echocardiography
TSP	trans-septal puncture
TTE	transthoracic echocardiography
TV	tricuspid valve
VA	ventricle-atrium
VE	ventricular ectopic
VF	ventricular fibrillation
VPB	ventricular premature beat

VPC	ventricular premature complex
VSD	ventricular septal defect
VT	ventricular tachycardia
WACA	wide-area circumferential ablation
WPW	Wolff-Parkinson-White
WSDP	widely split double potentials

Part 1

Essential background information

Chapter 1

Introduction to cardiac electrophysiology – a brief historical perspective

Within a few decades, clinical cardiac electrophysiology has evolved from an esoteric off-shoot, largely of theoretical interest to a few academic cardiologists, into one of the major sub-specialties of modern cardiology, threatening to eclipse coronary intervention in many tertiary centres in terms of workload and budgetary/resource allocation. The complexity, scope and technology of cardiac electrophysiology continue to change at a breathtaking pace and new trainees may benefit from a brief historical perspective on how the discipline has reached the current 'state of the art' and might evolve.

Early years

Following the first description of His bundle recording in the 1960s, invasive cardiac catheterization methods were rapidly adapted for routine intracardiac recording and programmed stimulation and the electrophysiological study (EPS) was born. Within a few years, these techniques had been used to unravel the mechanisms of all the common forms of supraventricular and ventricular tachycardia, and the key role of re-entry in arrhythmogenesis had been established. An early therapeutic application was surgical cure of Wolff-Parkinson-White Syndrome. During the 1970s arrhythmia surgery was extended to treat other forms of SVT refractory to medical therapy, as well as subsequently map-guided endocardial resection for VT. In addition, the insights gained from EPS provided the basis for anti-tachycardia pacing, which has been incorporated into the modern tiered-therapy ICD (it was also tried as a treatment for SVT).

The advent of catheter ablation

Despite these many important contributions, cardiac electrophysiology remained a marginal sub-specialty until the end of the 1980s – EPS was just required for the few patients undergoing surgery or receiving anti-tachycardia devices and only a small minority of tertiary centres considered it worth investing in the necessary medical expertise and facilities.

The situation was transformed by the emergence of catheter ablation. Closed chest ablation of the AV junction with standard diagnostic electrophysiology catheters and Lown defibrillators (under GA) was practised from the start of the decade but was very limited in its scope. The crucial advances were:

- Introduction of radiofrequency (RF) current as the standard power source for ablation, which was much safer and more controllable than DC shocks and obviated the need for GA in most cases.
- Commercial release of steerable ablation catheters to facilitate positioning within the heart.
- Development of detailed electrophysiological mapping techniques for identifying target sites, for example for ablation of accessory pathways.

By the early 1990s, catheter ablation of the common forms of SVT had become so straightforward and successful that arrhythmia surgery was largely supplanted; the threshold for referral of patients with this condition dropped, and almost all tertiary centres were prompted to develop their own cardiac electrophysiology services for the first time.

Era of consolidation

After an initial phase of rapid expansion, the 1990s were characterized by steady incremental progress in cardiac electrophysiology and ablation rather than further sea changes. Developments included:

- Extension of catheter ablation to common atrial flutter (cavo-tricuspid isthmus ablation) and scar-related VT.
- Replacement of traditional paper-based EPS recorders with modern digital, split-screen, multi-channel recorders offering superior performance.
- Greater customization of mapping and ablation catheters, support sheaths etc.
- Introduction of new power sources, especially saline-irrigated RF and cryoablation.

Emergence of catheter ablation for AF and VT

Although the surgical Cox-Maze procedures were developed and success-fully used to treat AF by the early 1990s, palliative AV junction ablation and pacing remained the mainstay of non-surgical treatment until recently. Nevertheless, catheter ablation for AF, the commonest arrhythmia, has always been a holy grail for electrophysiologists and the emergence of effective techniques within the past decade prompted a second phase of exponential expansion in arrhythmia services. Some of the key advances have been:

- Identification of the major role of the pulmonary veins in arrhythmogenesis and development of techniques for PV isolation and wide area circumferential ablation, and more recently linear ablation.
- Development of 3-D electroanatomic mapping techniques, more recently with image integration modalities.
- Remote navigation systems.

Over the same timeframe, ablation therapy has become increasingly important for VT associated with structural heart disease, particularly due to the inexorable growth of ICD populations, a significant propor-tion of who develop intractable ventricular arrhythmias, often resulting in multiple shock therapies. Many of the developments in 3-D mapping and power sources described above have also facilitated VT ablation but two other crucial developments have been:

- The concept of VT substrate mapping and ablation.
- The use of the epicardial route for VT mapping and ablation.

Conclusions

Current techniques for ablation of AF and VT are reasonably effective but still cumbersome and there are likely to be further technological and methodological advances over the coming years to address these short-comings. While awareness of newer developments is important, the priority for new trainees in cardiac electrophysiology is always to pick up (i) the basic principles underlying diagnostic EPS; (ii) how these techniques are applied to common presentations such as narrow complex tachycardia; (iii) a working knowledge of the electrophysiological features of the common cardiac arrhythmias; and (iv) the standard techniques for ablation of these arrhythmias. These four closely interlinked subjects constitute the major sections of this textbook.

Cardiac electrical system

Essential anatomy and physiology

The crista terminalis (CT)

This is a C-shaped muscular bundle that separates the flat-walled posterior part of the right atrium (RA) from the anterolateral trabeculated part that becomes the right atrial appendage. Superiorly it starts at the interatrial groove, anterior to the superior vena cava (SVC). It extends laterally and inferiorly to form the pectinate muscles that insert at the tricuspid valve (TV) anteriorly (Fig. 2.1).

• The CT acts as a barrier to electrical conduction (double potentials are identified along its course and it probably represents a functional rather than anatomical block – 📖 p. 310 on functional vs. anatomical block). This is critical for typical right atrial flutter (📖 p. 280).
• The CT (high, mid, or low) is often the site of origin of focal RA tachycardias in patients without structural heart disease (📖 p. 290).
• Catheter ablation of the CT has been used in patients with inappropriate sinus tachycardia (📖 p. 476).

The sino-atrial (SA) node

The sinus node is a crescent-shaped structure approximately 1.5 cm in size in the superior CT. It is mostly a subepicardial structure, separated from the RA endocardium by the CT itself, and rather than being just a discrete area as it is often depicted, it is a collection of nodal cells within a matrix of connective tissue. Complete ablation of the SA node (which is sometimes performed for inappropriate sinus tachycardia) is therefore very difficult.

The eustachian valve/ridge and the tendon of Todaro

The eustachian valve separates the inferior vena cava (IVC) from the inferior RA and is generally not seen on fluoroscopy but may often be appreciated on transoesophageal echocardiography. The eustachian ridge extends between the foramen ovale and the coronary sinus (CS) to the eustachian valve (Fig. 2.1). The tendon of Todaro lies within the eustachian ridge and runs superiorly to the AV node/His bundle. The tendon of Todaro is the lateral margin of the triangle of Koch (Fig. 2.2). Fluoroscopically the tendon runs between the upper borders of the CS os to the anteroseptal margin of the tricuspid valve annulus.

Atrio-ventricular (AV) node

The anatomy of the AV node is described in more detail in the AVNRT chapter (📖 p. 234).

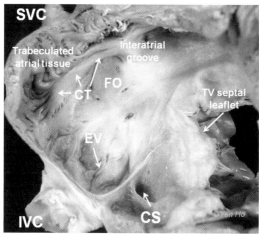

Fig. 2.1 Human right atrium with some important anatomical features labelled. The tricuspid valve (TV) orifice is seen on the right. The coronary sinus (CS) os, the eustachian valve (EV), and the fossa ovale (FO) are marked. The crista terminalis (CT) is a curved ridge that runs from the interatrial groove between the smooth posterior wall and the anterior trabeculated atrial tissue. Orientation of the specimen is almost equivalent to a straight antero-posterior projection with the superior vena cava (SVC) at the top and the inferior vena cava (IVC) at the bottom. (Image kindly provided by Professor S. Yen Ho, Imperial College, London, UK.) (📖 Plate 1 for colour version.)

The triangle of Koch

This region contains the AV node and its inferior extensions as well as the transitional fibres inserting into the compact AV node (📖 p. 234). The anatomy of the triangle is as follows:

- The tendon of Todaro makes one lateral margin.
- The septal leaflet of the TV is the other lateral margin.
- The membranous septum is located at the apex of the triangle.
- The base of the triangle is made up of the CS os and the tissue from the CS os to the TV annulus.

The triangle is particularly important in the ablation of:

- AVNRT – where anatomical variation is important to appreciate as this may affect the optimal site of ablation and minimize the risk of AV block (📖 p. 352).
- Septal and parahisian pathways – often have the atrial insertion located within the triangle.

Fossa ovale

The importance of the fossa ovale and its anatomy are described in the trans-septal puncture section (📖 p. 89).

His-Purkinje fibres

The His-Purkinje system consists of the His bundle, the left and right bundle branches, and the Purkinje network. The proximal portion of the His bundle is located on the atrial aspect of the tricuspid valve in the membranous atrial septum. The His bundle then penetrates the septum between the central fibrous body (fibrous tissue formed by the membranous septum and its confluence with the fibrous edges of the mitral and aortic valves) and the septal tricuspid valve leaflet to divide into the left and right bundle branches. The left bundle branch begins in the membranous septum below the right and non-coronary aortic cusps and divides into the left anterior (anterolateral) and posterior (posteromedial) fascicles. The right bundle is an insulated sheath of fibres that runs in the septum to the base of the RV papillary muscles and then fans out into the myocardium at the apex. The subsequent Purkinje network extends throughout the ventricular endocardium and its properties enable rapid propagation of the cardiac impulse to the ventricles simultaneously. Once the impulse leaves the Purkinje network it proceeds more slowly through the endocardium to the epicardium.

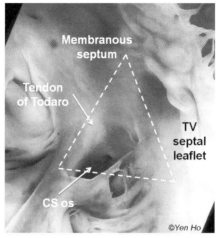

Fig. 2.2 Human necropsy specimen showing the anatomical landmarks that make up the triangle of Koch (dashed lines). The compact AV node lies at the apex of the triangle with the slow pathway fibres running along the right side of the triangle (📖 Chapter 11 on AVNRT). Note the Thebesian valve at the CS os, which is a fenestrated structure and can sometimes obstruct access to the CS. TV – tricuspid valve; CS – coronary sinus. (Image kindly provided by Professor S. Yen Ho, Imperial College, London, UK.) (📖 Plate 2 for colour version.)

The coronary sinus (CS) and the pyramidal space

The coronary sinus plays a critical role in performing electrophysiology studies. The CS os is located in the right atrium, and a diagnostic catheter can be positioned in the CS from the right atrium (either from a superior or inferior approach). As this lies in the atrio-ventricular groove, both atrial and ventricular activation can be measured. More distal positions measure lateral left-sided activation whilst more proximal positions measure septal activation (both right and left). Ablation may also be performed within the CS, both to ablate some atrio-ventricular accessory pathways, and more recently as part of some ablation strategies for atrial fibrillation. The pyramidal space is an area of the heart with the central fibrous body at the apex, the right and left atria on the lateral sides, the CS os at the base, and the muscular ventricular septum forming the floor. This space is important for mapping and ablation of septal/paraseptal pathways. Appreciation of this anatomical setup is important to explain the way that septal pathways cross the area, and it means that successful ablation of such pathways may be from the septum, in and around the CS os, on the right atrial side, or on the left atrial side (📖 p. 368).

The left atrium (LA)

Understanding of LA anatomy has increased in importance with the rapid increase in catheter ablation of atrial fibrillation (Fig. 2.3). The atrium consists of the body (which is separated from the right atrium by the foramen ovale), the LA appendage (which has pectinate muscle, unlike the smooth endocardium of the body), and the pulmonary veins (PVs) (which drain into the left atrium, and have muscular sleeves extending from the atrial body into the veins). In most individuals there are two left-sided and two right-sided PVs (Fig. 2.3) but anatomical variation is common, including a common left-sided os (short or long), which then divides into the upper and lower branches. A third PV on the right side is also seen in 10–15% of cases. Another important structure in the LA is the Bachmann bundle – this is a muscular connection between the left and right atrium anteriorly running from the level of the superior PVs to the right atrial appendage, superior to the His bundle. It is this interatrial myocardial bridge that sometimes accounts for a non-midline pattern on the CS catheter if it is advanced further round towards the left atrial appendage. The ligament of Marshall is also a left atrial structure, albeit epicardial. This neuromuscular bundle is the remnant of the left superior vena cava, and runs from the left superior PV along the AV groove to the distal CS. It has been shown to have sympathetically driven automaticity and may be implicated in the initiation and maintenance of arrhythmias such as AF.

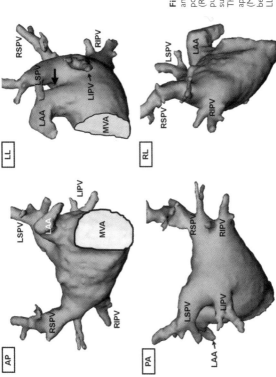

Fig. 2.3 Cardiac MR scans showing typical left atrial anatomy in four views – antero-posterior (AP), postero-anterior (PA), left lateral (LL), and right lateral (RL). Four pulmonary veins are seen: the left superior pulmonary vein (LSPV), left inferior PV (LIPV), right superior PV (RSPV), and right inferior PV (RIPV). The left atrial appendage (LAA) is marked, as is the approximate position of the mitral valve annulus (MVA). An important region for AF ablation is the ridge between the left-sided PVs and the LAA (black arrow on LL view) as this is highly variable in its thickness and this may affect the strategy for ablation in this area.

The right ventricle (RV)

The RV is the most commonly catheterized cardiac chamber at EP study. The anatomical relationship between the right atrium and RV with the tricuspid annulus is important to understand for accessory pathway mapping. The anatomy of the outflow tract is also important as this may be the site of origin for idiopathic VT (📖 p. 318).

The left ventricle (LV)

Like the RV, understanding the LV inflow (mitral valve annulus) anatomy assists with mapping and ablating left-sided accessory pathways (📖 p. 246). In the normal individual the LV cavity is more compact than the RV cavity and more trabeculated, so catheter manipulation may be more difficult.

Cardiac arrhythmia mechanisms – essential concepts

Action potential

The action potentials of cardiac myocytes are largely divided into two types:

- Normal myocytes (dependent on Na^+ influx for depolarization).
- Myocytes involved in the specialized conduction system (dependent on Ca^{2+}).

Sodium channel-dependent action potential (Fig. 3.1)

- Phase 0: rapid influx of Na^+ ions.
- Phase 1: efflux of K^+ ions.
- Phase 2: efflux of K^+ ions balanced by influx of Ca^{2+} ions (plateau).
- Phase 3: efflux of K^+ ions ('delayed rectifier' current).
- Phase 4: efflux of Na^+ and influx of K^+ (Na^+-K^+ ATPase pump).

Calcium channel-dependent action potential (Fig. 3.2)

- Phase 0: influx of Ca^{2+} ions.
- Phase 1/2/3: efflux of K^+ ions.
- Phase 4: unstable electrical property due to Ca^{2+} and K^+ rectifier currents, resulting in spontaneous depolarization.

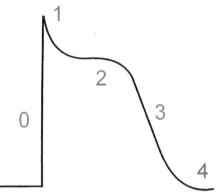

Fig. 3.1 Na^+ channel-dependent action potential. (📖 p. 16).

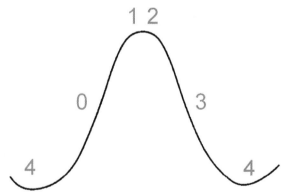

Fig. 3.2 Ca^{2+} channel-dependent action potential. (📖 p. 16).

Re-entry

Re-entry

Every cardiac cell is able to transmit impulses in every direction, but will only do so once within a short period of time – the period of time during which the cell is not able to conduct another impulse is known as the refractory period. Normally, the action potential impulse will spread through the heart quickly enough such that each cell will only respond once. However, if conduction is abnormally slow in some areas, part of the impulse will arrive late and potentially be treated as a new impulse. In other cases two limbs of the circuit have different conduction properties, e.g. the AV node and an accessory pathway. A critically timed premature beat (either atrial or ventricular) initiates the tachycardia and an excitation wave spreads around the circuit. This is maintained by the different properties of the various components of the circuit (Fig. 3.3). Depending on the timing, this can produce a sustained abnormal circuit rhythm. These re-entrant circuits are responsible for arrhythmias such as atrial flutter, atrio-ventricular nodal re-entrant tachycardia, atrio-ventricular re-entrant tachycardia, and many forms of ventricular tachycardia.

In summary, re-entry describes depolarization occurring in a closed circuit and depends on certain conditions:

- Presence of two 'pathways' with different electrophysiological properties, i.e. conduction velocities and refractory periods.
- Presence of a barrier, which may be anatomic (tricuspid valve, blood vessels, scars due to myocardial infarction, iatrogenic causes) or functional (e.g. crista terminalis).
- Path of slow conduction to prevent the depolarizing wave from catching up with the tail of repolarization, e.g. AV node, cavotricuspid isthmus, scar tissue.

The following terms may be used to describe the re-entrant circuit (Fig. 3.3):

- Cycle length is the time taken for the depolarization impulse to complete the circuit.
- Wavelength is the spatial distance of the circuit that is refractory to excitation. It is the product of the refractory period and conduction velocity.
- Temporal excitable gap is the time interval during the cycle length when the circuit may be 'excited' by an impulse/stimulus from outside the circuit.
- Spatial excitable gap is the spatial distance within the re-entrant circuit that is 'excitable'. It is the difference between the total length of the circuit and the wavelength.

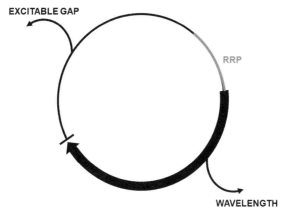

Fig. 3.3 Spatial characteristics of a re-entrant wave/circuit. (📖 p. 18). (RRP – relative refractory period.)

Automaticity and triggered activity

Automaticity

Automaticity refers to the spontaneous nature of cardiac muscle cell depolarization. It is driven by spontaneous phase 4 depolarization. All cardiac tissue has the ability to initiate an action potential; however, only some of the cells are designed to do so routinely, including the SA node, AV node, His bundle, and Purkinje fibres. Any other part of the heart that initiates an impulse is an ectopic focus. This may cause a single premature beat or produce a sustained arrhythmia. Conditions that increase such ectopic automaticity include sympathetic nervous system stimulation and hypoxia. At a cellular level it is probably a reduction in intercellular coupling that removes the inhibitory influence of ion flow and enables cells to fire at their intrinsic rate. Fibrosis may enable uncoupling at a structural level. An increase in intracellular Ca^{2+} may decrease gap junction conductance and again increase uncoupling.

Triggered activity

Triggered activity occurs by a non-re-entrant mechanism that appears to be primarily due to after-depolarization, which may be classified as early after-depolarization (EAD) if it occurs in phases 2 or 3 of the action potential, and delayed after-depolarization (DAD) if it occurs in phase 4 of the action potential (Fig. 3.4). They are thought to arise from altered cellular calcium handling and ionic currents. They are responsible for arrhythmia in long QT syndromes and digitalis toxicity.

Practical note

The differentiation between automaticity and triggered activity 📖 Table 3.1, p. 22 in the clinical setting may be relatively unimportant. Where catheter ablation is being performed for either type of arrhythmia, the aim is to initiate the tachycardia and identify its origin, which will be at the site of earliest activation. Ablation at this site should render the arrhythmia non-inducible whatever the mechanism.

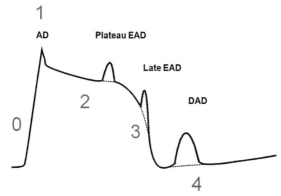

Fig. 3.4 The same Na$^+$-dependent action potential as in Fig. 3.1. is shown. Triggered activities are caused by after-depolarization (AD) currents. These may be early (EAD) or delayed (DAD) and can be responsible for both automatic and re-entrant arrhythmia.

Re-entry vs. automaticity vs. triggered activity

Differentiating the arrhythmia mechanisms

Table 3.1 Differentiating the arrhythmia mechanisms

	Re-entry	Triggered activity	Automaticity
Initiation by programmed stimulation	yes	yes	no
Termination by programmed stimulation	yes, abruptly	yes, usually gradually	no
Resetting	yes	yes	yes, usually flat response
Entrainment	yes	no	no
Site specificity of entrainment	yes	no	no
Overdrive suppression	no	yes	yes
Overdrive acceleration	yes	yes	yes
Adenosine sensitivity	yes/no	yes	no
Catecholamine sensitivity	yes/no	yes	yes

Role of programmed stimulation and intracardiac recording

Introduction

In the electrophysiology laboratory, programmed stimulation is important in the study of arrhythmia mechanisms and their treatment. It may be in the form of single, double, or multiple extrastimuli or rapid burst pacing. It may be useful for the following:
- Initiation of arrhythmia.
- Termination of arrhythmia.
- In cases of sustained arrhythmia that are well tolerated clinically, programmed stimulation is used to interact with the arrhythmia. The responses to extrastimuli testing and overdrive pacing (i.e. patterns of reset, entrainment, overdrive suppression/acceleration) provide further information on the arrhythmia.

During sustained arrhythmia, the ability of programmed stimulation to affect or interact with the arrhythmia depends on the following factors:
- Tachycardia cycle length.
- Refractory periods at the sites of stimulation.
- Distance to the area responsible for the arrhythmia.
- Conduction times to and from the area responsible for the arrhythmia.
- In cases of re-entrant tachycardia, the duration of the temporal excitable gap.

Inducibility

Programmed stimulation using the extrastimulus technique or incremental pacing is used to induce arrhythmia. This is usually performed sequentially in the ventricles and atria. Arrhythmia that is initiated by programmed stimulation is due to re-entry or triggered activity. The latter is often induced by incremental pacing. Sometimes, pharmacological adjuncts are required.

Initiating re-entrant arrhythmia (Fig. 3.5)

An impulse may block antegradely in one limb of the pathway with a longer refractory period. It then travels antegradely down the other pathway with shorter refractory period and slower conduction velocity before conducting retrogradely up the first pathway, which has recovered, thus forming a closed re-entry circuit.

Inducing arrhythmia is important for the following reasons:
• Mode of initiation may give a clue to the mechanism of the arrhythmia.
• To confirm that it is clinical arrhythmia in terms of ECG and patient's symptoms.
• To assess the haemodynamic consequences of the arrhythmia (albeit under controlled laboratory conditions).
• To act as a baseline for comparison after delivery of ablation treatment, i.e. so that there is an appropriate endpoint for treatment.
• To allow us to study different ways to terminate the arrhythmia.
• To search for any other arrhythmias.
• In paroxysmal AF ablation as a possible endpoint.

Sometimes, sustained arrhythmia may not be inducible and treatment may not be offered on that occasion. In some cases, a substrate for arrhythmia may be found and it may be appropriate to perform definitive treatment (e.g. evidence of AV nodal duality with echoes in a patient with clearly documented adenosine-sensitive narrow complex tachycardia).

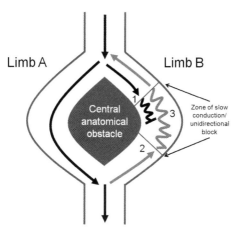

Fig. 3.5 Diagram showing initiation of re-entrant arrhythmia. Limbs A and B represent two pathways with different electrophysiological properties, surrounding a central anatomical obstacle, with a zone of slow conduction/unidirectional block in limb B. Classically limb A has slower conduction velocity but a shorter refractory period. The initial antegrade impulse (1) therefore propagates antegradely down limbs A and B, blocks in limb B (1), but continues down the slower limb A. If there is enough of a delay then the slow impulse excites limb B retrogradely (2) and returns to the zone of slow conduction, which allows excitation and propagation of the wavefront in this direction (3). As the wavefront returns, if limb A is no longer refractory then the wavefront is again propagated down this limb and a re-entrant circuit is formed.

Resetting

Resetting (Fig. 3.6)

During sustained re-entrant arrhythmia, a premature impulse may enter the excitable gap of the circuit before dividing into two wavefronts: the antidromic/retrograde wavefront (opposite in direction to the re-entrant tachycardia) collides with the preceding tachycardia wavefront, while the other wavefront is conducted orthodromically through the re-entrant circuit and exits at an earlier time (compared to the next expected beat of the re-entrant tachycardia). This phenomenon is termed resetting. Resetting is defined by the tachycardia being advanced by at least 20 ms.

For resetting to happen, the following conditions must be satisfied:
- The return tachycardia should have the same morphology and cycle length as before.
- The premature impulse should find the excitable gap and 'invade' the re-entrant circuit.

Resetting depends on 'invasion' of the re-entrant circuit by a premature impulse. This can be achieved with single, double, or multiple extrastimuli and can happen over a range of coupling intervals. In practice, introducing two or more extrastimuli and pacing near the re-entrant circuit facilitates the invasion of the re-entrant circuit by the premature impulse.

Post-pacing interval (📖 Chapter 22)

The post-pacing interval (PPI) is the return cycle length as measured from the last stimulus to the return electrogram in the pacing electrode. It represents the time taken for the impulse to travel from the pacing site to the tachycardia focus/circuit, around the circuit, and back to the pacing site. Hence, pacing sites that are remote from the tachycardia circuit exhibit long PPIs and those within the circuit will have PPIs within 30 ms of the tachycardia cycle length.

Note

- The range of coupling intervals from the onset of resetting to termination of the tachycardia reflects the duration of the excitable gap.
- Resetting response may be characterized by plotting the return cycle length against the coupling intervals (especially in VT):
  - Flat, increasing (increasing return cycle lengths with decreasing coupling intervals), or mixed flat and increasing curves are typical for re-entrant tachycardia.
  - Flat or decreasing curves may be seen in arrhythmia secondary to triggered activity.
  - Flat response for automatic tachycardia.
- Pacing from different sites may affect the resetting response in a re-entrant tachycardia, but site specificity of resetting is not a feature of automaticity or triggered activity.

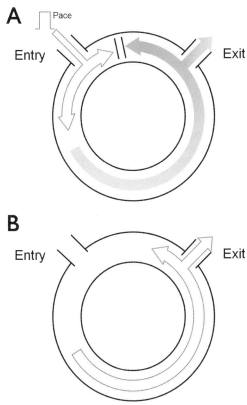

Fig. 3.6 Schematic diagram showing the principle of resetting. In (A) a re-entrant impulse is shown in grey, which has an entry and exit site. A paced stimulus (Pace) is introduced prematurely and collides retrogradely with the advancing impulse terminating this. However, the antegrade pacing stimulus enters the circuit at a point where the tissue is excitable and follows the original re-entrant circuit (B), but earlier than would have been the case had the original re-entrant impulse continued, i.e. reset.

Entrainment

Entrainment

A re-entrant tachycardia may be reset by premature extrastimuli. If a train of pacing stimuli is delivered with a pacing cycle length shorter than the tachycardia cycle length, the tachycardia may be continuously reset with each successive pacing stimulus. This phenomenon of continuous resetting is termed entrainment. Entrainment is present when at least two consecutive stimuli are conducted orthodromically through the circuit with the same conduction time.

Any one of the following criteria, if present, is widely used as support for entrainment being present, although they are not essential:
• Fixed fusion of paced complexes at constant pacing rate.
• Progressive fusion with faster pacing rates.
• Resumption of the tachycardia with a non-fused complex at a return cycle length that is equal to the pacing cycle length (when measured from the local pre-systolic electrogram).

While these criteria do support entrainment, absence of these criteria does not absolutely indicate the absence of entrainment. Resetting is the physiologic basis for entrainment.

Fusion (manifest/local/concealed, 📖 Chapter 22)

Fusion occurs when two wavefronts of activation (one from the pacing stimulus and the other exiting from the re-entrant circuit) occur at the same time. The QRS morphology, P wave morphology, or activation sequence is intermediate, representing a fusion of the fully paced rhythm and the re-entrant tachycardia.

Fusion that is evident on ECG depends on the following factors:
• Significant dissimilarity between the paced rhythm and the re-entrant tachycardia.
• Significant proportion of the myocardium activated by both wavefronts, sufficient to have an effect on surface ECG.
• Pacing cycle length that is necessary for resetting (the shorter the cycle length, the more it resembles the fully paced rhythm, i.e. progressive fusion).

Local fusion occurs when there is resetting of the tachycardia and when the local electrogram within the re-entrant circuit (usually involving a pre-systolic component) is unchanged in morphology. Local fusion may be demonstrated when there is no apparent ECG fusion.

When the pacing site is either within the re-entrant circuit or a bystander location arising from the circuit, the pacing impulse is conducted orthodromically within the circuit before exiting into the myocardium. Hence, QRS or P wave morphologies and activation sequences will be identical to the re-entrant tachycardia. This is termed concealed fusion. Sometimes, the orthodromic conduction time is long, resulting in a long stimulus to QRS time, i.e. latency (📖 Fig. 22.6, p. 493).

Entrainment is useful because:
• It proves that the arrhythmia mechanism is re-entry.
• It is used to find out if a location is part of the re-entrant circuit, i.e. PPI within 30 ms of tachycardia cycle length.
• It may also help determine if a site is likely to be a good target for ablation, e.g. concealed fusion with latency and good PPI for VT ablation.

Uses of entrainment/resetting manoeuvres

Atrial flutter	Entrainment at the cavotricuspid isthmus is important to show that it is part of the circuit. If not, other atypical flutters such as lower loop re-entry and left atrial flutter should be considered (📖 p. 282).
Atrial tachycardia/ AVNRT/AVRT	Ventricular entrainment is useful to distinguish atrial tachycardia (VAAV response) from AVNRT/AVRT (VAV response). His synchronous ventricular premature beat does not reset AVNRT but may reset AVRT (📖 p. 172).
Ventricular tachycardia	Entrainment mapping is used to complement activation mapping, substrate mapping, and pace mapping. The diastolic pathway is a target for ablation and may be identified by concealed entrainment with latency and good PPI (📖 p. 492).

Pace termination/ anti-tachycardia pacing

Pace termination (Fig. 3.7)

Pace termination may be used effectively to terminate a re-entrant tachycardia. This may be achieved by extrastimulus or rapid pacing. The principle of pace termination is that an impulse enters the re-entrant circuit and collides antidromically with the depolarizing head of the preceding wavefront and orthodromically with the refractory tail at a critical point in time. Resetting usually precedes termination if there is more than one extrastimulus.

The factors that may affect the effectiveness of pace termination are:
- The tachycardia cycle length (most important).
- Duration of the excitable gap.
- Distance of pacing site from the re-entrant circuit.
- Conduction velocity and refractory period of the tissue between the pacing site and the re-entrant circuit.
- Size of the re-entrant circuit.

In general:
- Success of pace termination is directly related to the number of extra-stimuli and rapid pacing is the most effective. However, rapid pacing may also terminate and reinitiate tachycardia.
- The shorter the cycle length, the lower the chance of pace termination, i.e. VT < 300 ms.
- Combination of overdrive pacing and extrastimuli may be effective.
- VT with short cycle lengths and rapid pacing may result in acceleration of VT.
- A steeper slope of an increasing resetting response pattern and resetting with long coupling intervals predict greater success of pace termination.
- May be site dependent.
- Increasing the pacing current may improve the chances by decreasing the measured local refractoriness.
- Pharmacological adjuncts may be considered.
- In cases of haemodynamic compromise, DC cardioversion should be used.

Anti-tachycardia pacing (ATP)

Two methods commonly used in devices for treating VT:
- Burst pacing (set number of impulses at a constant cycle length).
- Ramp or auto-decremental pacing (a set number of impulses with decreasing cycle lengths).

Both modalities seem to be equally effective, although some studies have shown that ramp pacing is better. Newer pacing modalities with rate-adaptive characteristics (i.e. varying the coupling intervals according to the tachycardia cycle length) may reduce the incidence of acceleration. ATP is always used with a back-up defibrillator. ATP for atrial arrhythmia has been largely abandoned.

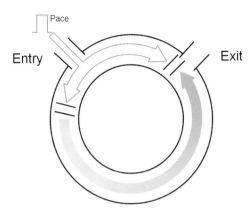

Fig. 3.7 Schematic diagram showing termination in a re-entrant circuit with pacing. The stimulated impulse (Pace) collides with the re-entrant impulse (grey) retrogradely before it exits, but unlike with resetting (Fig. 3.6) the antegrade stimulus arrives at the tissue when it is still refractory and the stimulus is blocked.

The diagnostic intracardiac electrophysiology study: essential information and basic principles

Introduction

Diagnostic intracardiac EPS is the foundation stone of modern arrhythmia management. Until the 1990s it was performed as a stand-alone procedure, usually to guide drug therapy or arrhythmia surgery. It could be conducted in detail without time constraints, followed by careful postoperative analysis of the paper traces, an arrangement conducive to training new specialists. The learning process has grown more challenging due to:
- Time pressures to limit diagnostic EPS now that combined diagnostic/ablation procedures have become the norm.
- Cost pressures to sacrifice the number of multi-polar catheters used.
- Digital recording systems, which allow limited time for off-line analysis.

A thorough knowledge of standard EPS techniques and understanding of the underlying principles remains crucial for trainees aspiring to undertake catheter ablation. They should always follow a systematic approach with basic checklists to avoid diagnostic pitfalls – substantial experience is needed to conduct EPS to a high standard under time pressure, with the ability to take shortcuts safely where appropriate but also to recognize unexpected/unusual patterns promptly and adapt accordingly.

Expertise in EPS develops through following standard procedures and pattern recognition but also depends on an appreciation of key concepts:
- Distinction between **refractoriness** and **conduction velocity** as the fundamental electrical properties of excitable cardiac tissues.
- **Decremental** vs. **non-decremental conduction** dynamics, the former being a characteristic property of the AV node (📖 p. 62).
- The role of **re-entry** in most cardiac arrhythmias and the significance of the **excitable gap** – this underpins our ability to initiate and terminate tachycardias by **programmed stimulation**, and the utility of pacing manoeuvres such as **resetting** and **entrainment** (📖 pp. 18, 23, 26, 28).

Indications for EPS
- Diagnosis of narrow complex tachycardia (📖 p. 130) to establish the arrhythmia mechanism, generally as a prelude to catheter ablation.
- Diagnosis of broad complex tachycardia (📖 p. 190) to establish the arrhythmia mechanism, particularly differentiating SVT, VT, and pre-excited tachycardias, to enable selection of appropriate treatment.
- Risk stratification for sudden death (📖 pp. 212, 257):
  - post-infarction patients
  - Brugada syndrome
  - WPW syndrome.

Rarely:
- Investigation of bradyarrhythmias:
  - sinus node function
  - AV conduction ('His bundle study').
- Investigation of undiagnosed syncope or paroxysmal tachycardia.
- To test and fine-tune anti-tachycardia pacing algorithms.

'Electropharmacological testing' to assess the efficacy of anti-arrhythmic drugs in VT patients was once widely practised but has now largely been discredited.

Patient preparation

The exact preparation required depends upon the type of procedure (diagnostic ± ablation) being performed and is detailed in each of the relevant chapters. However, there are some general principles as outlined below.

Anti-arrhythmic drugs

Where arrhythmia inducibility is important for diagnosis at EP study these should be stopped 4–5 half-lives before the procedure. The long half-life of amiodarone means either that it needs to be stopped 6+ weeks before the procedure, or else a decision must be made that it is simply continued through to the procedure. For all anti-arrhythmics the possibility that discontinuation may provoke arrhythmia must be considered and the patient warned appropriately.

Anticoagulant drugs

In general, performing an ablation in a patient taking anti-platelet agents, e.g. aspirin, is not a problem. The combination of aspirin and clopidogrel may increase the risk of bleeding and the decision to stop one (normally clopidogrel) depends upon the risk for the patient, e.g. have they had a recent PCI with a drug eluting stent? Warfarin may be continued for ablation of persistent atrial flutter, and increasingly also for persistent atrial fibrillation. If the patient is already in sinus rhythm, or has paroxysmal arrhythmia then the warfarin can be discontinued.

Informed consent

The name of the procedure (do not use abbreviations on consent forms) and the specific indication for the procedure need to be explained in non-medical terms to the patient and documented. Complications and the approximate risks of these for the specific procedure must also be documented. The specific frequencies of complications are listed in the individual ablation chapters but there are some general categories to consider:

- Vascular access: haematoma; DVT; AV fistula; arterial pseudoaneurysm; pneumothorax (if subclavian approach used).
- Catheter manipulation: vascular damage; microemboli, particularly in the left ventricle, and risk of stroke; coronary artery dissection if retrograde aortic approach used; cardiac perforation and tamponade.
- Radiation exposure: with careful management this can be kept to a minimum and therefore need not be specifically commented upon. In patients of child-bearing age, the possibility of pregnancy must be specifically checked.
- RF application: AV nodal damage requiring permanent pacemaker implantation; cardiac tamponade; coronary artery damage if an epicardial approach is used; chest pain (both acutely and, in a very small proportion of patients, chronically).
- Myocardial infarct, stroke, or death. Mortality is uncommon in 'normal heart' ablation (<0.1%) but may be up to 2% in some ablations (e.g. ischaemic VT). Similarly myocardial infarct and stroke risk are very low in most patients, but some procedures carry higher risk, e.g. extensive left atrial ablation for AF carries a higher stroke risk.

Sedation and general anaesthesia

The use of sedation or general anaesthesia for procedures depends upon a number of factors including local protocols. Conscious sedation can be used for most procedures, particularly as general anaesthesia may be more likely to render arrhythmia non-inducible. An example of sedation/analgesia protocols is:

• Midazolam (up to 0.2 mg/kg/hr); and
• Fentanyl (up to 2 mcg/kg/hr) IV.

Other drugs used include diazemuls, diamorphine, morphine, and propofol.

General anaesthesia is more frequently used for ablation in patients for VT ablation with significant structural heart disease, atrial fibrillation ablation, or in those undergoing epicardial ablation. All of these may also be safely performed with conscious sedation. Paediatric EP studies and ablation are also normally performed under general anaesthesia.

Intravenous access and monitoring

Peripheral IV access is needed before commencing any EP study. This may be for administration of sedation/analgesia, or for other drugs such as provocation agents. Because of the use of sedation or general anaesthesia, patients are usually fasted for at least six hours. Once in the lab the patient is connected to various monitors (commonly non-invasive blood pressure, oxygen saturation, and if necessary remote defibrillation electrode pads). Twelve-lead ECG recording is continuous and normally through the EP recording system so radiolucent electrodes are attached in the standard surface positions so that they do not interfere with fluoroscopic imaging.

Equipment setup and laboratory design

Trainees in cardiac electrophysiology should be familiar with the essential and desirable equipment list for a functioning EP lab and ensure that they are fully conversant with the operation of the units in their own department, rather than relying entirely on technical and nursing staff. In addition, it is important to understand the issues surrounding lab design and layout. Although often dismissed as self-evident, these are frequently overlooked in the commissioning of new facilities, resulting in significant inconvenience and/or clinical risk. After installation, it can be very difficult to correct any problems with the layout.

Equipment checklist

- General catheterization lab equipment (radiographic table, fluoroscopy/cine unit, haemodynamics, external defibrillator etc.).
- Multi-channel electrophysiological recording system:
  - digital with optical drive for archiving, plus selected paper printouts
  - dual screen, one for real-time display, other for review/analysis
  - usually 20+ channels in modern systems
  - slaved display screens for operator (gantry) and control room.
- Programmable stimulator for pacing and extrastimulus techniques:
  - integral to the recording system or interfaced
  - minimum two channels (e.g. for pacing A and V simultaneously).
- Junction box to interface the catheter connections with the recorder and stimulator.
- 3-D electro-anatomical mapping system (CARTO or NavX) (📖 CARTO mapping p. 100 and NavX mapping, p. 104), interfaced with standard electrophysiological recording system.
- Radiofrequency (RF) current ablation generator, including irrigation facility for cooled-tip ablation.
- Optional but desirable equipment includes facilities for internal DC cardioversion, cryoablation, and intracardiac echocardiography (ICE).

Laboratory layout/design

This partly depends on availability of space and whether the lab is also being used for device implantation and/or general cardiac catheterization. Important features include:
- Clear operator view of gantry screens including fluoroscopy (active and image-reference), haemodynamics, electrophysiological recorder (dynamic and review), and 3-D system. Also the ability to switch gantry to either side of the table, e.g. operating from left subclavian approach.
- Sufficient room and adjustable lighting to facilitate access to the head/neck areas for subclavian or jugular procedures. Ideally the radiographic table should be adjustable for head-down tilt.
- Reliable two-way intercom with control area.
- Protective shielding of equipment cables to limit risk of physical damage and electromagnetic interference (but ideally still accessible for repair or replacement).
- Space for GA procedures or other bulky equipment such as ICE machine or cryoablation generator.

Equipment specifics

Stimulator and EP recording system

The basic requirements of the electrophysiology laboratory include a means of measuring and displaying the electrograms, recording these for interpretation both in real-time and review, and the ability to stimulate the myocardium. The *stimulator* provides a means of introducing paced beats into the cardiac chamber of choice. It is common for both the current and the pulse width to be adjustable, with the output set at twice the diastolic threshold (the minimum current in milliamps for a given pulse width that will capture the myocardium). The stimulator is able to provide different pacing options – standard pacing at a fixed rate or programmed stimulation. The *EP recording system* provides a means of acquiring the intracardiac signal recorded by an appropriately positioned catheter. This is then amplified and filtered to remove unwanted components of the signal (see 📖 p. 54). Caution needs to be exercised with filtering to avoid inadvertently altering the signal in such a way that either the useful information is removed or the resulting signal leads to misinterpretation.

Imaging
Fluoroscopy
Imaging during EP studies is mostly with conventional radiographic fluoroscopy. The radiation dose that both the patient and the operator are exposed to is an important safety consideration of any procedure. The use of low frequency pulsed imaging enables visualization of the catheters with sufficient accuracy whilst minimizing the dose. Also, by operating in the PA projection the scattered dose to the operator is kept low (the LAO projection being worst for scatter to the operator). The use of biplane fluoroscopy may minimize movement of the image intensifier but many labs use monoplane routinely.

Intracardiac echocardiography
This technique is used by some operators routinely in certain procedures, e.g. AF ablation. Although it can be very helpful in delineating anatomy very precisely and in monitoring ablation for potential complications (microbubble formation during excessive heating). Because of its expense this may not be cost-effective.

3D Mapping systems
Recent developments have enabled mapping of more complex arrhythmias other than with conventional electrogram recording and fluoroscopy alone. For a more detailed description 📖 Chapter 6.

Remote navigation systems
There are currently two systems that can be used to remotely manipulate catheters within the heart. The Stereotaxis system (Stereotaxis, Inc., St. Louis, MO) uses computer-controlled, externally applied magnetic fields that precisely and directly govern the motion of the internal working tip of the catheter. This requires two large magnets (one on either side of the patient) and specifically designed catheters with a 'magnetic' tip. The Sensei X Robotic Catheter System (Hansen Medical Mountain View, CA)

uses a specially designed catheter manipulation system that can guide a standard proprietary catheter tip within the heart, again accurately and with stability that may be superior to manual catheter manipulation.

Practical tips: common settings on an EP system

His bundle and most intracardiac electrograms are best visualized when the signal is filtered at 30–40 Hz (high pass) and 400–500 Hz (low pass). If the filter settings are too high then critical components of the signal may be filtered out, whereas if the filters are too low the signal may be very 'noisy' and small deflections (such as the His) may be obscured (📖 p. 54).

Catheter technology

Catheter design varies greatly. The simplest diagnostic catheters have a fixed shape and a small number of poles for both recording and pacing, whilst other catheters may be steerable, have multiple poles, or allow irrigation of fluid to the tip during ablation. The choice of which catheter to use depends upon the indication. For diagnostic studies the catheters vary from 5 to 7 French. The simplest are quadripolar (four poles arranged as two pairs). Those with smaller interelectrode spacing enable recording of signals over a small, specific area. Larger electrode spacing allows more rapid acquisition of information over a larger area. Ablation catheters are usually larger (7 or 8 French) and have a variety of designs depending on the arrhythmia being ablated. The distal electrode size and the energy source used are two of the design features that can affect lesion efficacy and size.

Radiofrequency energy

Radiofrequency (RF) energy is the commonest form of ablation energy used. Electromagnetic energy is converted to thermal energy. The principle is known as 'resistive heating': as electrical current passes through a medium (in this case tissue) the voltage drops and heat is generated. Usually the electrical current is unipolar, i.e. an indifferent electrode (commonly an adhesive patch on the skin) is needed to complete the circuit. Typically the frequency used is 500 kHz – lower frequencies are more likely to stimulate cardiac muscle/nerves; higher frequencies do not cause resistive heating and conventional catheters do not transmit this 'microwave' energy efficiently. Resistive heating only occurs within a few millimetres of the tissue surface. Further heating is 'conductive' and the depth depends on the size of the initial resistive heat source. The size of the initial heat source depends upon the power, the electrode diameter and length, and the area of contact. Convective cooling of blood flowing over the tissue dissipates the heat and reduces energy delivery to the tissue.

Conventional vs. cooled-tip catheters

The heating of tissue with RF at high temperatures is limited by an associated rise in impedance. Ablation that is temperature limited, i.e. limited to a pre-specified upper temperature limit, may therefore limit power delivery. If the catheter tip temperature can be kept lower, then more power can be delivered to the tissue and a larger lesion created. This theory underpins the use of cooled-tip catheters, where the tip of the catheter is kept at a lower temperature, usually through the irrigation of fluid around the tip (either in a closed loop around the inside of the catheter tip electrode, or through open irrigation ports at the catheter tip). Experimental studies have demonstrated that this results in the maximum temperature during ablation occurring deeper in the myocardium rather than at the surface. This may be particularly helpful in areas where there is relatively little blood flow to provide natural convective cooling and the temperature at the tip of the catheter would otherwise rise quickly, preventing power delivery.

Distal electrode size

The distal electrode size will vary depending upon the type of energy delivery but they range from 3 to 10 mm, with 4 mm being a common size for radiofrequency (RF) ablation catheters.

Table 4.1 Factors affecting lesion size

Factor	Effect on lesion size
Power	Directly proportional
Electrode temperature	Directly proportional
Energy delivery duration	Exponential (5–10 second $t_{1/2}$)
Contact pressure	Directly proportional
Electrode size	Directly proportional
Blood flow	May reduce lesion size if flow acts as a heat sink (either around the electrode–tissue interface or within the tissue below the surface of the electrode)
Scar	Smaller lesions

Cryoablation

Cryothermal energy was previously used in non-cardiac applications and is now used for catheter ablation routinely. In order to create a lesion the tissue must first go through a 'freeze' phase with intracellular and extracellular ice crystal formation. 'Thawing' then causes cell swelling and membrane rupture, creating irreversible damage. Over the next 48 hours there is then a haemorrhagic/inflammatory phase and finally a fibrotic phase (both similar to RF). The benefits of cryoablation are:

• It is painless (unlike RF, which can be very painful) and may be used in patients where ablation would normally require significant sedation/ analgesia (e.g. cavotricuspid isthmus ablation) but is not desirable for medical reasons (e.g. respiratory depression).
• The tissue can be cooled to a temperature (approx. −30°C) at which the effect can be monitored ('freeze mapping'). If there are adverse signs then the cooling is stopped and the effect is still reversible. If the effect is desirable then the catheter tip is cooled to a temperature at which irreversible damage occurs (−80°C). An example of where this is useful is ablation of anteroseptal accessory pathways (📖 p. 370 in AP section). Some operators also use cryoablation for slow pathway ablation because they believe it reduces the risk of causing AV block (📖 p. 358 in AVNRT section).
• Once the catheter tip is cooled below −20°C the tip becomes firmly adherent to the tissues. This can be helpful in providing stability during ablation, e.g. if ablating during tachycardia the catheter will not displace as sinus rhythm resumes, or can allow programmed stimulation to be performed whilst 'freeze mapping' without displacing the catheter.
• Cryoablation is also used for atrial fibrillation using special balloon catheters that ablate circumferentially around the pulmonary vein ostium/antrum.

Other ablation energy sources

A number of alternative energy sources have been used to try to overcome some of the limitations of RF, particularly the need for good tissue contact with the latter:

Microwave – creates thermal energy like RF but unlike RF the mechanism is dielectric. Electromagnetic radiation is converted to kinetic energy. These waves can get into tissue from virtually any distance and therefore this is particularly useful for penetrating scar tissue.

High intensity frequency ultrasound (HIFU) – vibration energy is propagated as a mechanical wave. When this wave hits an absorbing medium such as tissue it is converted to heat. HIFU may be used to focus energy and create lesions at a particular distance from the transducer, penetrating through any tissue in between.

Laser (Light Amplification by Stimulated Emission of Radiation) – the ability of laser light to be highly focused means that large, deep lesions can be created by subsequent energy scatter within the tissue. A number of different lasers have been tried including argon, YAG, and diode.

Bipolar RF – this type of RF has been particularly used in the ablation of atrial fibrillation.

Vascular access

General

In order to position the catheters at various intracardiac positions, access to the vascular tree is required. The modified Seldinger technique is used to gain access to the vascular tree, either from the upper or lower extremity. In most cases, venous access is obtained from the femoral vein and would allow catheter placement in the right atrium (RA), right ventricle (RV), coronary sinus (CS), and the left side of the heart after a transseptal puncture. Some groups routinely use venous access from the upper extremity (jugular/subclavian) for the coronary sinus catheter, or if positioning of the catheters is difficult or impossible, use the inferior approach. Arterial access is needed when using the 'retrograde' approach to map or ablate on the left side of the heart. It is also useful for haemodynamic monitoring during procedures.

Operators differ regarding the maximum number of catheters introduced via a single vein (two to four in adults, usually no more than two in children), and whether to perform a single puncture and 'multi-wire', or to perform multiple punctures (possibly less risk of bleeding).

Lower extremity (Fig. 4.1)

Both right- or left-sided vessels may be used. Right is often easier as most operators are right-handed. The groins may need to be shaved and legs should be slightly adducted and externally rotated.

Femoral artery

- The inguinal ligament extends from the anterior superior iliac spine (ASIS) to the pubic symphysis.
- The artery is located by palpating just below the midpoint of the inguinal ligament.
- Advance the cannulation needle about 2 cm below the inguinal ligament (usually at the groin crease) at 30–45° to the skin surface.
- Sometimes it may be helpful to use fluoroscopy to guide puncture over the femoral head.

Femoral vein

- The femoral artery is palpated as above.
- The femoral vein runs parallel and within 2 cm medial to the femoral artery.
- Advance the cannulation needle at 30–45° to the skin surface at or just below the level of the skin crease.
- The femoral vein usually lies about 2–4 cm below the skin surface.
- Usually limit to two to three catheters in each vein.

Practical tips

• Inadvertent puncture of the femoral artery happens when the needle is directed too laterally, especially at the level of the groin crease when the artery and veins lie close together.
• If arterial and venous access is needed on the same side, ensure that the venous and arterial punctures are adequately separated. If there is inadvertent arterial puncture, ensure that there is haemostasis before getting venous access. This is to reduce the risk of arterio-venous fistula.

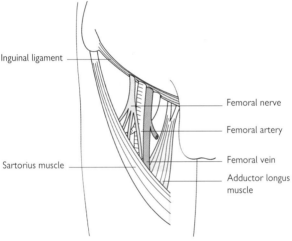

Fig. 4.1 Right femoral vein anatomy. Reproduced from Myerson S, Choudhury RP, and Mitchell ARJ (2006) *Emergencies in Cardiology*, Oxford University Press.

Upper extremity (Figs. 4.2 and 4.3)
Needed when an inferior approach is unavailable (e.g. anomalous IVC) or to facilitate the positioning of certain catheters (e.g. coronary sinus).

Subclavian vein
- Identify the junction between the medial third and lateral two-thirds of the clavicle (usually the apex of the medial convex curve of the clavicle).
- Starting 2 cm inferior and lateral to this point, aim towards the clavicle.
- After hitting the clavicle, move the needle stepwise down the clavicle until the needle tip is just below the clavicle.
- Swing the needle to aim at the nadir of the suprasternal notch, keeping the needle horizontal to the bed.
- There is a 1–2% risk of pneumothorax.

Axillary vein/extrathoracic subclavian vein
- The axillary vein becomes the subclavian vein at the lateral border of the first rib.
- Under fluoroscopy, the needle is advanced towards the junction between the lateral margin of the first rib and the inferior border of the clavicle (usually angled at 45–60° to the horizontal).
- Care is taken not to advance the needle past the medial border of the first rib to avoid risk of pneumothorax.
- If the extrathoracic subclavian vein is not encountered on hitting the rib, the needle is pulled back and angled differently to 'walk' along the first rib until the vein is encountered.
- Venogram of the veins can be performed by injecting contrast through an ipsilateral vein in the forearm and the 'roadmap' of the veins may be used to guide puncture of the extrathoracic vein or the axillary vein.
- The axillary vein puncture is performed under fluoroscopy with the needle almost vertical over the second rib where the venogram demonstrates the vein to pass.
- The tip of the needle should remain over the silhouette of the second rib to prevent risk of pneumothorax.

Internal jugular vein
- Identify the apex of the triangle between the clavicular and manubrial heads of the sternomastoid muscle.
- Palpate the carotid artery and insert the needle lateral to the artery at the apex of the triangle, aiming for the ipsilateral nipple or anterior superior iliac spine.
- The vein is usually fairly superficial.
- There is a 1% risk of pneumothorax.

Practical tips
- Contrast injection through the ipsilateral arm vein can help in localizing the subclavian and axillary veins.
- Head-down tilt may be helpful to fill the veins in patients who are dehydrated.
- The subclavian artery lies superior to the vein.

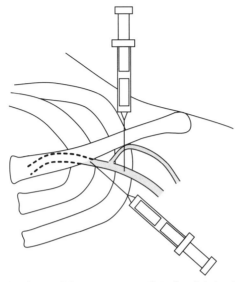

Fig. 4.2 Extrathoracic subclavian vein puncture with tip of needle in the triangle formed by the clavicle, first rib, and subclavian vein. Vertical axillary vein puncture over second rib after venography. Reproduced from Timperley J, Leeson P, Mitchell ARJ, and Betts T (eds.) (2008) *Pacemakers and ICDs*, Oxford University Press.

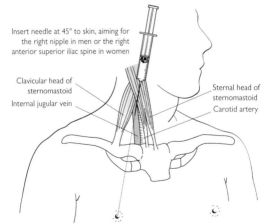

Insert needle at 45° to skin, aiming for the right nipple in men or the right anterior superior iliac spine in women

Clavicular head of sternomastoid

Internal jugular vein

Sternal head of sternomastoid

Carotid artery

Fig. 4.3 Internal jugular central line insertion. Reproduced from Myerson S, Choudhury RP, and Mitchell ARJ (2006) *Emergencies in Cardiology*, Oxford University Press.

Standard catheter placement

Catheters are positioned under fluoroscopic guidance but may be introduced non-fluoroscopically with NavX (📖 p. 104) to reduce radiation exposure. The standard four-catheter electrophysiology study involves positioning the catheters at four different sites (Fig. 4.4) as outlined below.

High right atrium (HRA)

- Josephson or Cournand shape.
- Quadripolar for simultaneous stimulation/recording.
- High posterolateral wall at the junction of the superior vena cava approximating SA node exit site. In difficult cases, the RA appendage (more anterior structure) may be used.
- The catheter is advanced under fluoroscopy (in the AP projection) to high RA and torqued to position the catheter tip posterolaterally or more anteriorly for the appendage.
- Repositioning may be needed for poor stability/capture or phrenic nerve stimulation.

Right ventricle (RV)

- Josephson or Cournand shape.
- May use bipolar to reduce cost as V-capture can be inferred from ECG.
- Usually positioned at the RV apex, although the RV outflow tract is useful in a few difficult cases or for two-site ventricular stimulation protocols (📖 p. 78) to increase sensitivity.
- Catheters are advanced under fluoroscopy (usually in the RAO or AP projection) into the RV apex.
- From the RV apex, withdrawing the catheter gradually and applying clockwise torque will allow the catheter to be positioned in the RVOT.
- Repositioning may be needed because of poor stability/capture or intractable ventricular ectopy.

His bundle catheter (His aka 'low RA')

- Multi-polar catheter (≥4 electrodes) is always required for continuous recording of the local A and V signals as well as His deflection, notwithstanding the effects of respiration and changes in orientation due to pacing or tachycardia. A pre-shaped catheter ('His-hugger') may be preferred to a Cournand to improve stability. The standard technique is to position the catheter across the antero-superior aspect of the tricuspid annulus under fluoroscopy (RAO or AP projection). It is helpful to look at the intracardiac electrograms while positioning the His catheter. The catheter is withdrawn slowly with clockwise torque (to improve septal contact) until the characteristic A-H-V signal is obtained. An LAO view is helpful to check that the catheter tip is near the 1–2 o'clock position on the tricuspid annulus.
- Repositioning is frequently needed due to poor stability. **If the H signal is lost during EPS, catheter dislodgement should always be assumed**.
- Excessive 'ventricularization' of the catheter position (no A electrogram) may record the right bundle (RB) potential rather than His deflection and underestimate the HV interval.

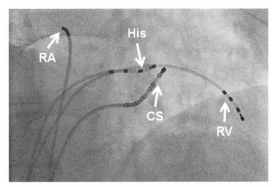

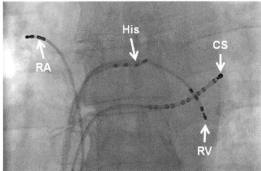

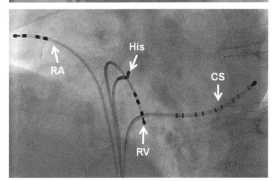

Fig. 4.4 High right atrium (RA), His bundle (His), coronary sinus (CS), and right ventricular (RV) catheters are shown in RAO (top), AP (middle), and LAO (bottom) fluoroscopic projections for a standard four-wire electrophysiology study catheter setup.

Coronary sinus (CS) (Fig. 4.5)

Multi-polar catheter (8–10 electrodes) to record LA activation sequence. The CS ostium lies slightly infero-posterior to the tricuspid annulus and is 'shielded' by the eustachian ridge making it easier to enter from a superior approach. Using a steerable catheter means CS cannulation can be accomplished via a femoral approach in >95% of cases:

• The catheter is initially placed just across the tricuspid annulus, deflected inferiorly, and withdrawn with *clockwise* torque until equal A and V signals are recorded (Fig. 4.5, panel 1).

• Use the LAO projection to manoeuvre the catheter tip into the CS ostium (indicated by a 'jump' across the cardiac margin but still obtaining A and V signals) (Fig. 4.5, panel 2).

• Release the deflection of the catheter and clockwise torque to allow the tip to turn superiorly and follow the course of the great cardiac vein until the proximal poles are just inside the CS ostium (Fig. 4.5, panel 3).

• If the distal tip is directed more inferiorly with a pure V signal, it has probably entered an LV branch and should be withdrawn into the mid-CS and advanced with the tip directed superiorly (may require counter-clockwise torque) (Fig. 4.5, panel 4).

CS cannulation from a superior approach can usually be accomplished with a non-steerable catheter. The catheter is positioned across the tricuspid annulus and then slowly withdrawn and advanced alternately with *counter-clockwise* torque until the tip engages the CS ostium. In most cases the catheter will then pass freely into the great cardiac vein.

Problems with CS catheter placement include:

• Failure to cannulate.

• Partial introduction with the distal poles at the mid-CS position and the proximal poles outside the ostium, potentially resulting in misclassification of midline activation as eccentric.

• Recurrent catheter dislodgement, usually only a problem with the inferior or transfemoral approach.

Possible solutions include switching to a superior approach (rarely vice versa) or using a support sheath (e.g. SR0) to facilitate catheter placement via the inferior approach (occasionally a steerable ablation catheter is needed to intubate the CS and then 'railroad' the long sheath before exchanging to the CS multi-polar catheter).

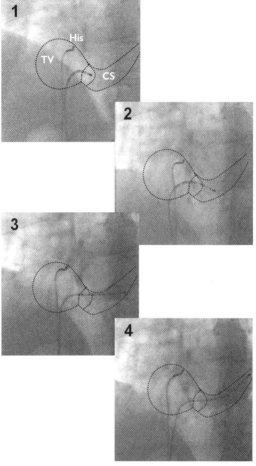

Fig. 4.5 Positioning the coronary sinus (CS) catheter from the femoral approach. See text for details. LAO projections are shown. TV – tricuspid valve. His catheter is shown for reference.

Intracardiac recording techniques

An intracardiac electrogram (EGM) is a recording of the localized electrical activity by electrode(s) positioned in the heart. Recordings are generated by voltage differences recorded by two electrodes, the anode and cathode. The EGM may be unipolar or bipolar. It undergoes signal processing to remove unwanted electrical activity ('high pass' and 'low pass' filters) and gain modification (usually adjusted manually according to signal amplitude). Understanding the fundamental aspects of recording techniques, their strengths and limitations, aids in the interpretation of intracardiac EGMs.

High pass filtering
- Attenuates frequencies *lower* than the specified cut-off.
- Low frequency oscillations due to respiration or catheter movements are removed by high pass filtering.
- Far-field signals are of lower frequency because the high frequency content attenuates more rapidly with distance from the recording site.
- Hence high pass filtering of a unipolar electrogram reduces far-field signals and may improve the detection of lower amplitude local signals.

Low pass filtering
- Attenuates frequencies *higher* than the specified cut-off.
- Removes electrical noise etc.

Band pass filtering and the notch filter
- Most commonly used band is with filters set to 30 Hz (high pass) and 250 Hz (low pass).
- The 'notch filter' is specifically used to attenuate signals around 50–60 Hz to attenuate noise due to AC current.

Correlation of intracardiac electrogram and surface ECG
- A bipolar intracardiac EGM only measures the electrical activity in a localized area of the heart where the recording electrode is placed. Hence a series of electrodes placed in the standard positions for EPS will give information about conduction velocities and the activation pattern, i.e. the sequence of depolarization in those positions.
- *High RA* – the electrogram corresponds to the depolarization wavefront arriving at the atrial cells at the superior region of the RA. As the SA node has a superior position in the RA, the timing of the HRA electrogram is very close to the beginning of the P wave on the surface ECG.
- *His (low RA)* – the atrial EGM corresponds to the depolarization wavefront arriving at the atrial cells in the low right atrium, adjacent to the AV node. The His bundle EGM corresponds to the depolarization of the proximal His-Purkinje system after the depolarization exits from the AV node. Hence it falls between the A and V deflections. The ventricular EGM corresponds to the depolarization of the ventricular cells adjacent to the AV node. As the septal area of the RV is one of the first areas to depolarize, the timing is usually close to the onset of QRS.

- **CS** – the atrial EGM corresponds to the depolarization of left atrial cells adjacent to the mitral annulus. As the depolarization wavefront travels leftward from the SA node, the activation pattern will be from proximal to distal CS. The ventricular EGM corresponds to the depolarization of left ventricular cells adjacent to the mitral annulus.
- **RV** – the ventricular EGM corresponds to the depolarization of the right ventricular apex after the depolarization has exited the His-Purkinje system. The timing is close to the onset of QRS.

Unipolar electrograms

- Recorded via a single exploring electrode within the heart and a second electrode remote from the heart (also called the **'indifferent electrode'**), which has little or no cardiac signal).
- Usually, the intracardiac electrode is the anode and the indifferent electrode is the cathode (preferred to Wilson's central terminal because the latter causes much more electrical noise).
- High pass filter is normally set at 0.5 Hz.
- The morphology of the unipolar electrogram indicates the direction of waveform propagation (📖 Fig. 4.6).
- The maximum negative slope (−dV/dt) of the electrogram corresponds to the depolarization wavefront arriving at the electrode.
- At the site of initial activation, the electrogram shows a 'QS' complex as the depolarization wavefront spreads away from the recording electrode (typical of a successful ablation site for focal arrhythmias).
- Shallow initial negative slope of the 'QS' complex suggests deep origin of the activation focus, i.e. away from the endocardial surface.
- 'RS' complex indicates that the site is remote from the arrhythmia focus.
- Unipolar electrograms may contain far-field signals that obscure the local potentials, especially when the local potentials are of small amplitude, e.g. scar tissue.
- A high pass filtered unipolar electrogram (30 Hz) resembles a bipolar electrogram.

Bipolar electrograms

- Recorded via two electrodes (dipole) in close proximity in the heart.
- Conventionally, the distal electrode is the cathode and the proximal electrode is the anode.
- The bipolar EGM is generated by summation of the potentials from the two electrodes at each point in time, i.e. the sum of the two unipolar EGMs.
- The bipolar EGM (Fig. 4.6) represents the local electrical signal as far-field signals are largely removed.
- The initial peak of the bipolar signal ('intrinsic deflection') corresponds to depolarization beneath the electrodes.
- Timing of the bipolar signals at different intracardiac locations is of crucial importance during EPS and mapping of arrhythmias.
- Amplitude and morphology of the bipolar EGM depend on the direction of wavefront propagation, but are generally unhelpful in clinical use.

Table 4.2 Bipolar vs. unipolar electrograms

Bipolar electrograms	Unipolar electrograms
Timing is more important; morphology is less useful	Signal morphology is important, i.e. QS vs. RS
Represents local electrical activity	Affected by far-field electrical signals
Widespread use in EPS	Useful for activation mapping
Able to map small fractionated electrograms in scar tissue	Less useful when mapping scar tissue

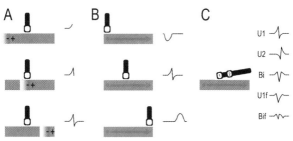

Fig. 4.6 (A) **Derivation of the unipolar electrogram**. With the recording electrode at a fixed site, an electrical wavefront (shown as –/+) spreads past. As activation approaches the electrode (top panel) and leaves it (bottom panel), the unipolar electrogram shows relatively slow (shallow) positive and negative deflections respectively. The steepest negative deflection (max. dV/dt) occurs as the wavefront passes the tip (middle panel). (B) **Unipolar electrogram for activation mapping**. With the recording electrode positioned at the site of a focal electrical source (top panel), the unipolar electrogram shows a totally negative QS deflection. As the recording electrode is positioned progressively further from the source, the unipolar signal becomes equiphasic (middle panel) and eventually positive (bottom panel). (C) **Derivation of the bipolar electrogram**. The recording electrode is positioned some way from a focal electrical source. The distal pole is slightly closer, so its unipolar electrogram U1 is equiphasic, whereas the proximal pole is slightly further away and its unipolar electrogram U2 is more positive. The bipolar signal (Bi) is derived by summing U1 and U2 and the effect of filtering (U1f and Bif) is also shown.

Outline of the standard electrophysiology study

The electrophysiology study (EPS) involves recording electrical activity (**'intracardiac electrograms'**) and pacing (**'programmed stimulation'**) from different positions within the heart. Although each EPS should be tailored to individual patients to answer specific questions, it should be done in a systematic fashion.

Outline of basic EPS

1. Placement of catheters (📖 p. 50).
2. Measurement of baseline intracardiac conduction intervals (📖 p. 60).
3. Conduction curves using extrastimulus technique:
   • Ventricle: retrograde curve (📖 p. 72).
   • Atrium: antegrade curve (📖 p. 68).
4. Evaluation of antegrade and retrograde conduction using incremental pacing.
5. Induction and termination of tachyarrhythmia (📖 p. 154).
6. Pattern of antegrade and retrograde myocardial activation during tachyarrhythmia (📖 p. 154).
7. Pacing manoeuvres during tachyarrhythmia (📖 p. 166):
   • Resetting by extrastimuli.
   • Entrainment.
8. Use of adjunctive drugs to help with induction or termination of arrhythmia (📖 p. 84).
9. Other techniques:
   • Parahisian pacing (📖 p. 150).
   • Ventricular stimulation protocols (📖 p. 78).
   • Assessment of sinus node function (automaticity and conduction) (📖 p. 220).
   • Assessment of AV conduction (📖 p. 224).

Basic intervals

Cycle length (CL)
Length of time between each heart beat, measured in milliseconds (ms).
It is a measure of heart rate.
i.e. 60 000/CL (ms) = heart rate (bpm)

PA interval (normal: 25–55 ms)
This is an estimation of intra-atrial conduction time. It is measured from
the earliest atrial activity (usually onset of P wave) to the intrinsic deflection of the atrial electrogram on the His catheter.

AH interval (normal: 55–125 ms) (Fig. 4.7)
This is a measure of conduction time from low right atrium through the
AV node to the His bundle. It reflects AV nodal conduction time. It is
measured from the intrinsic deflection of the atrial electrogram to the
onset of the His electrogram on the His catheter.

HV interval (normal: 35–55 ms) (Fig. 4.7)
This is the conduction time from the proximal His bundle, through the
His-Purkinje system to the ventricular myocardium. It is measured from
the onset of the His electrogram to the earliest recorded ventricular activation (usually the onset of QRS).

PR interval = PA interval + AH interval + HV interval.

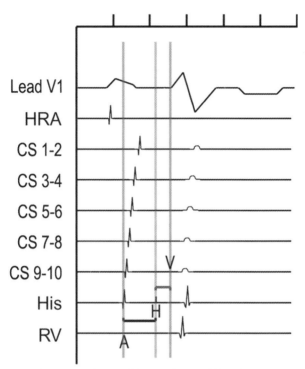

Fig. 4.7 Measurement of AH and HV intervals. A single ECG lead (V1), high right atrial (HRA), coronary sinus (CS), His, and right ventricular (RV) intracardiac recordings are shown. Note the pattern of antegrade conduction during sinus rhythm (📖 Normal activation patterns, p. 62).

Normal activation patterns

Antegrade conduction during sinus rhythm (Fig. 4.7) or high RA pacing (Fig. 4.8)

- Atrial activation starts from the SA node and spreads in a radial fashion, i.e. inferiorly to the AV node and from RA to LA.
- The atrial EGM recorded at the HRA is earlier than the His or CS.
- The timing of atrial EGMs recorded by the CS catheter shows a proximal to distal progression, reflecting left atrial activation spreading from the interatrial septum.
- Activation then proceeds through the AV node, His-Purkinje system, and the bundle branches through to the ventricles. The His electrogram is clearly recorded before the earliest ventricular activity.
- IVS is depolarized first followed by the apical regions, then the ventricular free walls, and finally the posterobasal region.
- The left posterobasal region is the last to be activated, and hence the timing of the ventricular EGM is usually latest in the mid- to distal CS.

Retrograde conduction during RV pacing (Fig. 4.8)

- The electrical impulse travels from the ventricular myocardium to the bundle branches and up the His-Purkinje system and AV node before spreading radially to the atria (i.e. from the atrial septum to the right and left atria).
- The His EGM is often lost in the ventricular EGM.
- The earliest atrial EGM will be located at the inferior atrial septum ('midline') and is most commonly recorded on the His catheter but sometimes on the proximal CS electrodes.
- Activation then spreads caudo-cranially to the high RA.
- The timing of atrial EGMs recorded by the CS catheter shows a proximal to distal progression, reflecting atrial activation spreading from the septum to the left.
- Normal activation through the AV node (located at the septum) then spreading out radially is termed 'midline' activation (often misleadingly referred to as 'concentric' activation). As the AV node exhibits a decremental conduction property, normal activation will be decremental and midline.

Decremental vs. non-decremental conduction (Fig. 4.9)

Conduction velocity of impulses through certain myocardial tissues may decrease with increasing heart rate or decreasing coupling intervals. This phenomenon of rate-related prolongation of conduction is termed **decremental conduction**. This applies particularly to the AV node. Hence, there is clear AH interval prolongation following extrastimuli with short coupling intervals, accounting for the characteristic appearance of the antegrade and retrograde conduction curves (Figs. 4.9 and 4.15). The atrial, ventricular, and His-Purkinje cells show **non-decremental** or very little decremental conduction. The majority of accessory pathways also exhibit non-decremental conduction, but about 8% demonstrate decremental conduction, particularly Mahaim atrio-fascicular and atrio-ventricular bypass tracts (📖 p. 376).

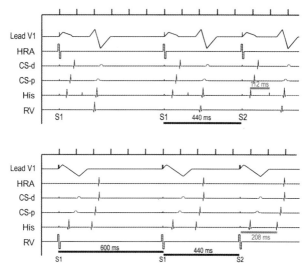

Fig. 4.8 Normal antegrade activation (upper panel) during HRA pacing at S1S1 600 ms with extrastimulus S2 at coupling interval S1S2 440 ms, resulting in slight decremental conduction delay within the AV node, manifesting as prolongation of the AH interval (112 ms). Normal retrograde activation (lower panel) during RV pacing at S1S2 600 ms, earliest at His and then PCS, later spreading to DCS and high RA. Extrastimulus S2 at coupling interval S1S2 440 ms results in slight decremental conduction delay via the AV node, manifesting as prolongation of the VA interval (208 ms). The retrograde His deflection is often *not* visible.

Extrastimulus technique

The extrastimulus technique is the most important form of programmed stimulation. One or more extrastimuli are delivered across a range of coupling intervals (timings) at various intracardiac sites.

Objectives

- To evaluate AV and VA conduction (**antegrade** and **retrograde conduction curves**).
- To study the electrophysiological properties (especially **refractoriness**) of the AV conduction system, atria, ventricles, and accessory pathways.
- To induce/terminate re-entrant tachyarrhythmias and analyse their mechanisms.

Basic technique

- Stimulation is carried out at current strength twice diastolic threshold.
- One or more premature impulses or **extrastimuli** are introduced, following a series of impulses at a fixed cycle length, the **drive train**.
- The drive train usually consists of eight paced beats (each termed **S1**) to achieve reasonable steady state.
- The first extrastimulus (termed **S2**) is delivered after a fixed interval following the final S1. This is the **coupling interval**.
- The coupling interval of S2 is progressively reduced in 20 ms decrements until 300 ms, then in 10 ms decrements until refractoriness.
- Extrastimulus technique is used to perform antegrade and retrograde curves (📖 pp. 68, 72) pacing from HRA and RV respectively.
- A second extrastimulus is termed **S3** and a third extrastimulus is termed **S4**.

The extrastimulus may be coupled to intrinsic cardiac impulses, e.g. stages 1 and 2 of the Wellens VT stimulation protocol (📖 p. 80) or His-synchronous VPBs during narrow complex tachycardia (📖 p. 166).

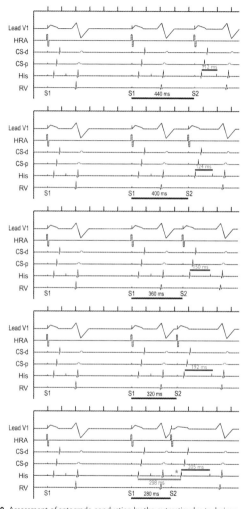

Fig. 4.9 Assessment of antegrade conduction by the extrastimulus technique. Following a drive train (S1S1) of high RA pacing at constant CL 600 ms, the extrastimulus (S2) is delivered at progressively earlier coupling intervals (S1S2) on each successive panel, from 440 ms in the top panel down to 280 ms in the bottom panel. The extrastimulus results in decremental conduction delay in the AV node manifesting as progressive prolongation of the A2H2 interval (shown in red) from 112 ms to 205 ms without any sudden jump, and without any prolongation of the HV interval. These findings are consistent with normal decremental antegrade conduction.

Refractory periods

(See Fig. 4.12)

After a cardiac cell is depolarized, the period of time during which it cannot be depolarized again (from phase 0 to late in phase 3 of the cell's action potential) is termed the **refractory period**. As the monophasic action potential is not recorded routinely, electrophysiologists have defined three different refractory periods based on the cardiac cell's response to premature stimuli.

Effective refractory period (ERP) (Figs. 4.10 and 4.11)

This is defined as the longest coupling interval (S1S2) that fails to capture or propagate through the tissue.

For example, ERP of the AV node is the longest A1A2 that does not result in H2.

Relative refractory period (RRP)

This is defined as the longest coupling interval (S1S2) that results in a delay of capture (**latency**) or slowed conduction through the tissue, i.e. when the 'output' interval is just greater than the 'input' interval.

For example, RRP of the AV node is the longest A1A2 that results in H1H2 (output interval) being greater than A1A2 (input interval).

Functional refractory period (FRP)

This is defined as the shortest 'output' interval from the tissue.

For example, FRP of the AV node is the shortest possible H1H2 interval.

Refractory period is closely related to heart rate or drive train. For most cardiac tissue, faster heart rate or shorter cycle lengths result in shorter refractory periods. However, the opposite applies to the AV node, i.e. shorter cycle lengths result in longer refractory periods.

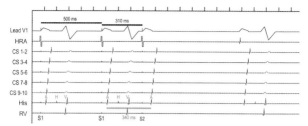

Fig. 4.10 The most common type of block with programmed electrical stimulation from the atrium is block in the AV node. The drive train CL is 500 ms. The last two paced beats of the drive train (S1) are shown followed by an atrial extrastimulus (S2) with a coupling interval of 310 ms. The atrium is captured 340 ms later but there is no conduction through the AV node (no His deflection). If a coupling interval of 320 ms is conducted through the AV node then 310 ms is the AV node effective refractory period (AVN ERP).

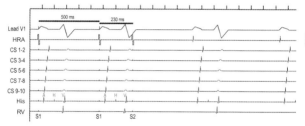

Fig. 4.11 The 'block' with programmed electrical stimulation from the atrium is in the atrium itself in this example. The drive train CL is 500 ms. The last two paced beats of the drive train (S1) are shown followed by an atrial extrastimulus with a coupling interval of 230 ms. The atrium is not captured. If a coupling interval of 240 ms captures the atrium (as in Fig. 4.10) then the atrial effective refractory period (AERP) is 230 ms.

Antegrade curve

Technique

- Pacing (8-beat drive train plus S2 extrastimulus) delivered at HRA:
  - May use multiple drive cycle lengths, e.g. 600 ms and 400 ms.
  - S2 delivered from initial coupling interval shorter than drive cycle, adjusted in 20 ms decrements until 300 ms, then in 10 ms decrements until failure of atrial capture.
  - If atrial ERP is reached before AV nodal ERP, using a drive train with a shorter cycle length may ↓ atrial ERP and ↑ AV nodal ERP.
- Plot A1A2 interval at low RA (i.e. His catheter) vs. output interval H1H2 and/or V1V2 (earliest V activation surface or intracardiac).
- Plot A1A2 interval vs. A2H2 interval at low RA (i.e. His catheter).
- The ERP, RRP, and FRP of the AV node can be determined:
  - S1S2 should *not* be used as a surrogate for A1A2 – at short coupling intervals, intra-atrial conduction delay makes A1A2 progressively longer than S1S2.
  - May require double extrastimuli (S2S3) if too much intra-atrial conduction delay at short coupling.
  - Antegrade curve can be performed from other sites, e.g. CS.

'Normal' results (Figs. 4.12 and 4.13)

- Decremental AV nodal conduction, i.e. H1H2 and A2H2 prolong with decreasing A1A2.
- Normal HV interval with non-decremental response to A1A2.
- At short coupling intervals may observe A1A2↑ as S1S2↓ due to intra-atrial conduction delay.
- Decremental conduction rarely occurs in the His-Purkinje system.
- AH jump without echo beat may be seen in 30% of controls as normal variant (Fig. 4.14).

Abnormal results

- AH jump, especially if associated with atrial echo beat (⬜ Figs. 4.12, 4.13, 7.6).
- Pre-excitation (⬜ p. 264).
- Pathological AH or HV prolongation (⬜ p. 224).
- HV decrement (usually).

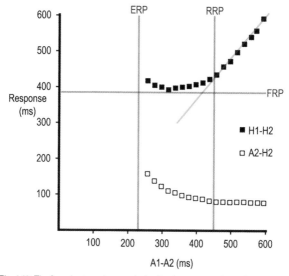

Fig. 4.12 The formal antegrade curve derived by the extrastimulus technique shown in Fig. 4.8. Note that the A1A2 interval is used rather than S1S2 to reflect the true coupling interval of the extrastimulus at AV nodal level, as there is often intra-atrial conduction delay at shorter S1S2 intervals. Normal, smooth decremental conduction is shown as evidenced by the gradual increase in A2H2 and divergence of H1H2 away from the unity line until AV nodal ERP is reached. The curve also shows the derivation of RRP and FRP, but these indices are seldom used outside research studies on anti-arrhythmic drugs.

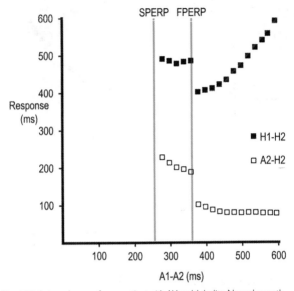

Fig. 4.13 Antegrade curve from a patient with AV nodal duality. Normal smooth decremental conduction is observed until A1A2 reaches the effective refractory period of the fast pathway (FPERP), whereupon conduction switches from fast to slow pathways with a concomitant 'jump' of >50 ms in A2H2 and H1H2, creating the discontinuity of the curve. Decremental conduction down the slow pathway then continues until its refractory period is reached (SPERP), whereupon AV nodal conduction blocks altogether.

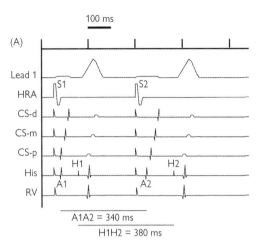

A1A2 = 340 ms

H1H2 = 380 ms

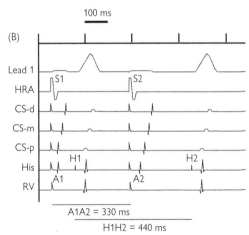

A1A2 = 330 ms

H1H2 = 440 ms

Fig. 4.14 Antegrade curve showing evidence of dual AV nodal physiology.
(A) Atrial pacing from HRA. Normal decremental antegrade conduction with atrial extrastimulus results in A1A2 of 340 ms and conducted H1H2 of 380 ms.
(B) Shortening the extrastimulus by 10 ms results in A1A2 of 330 ms and a 'jump' in H1H2 by 60 ms to 440 ms, reflecting antegrade block in the fast pathway and switch to slow pathway conduction. However, the impulse terminates in the ventricle with no echo beat back to the atria (see Fig. 7.6 for comparison).

Retrograde curve

Technique
- Pacing (8-beat drive train plus S2 extrastimulus) delivered at RV:
  - Usually done before antegrade curve as there is less chance of causing atrial fibrillation.
  - May use multiple drive cycle lengths, e.g. 600 ms and 400 ms.
  - S2 delivered from initial coupling interval shorter than drive cycle, adjusted in 20 ms decrements until 300 ms, then in 10 ms decrements until failure of ventricular capture.
- Plot V1V2 interval at LRA (i.e. His catheter) vs. output interval A1A2 (earliest A activation in any lead), as H1H2 often not measurable.
- Plot V1V2 against V2A2 (i.e. VA time):
  - Repeat after isoprenaline infusion if VA block or VA Wenckebach conduction at baseline.
  - Always continue adjusting S1S2 down to refractoriness to avoid missing **'gap phenomena'**.
  - Retrograde curve may be performed from other sites, especially LV.

'Normal' result
- Decremental VA conduction (i.e. V2A2 > V1A1); the decremental conduction mainly occurs at the His-Purkinje system, but may also involve the AV node. Unfortunately it is rare to record a His bundle electrogram, which is often buried within the ventricular electrogram.
- Atrial activation is midline (loosely referred to as 'concentric'), i.e. earliest A electrogram in His/LRA catheter. However, earliest activation is in proximal CS electrogram in 30–40% due to a more posterior retrograde exit site.

Other 'normal' findings
- No evidence of VA conduction despite pharmacological provocation.
- Gap phenomena – VA conduction blocks at relatively long V1V2 coupling interval but resumes after a 'gap' at shorter V1V2 coupling interval.
- Ventricular extra beats post-extrastimulus due to:
  - Bundle branch re-entry – i.e. retrograde right bundle branch block, so that S2 crosses the septum and conducts retrogradely via the left bundle. By then the right bundle recovers and conducts the impulse antegradely (in patients with cardiomyopathy, this may result in sustained bundle branch re-entrant VT).
  - Ventricular echo – implies that the AV node has dual retrograde pathways. Retrograde conduction via the fast pathway is blocked initially. The impulse then travels up the slow pathway before conducting down the fast pathway.

'Abnormal' results
- Non-decremental VA conduction (□ p. 142).
- Eccentric atrial activation (□ p. 145).
- VA 'jump' (□ p. 73).

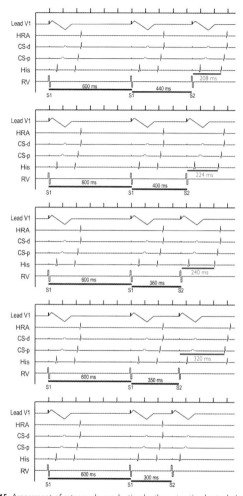

Fig. 4.15 Assessment of retrograde conduction by the extrastimulus technique. RV pacing at drive train (S1S1) 600 ms results in normal 'midline' retrograde atrial activation, i.e. His → PCS → DCS and HRA. The extrastimulus (S2) is brought in at progressively shorter coupling intervals (S1S2) and results in progressive decremental conduction delay in the AV node manifesting as prolongation of the V2A2 conduction time (shown in red), from 208 ms to 240 ms as S1S2 shortens from 440 ms to 360 ms. At S1S2 350 ms there is a retrograde 'jump' of V2A2 by 80 ms with a subtle change in earliest VA activation from His to earliest at PCS, consistent with a change from retrograde fast to slow pathway conduction. At S1S2 300 ms (bottom panel), the S2 is not conducted retrogradely as AV nodal refractoriness has been exceeded.

Incremental pacing

May provide complementary information to extrastimulus technique as it avoids the problem of intracardiac conduction delay at short coupling intervals, especially when assessing antegrade conduction.

- Incremental atrial pacing (IAP):
  - Regular pacing starting from 400 ms.
  - Gradually decrease in 10 ms steps until there is no 1:1 AV conduction, i.e. the AV Wenckebach point (normally <450 ms) (Fig. 4.16).
  - Is there any AH jump?
  - Is PR > or < RR at just above AV Wenckebach cycle length (Kay's sign, Fig. 4.17).
- Incremental ventricular pacing using similar protocol.
- Consider pharmacological adjuncts to help with arrhythmia induction.

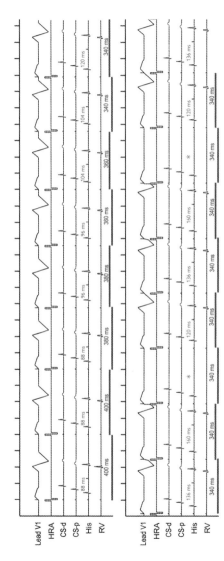

Fig. 4.16 Incremental atrial pacing (IAP). High right atrial pacing at progressively shorter cycle lengths from 400 to 360 ms (top panel) with preservation of 1:1 atrio-ventricular conduction and gradual increase in AH interval from 83 to 104 ms (shown in red). At pacing cycle length 340 ms, AV Wenckeback conduction occurs with progressive AH prolongation (120 → 136 → 160 ms) followed by block and then repeat of the same cycle.

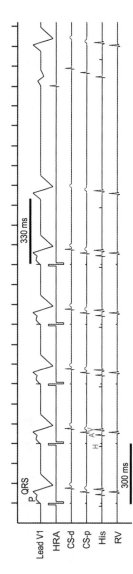

Fig. 4.17 Kay's sign. High right atrial pacing at cycle length 300 ms has resulted in 1:1 atrio-ventricular conduction but with marked AH prolongation, such that PR interval (330 ms) is greater than RR interval (300 ms), suggestive of AV nodal duality and antegrade conduction over a slow pathway. Bakes JH et al. (1996) *J Cardiovasc Electrophysiol* **7**(4): 287–94.

Ventricular stimulation protocols

Background

- Sudden cardiac deaths are most commonly secondary to ventricular arrhythmia (VT or VF).
- Previous myocardial infarction, poor LV systolic function, broad QRS complexes, and previous VT/VT are all risk factors for sudden cardiac death.
- The most common mechanism of ventricular tachycardia (VT) is re-entry (usually around scar tissue following MI).
- Less commonly, triggered activity and automaticity may be the underlying mechanism for VT.
- VT due to re-entry and triggered activity lends itself to be studied in the laboratory using programmed stimulation.
- It is indicated as part of the risk stratification of unexplained syncope or non-sustained VT in patients at risk of sudden cardiac death (e.g. previous MI, depressed LV EF, other forms of structural heart disease, e.g. HOCM).
- It is also used to study and characterize VT to aid in catheter ablation and programming of anti-tachycardia pacing (ATP) in ICDs.
- It is now rarely used to evaluate the efficacy of drug treatment.

General principles

- Different protocols are used in different laboratories but they are based on some basic principles.
- Programmed stimulation using multiple extrastimuli is used.
- A stepwise protocol is used whereby every subsequent stage represents a more aggressive stimulation (e.g. there are 12 stages in the Wellens protocol).
- Number of extrastimuli, drive train at different cycle lengths, pacing at more than one ventricular site, incremental pacing, and isoprenaline infusion increase the sensitivity.
- Increasingly aggressive stimulation reduces the specificity.
- Use of high stimulation outputs (≤ twice diastolic threshold) reduces specificity.
- Use of short-coupled (<200ms) extra stimulis reduces specificity.
- The use of three extrastimuli is optimal for sensitivity and specificity.
- Sustained monomorphic VT is considered a positive test.
- Non-sustained polymorphic VT or VF are considered non-specific, although interpretation of results needs to take into consideration the patient's background and the reason for performing the test.
- Generally, VT that is reliably initiated by extrastimuli is due to re-entry.
- VT secondary to triggered activity or automaticity usually needs isoprenaline and incremental pacing for induction.

Procedure

- Catheters are placed in the standard RV, His, and sometimes HRA positions.
- Output sets a twice diastolic threshold.
- Patients should have defibrillation pads attached in case of VF or haemodynamically compromising VT.
- Eight-beat drive train (S1) at a cycle length of 600 ms is followed by a premature extrastimulus (S2).
- The S1S2 coupling interval is reduced in 10 ms decrements until ventricular refractoriness.
- Then S1S2 is held just above the ventricular ERP and S3 introduced.
- Again S2S3 is gradually reduced to ventricular refractoriness.
- The process is then repeated with a drive train cycle length of 400 ms.
- Following that, S4 is introduced with drive trains of 600 ms and 400 ms.
- This protocol may be repeated with isoprenaline infusion.
- If VT is still not induced, consider:
  - Pacing at a different site (usually RVOT).
  - Incremental ventricular pacing until VA Wenckebach cycle length.
  - Long-short stimulus sequence.
  - Other pharmacological agents (e.g. atropine, adrenaline).

Initiation of sustained monomorphic VT

- Confirmation of VT with 12-lead ECG and comparison with ECG of clinical VT (if present).
- There should be clear dissociation of atrial/His electrograms and ventricular electrograms.
- Synchronized DC cardioversion if haemodynamic collapse.
- Pace termination with burst or ramp pacing beginning at just shorter than VT cycle length, then gradually reducing the paced cycle length.
- Sometimes this may lead to acceleration of VT requiring cardioversion.
- This is considered a positive test.

Initiation of VF or polymorphic VT

- Requires urgent defibrillation.
- This is usually considered non-specific, although interpretation must take account of clinical background (e.g. survival of cardiac arrest, suspected long QT/Brugada, etc.) and the aggressiveness of VT stimulation required to initiate the arrhythmia.
- Greater specificity associated with:
  - Induction by single or double extrastimuli vs. triple extrastimuli.
  - Late-coupled vs. short-coupled extrastimuli.
  - Output set at twice diastolic threshold.
  - No requirement for isoprenaline infusion.

How to do a VT stimulation study – Wellens protocol

The original stimulation protocol that is widely recognized is commonly referred to as the 'Wellens' protocol, named after one of the electrophysiologists who originally defined it.

- A single pacing catheter (usually a diagnostic quadripolar catheter) is placed in the right ventricular apex.
- The pacing protocol is then performed, consisting of 12 'stages' (see Fig. 4.18 for a template).
- The study is normally terminated if either sustained ventricular arrhythmia is induced (monomorphic VT/polymorphic VT/VF – 📖 p. 79 for interpretation) or if all 12 stages are completed with no inducible arrhythmia (a 'negative' study).
- The first two stages involve adding sensed extrastimuli – the delay of the first extrastimulus (S1) is progressively shortened, e.g. 500 ms, 450 ms, 400 ms, then decreased in 20 ms decrements to 300 ms, then decreased in 10 ms decrements to ERP or a minimum of 200 ms. The S1 delay is then fixed at 10–20 ms greater than ERP (or 200 ms if capture of the ventricle was still occurring), and a further extrastimulus (S2) is added and the delay again reduced in the same fashion until ERP or a minimum of 200 ms.
- Stage 3 onwards consists of basic drive trains (eight paced beats at a fixed cycle length, commonly 600, 500, and 400 ms – again referred to as S1), with up to three extrastimuli (S2, S3, and S4) added in sequence in the same fashion as the sensed extras above. As triple extrastimuli are most likely to induce non-specific polymorphic VT/VF, the S4 pacing protocols are performed after all the S2 and S3 ones have been completed if no arrhythmia has so far been induced.

Practical note

Be alert to the fact that capture may be lost by one or more of the extrastimuli at any time. If so then the delay on the non-captured extrastimulus should be increased by 10–20 ms and that stage of the protocol repeated again, confirming capture of the ventricle with all the extrastimuli.

	S1	S2	S3	S4	Outcome
Stage 1 (SR)					
Stage 2 (SR)	From stage 1				
Stage 3	600				
Stage 4	600	From stage 3			
Stage 5	500				
Stage 6	500	From stage 5			
Stage 7	400				
Stage 8	400	From stage 7			
Stage 9	From stage 2	From stage 2			
Stage 10	600	From stage 4	From stage 4		
Stage 11	500	From stage 6	From stage 6		
Stage 12	400	From stage 8	From stage 8		

Fig. 4.18 Wellens pacing protocol. SR – sinus rhythm, i.e. sensed extrastimuli; S1 is eight paced beats for stages 3 to 8, and 10 to 12, at the cycle length shown in milliseconds; Outcome – record whether VT/VF is induced or not.

How to do a VT stimulation study – protocol variations

Most electrophysiologists will use a modified version of the longer Wellens protocol. A modified version is shown in Fig. 4.19.

- This will often be performed from more than one site, commonly two (the RV apex and RV outflow tract).
- Where there is diagnostic uncertainty about the nature of a broad complex tachycardia, it is common to use at least one other quadripolar catheter in the His position and possibly also one in the high right atrium.
- Where the programmed electrical stimulation is being performed to induce VT with a view to ablation, variations may be used to increase the chances of actually inducing an arrhythmia:
  - Different cycles may be used (e.g. 'long-short-long' – rather than simply shortening the extrastimulus interval until the ventricular refractory period is reached and then introducing another one and shortening the interval again, a deliberately longer interval followed by a shorter and longer one for three extrastimuli are used, as this may be more likely to activate the critical component of the VT circuit in some cases).
  - 'Sensed' extrastimuli may be used – these are extrastimuli that are delivered at a defined coupling interval after the patient's own intrinsic ventricular activation, i.e. without a series of fixed cycle-length paced beats preceding them.
  - Pacing stimulation may be performed in the area thought to be critical to the arrhythmia, e.g. in and around the left ventricular scar in a patient with left ventricular VT.
  - Automatic/triggered forms of VT (📖 p. 308) are more often induced with burst pacing rather than programmed electrical stimulation.
  - Adjunctive pharmacological agents may be used in addition to pacing protocols in some cases (particularly the automatic/triggered types), e.g. isoprenaline, epinephrine, atropine, aminophylline, or calcium.

	S1	S2	S3	S4	Outcome
Stage 1 RV apex	600				
Stage 2 RV apex	600	From stage 1			
Stage 3 RV apex	400				
Stage 4 RV apex	400	From stage 3			
Stage 5 RVOT	600				
Stage 6 RVOT	600	From stage 5			
Stage 7 RVOT	400				
Stage 8 RVOT	400	From stage 7			
Stage 9 RV apex	600	From stage 2	From stage 2		
Stage 10 RV apex	400	From stage 4	From stage 4		
Stage 11 RVOT	600	From stage 6	From stage 6		
Stage 12 RVOT	400	From stage 8	From stage 8		

Fig. 4.19 A modified protocol example. Pacing is performed from either the right ventricular (RV) apex or RV outflow tract (RVOT); S1 is eight paced beats at the cycle length shown, in milliseconds; Outcome – record whether VT/VF is induced or not.

Role of adjunctive drugs

Drugs are used during EPS for the following reasons:
• Altering the autonomic tone.
• Blocking the AV node.
• Improving the chance of inducing arrhythmia.
• Treating arrhythmia.

Increasing sympathetic tone/decreasing parasympathetic tone

• In general, increase in sympathetic tone causes enhanced automaticity, increased conduction velocity, and decreased refractory period; the same happens for decrease in parasympathetic tone.
• SA and AV nodes are innervated by both sympathetic and parasympathetic fibres while the rest of the heart is mainly innervated by sympathetic fibres.
• Adrenaline and isoprenaline (ß-agonists) are used to increase sympathetic tone.
• Atropine (anti-muscarinic) decreases parasympathetic tone.
• They will cause an increase in the intrinsic heart rate and improve AV node conduction. They are also used to improve the induction of arrhythmia.

Blocking the AV node

• This is useful to check if the AV node is participating in the tachycardia.
• If the AV node is part of the tachycardia circuit, the tachycardia will be terminated (e.g. AVNRT, AVRT).
• Arrhythmia will continue if the AV node is not involved in the tachycardia (e.g. focal atrial tachycardia, atrial flutter, and VT); however, this may not always be true.
• Blocking the AV node may also reveal the presence of accessory pathways (i.e. latent pre-excitation).
• Adenosine is commonly used to block the AV node transiently.
• Some ectopic atrial tachycardias and idiopathic VTs may also be terminated with adenosine even though they are not dependent on the AV node.
• Occasionally, high doses of adenosine may provoke AF or even ventricular arrhythmias.
• ß-blockers or verapamil may be given as infusions for longer durations of AV block, e.g. for rate control in AF.

Treatment of arrhythmia

• Flecainide is the drug of choice for cardioverting AF (but not atrial flutter).
• VT stimulation formerly was used to test the efficacy of anti-arrhythmic drug treatment for VT (electropharmacological testing) but nowadays that is largely confined to investigation of new agents.

Table 4.3 Commonly used pharmacological agents during EPS

Drug name	Dose
Isoprenaline	May be given as an IV bolus (1–5 mcg)
	Usually given as an IV infusion (1.0–4.0 mcg/min)
Adrenaline	Usually given as an IV infusion (0.01–0.1 mcg/kg/min)
	Cardiac arrest dose (10 ml of 100 mcg/ml) as IV bolus
Esmolol	Urgent IV bolus 1 mg/kg over 30 seconds
	IV infusion 10 mg/mL in 5% dextrose or 0.9% saline. Load with 0.5 mg/kg/min for 1 minute only; maintenance with 0.05–0.3 mg/kg/min, starting at 0.05 mg/kg/min
Atropine	Given as an IV bolus (500 mcg–1 mg)
	Cardiac arrest dose 3 mg as IV bolus
Adenosine	Given as an IV bolus (up to 36 mg usually 6–18 mg)
Verapamil	IV 5–10 mg over 2–3 minutes; additional 5 mg after 5 minutes if necessary
Flecainide	IV 2 mg/kg to a maximum of 150 mg over 15 minutes
Amiodarone	Cardiac arrest dose 300 mg as IV bolus
	Slow IV bolus 150 mg over 10 minutes (in 100–250 mL 5% dextrose)
	IV infusion to total 1.2 g in 500 mL 5% dextrose over 24 hours through central line
Lidocaine	IV bolus 50–100 mg over 1–2 minutes
	Infusion 4 mg/min for 30 minutes, 2 mg/min for 2 hours, then 1 mg/min
Procainamide	IV 30 mg/min infusion up to a maximum total dose of 17 mg/kg; maintenance infusion 1–4 mg/min

Peri-procedural management

Day case vs. inpatient care

- Many ablations are now routinely performed as day case procedures (i.e. discharge on the same day as the procedure): AV node ablation; atrial flutter ablation; AVNRT; AVRT; WPW; atrial tachycardia; RVOT; and fascicular VT.
- Other more complex procedures often necessitate an overnight stay: AF ablation; VT ablation in structural heart disease; and ablation in patients with complex congenital heart disease.
- Some of the more complex procedures such as AF ablation are being performed in some centres as day case procedures. This has been facilitated by developments in technology (□ Chapter 20).

Complications

- Vascular access: haematoma; DVT; AV fistula; arterial pseudoaneurysm.
- Catheter manipulation: vascular damage; microemboli, particularly in the left ventricle, and risk of stroke; coronary artery dissection if retrograde aortic approach used; cardiac perforation and tamponade.
- RF application: AV block (depends upon procedure, □ specific ablation chapters in Part 4); cardiac tamponade; coronary artery damage if epicardial ablation is performed.
- Myocardial infarction, stroke, and mortality risk are again dependent upon the type of procedure: the majority of day case-type procedures carry a risk of <1:2000.

Discharge advice and follow-up arrangements

Advice regarding vascular access sites

- Gentle exercise for one week to minimize late bleeding from femoral puncture sites, particularly arterial (longer if patient is taking coumarin-type anticoagulation).
- If bleeding does occur at home then patient should lie down and apply pressure firmly just above puncture site (or get someone else to) for ten minutes, and then call for medical assistance.
- If there is sudden severe pain, sudden swelling, or loss of power in the limb then medical assistance should be sought urgently – however, bruising extending painlessly down the leg from a haematoma initially confined to the groin is to be expected.
- Driving is not recommended for two to seven days, and in some countries there are legal requirements not to drive for a certain period.
- Immersing in water, e.g. in a bath or swimming, is also not recommended for a week, but showering is fine after 12–24 hours.

Follow-up

- This will depend upon the type of procedure but normally patients are reviewed with at least a 12-lead ECG and assessment of symptoms approximately 6–16 weeks later.

Trans-septal puncture

General points

Trans-septal puncture is a key technique for the interventional electro-physiologist to allow access to the left atrium and left ventricle. In order to perform the procedure safely a detailed understanding of the technique and the anatomy of the septum is required. Techniques for trans-septal puncture vary and general principles will be covered in this section.

Indications for trans-septal puncture
- Ablation of left-sided accessory pathways.
- Ablation of atrial fibrillation and atrial tachycardias following previous ablation for atrial fibrillation.
- Ablation of focal tachycardia arising in the left atrium.
- Ablation of ventricular tachycardia – particularly where the origin is thought to be the LV free wall.
- Ablation of left-sided slow pathways in AVNRT (rarely required).

Complications of trans-septal puncture
- Aortic perforation.
- Pulmonary artery perforation.
- Pericardial tamponade.
- Stroke.
- Haemothorax.

The overall risk of significant complications is around 1%.

Tips to avoid complications with trans-septal puncture
- Never advance the trans-septal sheath over the needle unless you know where the tip of the needle is located. The trans-septal needle itself is very small and very rarely causes significant problems. Even if the needle enters the aorta, as long as the trans-septal sheath itself has not been advanced, this can usually be managed by withdrawing the needle.
- Never advance the trans-septal sheath and dilator into the SVC without a wire.
- Always confirm placement of the needle in the left atrium in at least two different ways: pressure measurement, withdrawal of oxygen-rich blood, and/or imaging.
- If in doubt, **STOP** and remove the trans-septal needle; replace with the guidewire and start again.

The anatomy

The true interatrial septum consisting of that part of the atria that is bordered by both the left and the right atrial cavities is relatively small and only makes up a minor part of the medial wall of the right atrium. It largely consists of the fossa ovale (📖 Fig. 2.1), which is formed from the septum secundum during embryonic life.

Anatomical relations of the interatrial septum

- Superiorly: superior vena cava.
- Antero-superiorly: aortic root.
- Postero-superiorly: pulmonary artery.
- Anteriorly: triangle of Koch and septal tricuspid annulus.
- Anteroinferiorly: coronary sinus os.
- Inferiorly: inferior vena cava.
- Posteriorly: fold of tissue between right and left atrium.

Equipment

Trans-septal sheath

Trans-septal sheaths are pre-formed sheaths that are designed to ease access to particular parts of the LA. They come with a dilator and guidewire. Both the sheath and dilator should be flushed fully before use to avoid air bubbles.

Trans-septal needle

Trans-septal needles are long, hollow needles with a pre-formed bend at the tip. Designs vary, but one of the most common is the Brockenbrough (BRK) needle. The curved end of the needle comes in various sizes, often labelled as BRK 0, 1, or 2 with increasing degrees of bend. For the majority of patients a BRK 0 needle is appropriate. Many operators feel that the BRK 0 needle does not have sufficient bend and manually increase the needle bend prior to performing a trans-septal puncture. The trans-septal needle comes with an inner guidewire designed to protect the tip of the needle as it is advanced through the dilator of the trans-septal sheath.

Pressure monitoring

Pressure monitoring of the trans-septal needle is used by many operators to allow correct positioning of the needle in the LA and to allow immediate detection of inadvertent aortic or pulmonary artery puncture.

Anatomical reference markers

The most feared complication of trans-septal puncture is inadvertent aortic puncture. In order to minimize the risk of this, many operators mark the aorta so that its position can be seen fluoroscopically. This can be done in two ways:

His catheter: The bundle of His lies just adjacent to the aortic root. A catheter detecting the His signal will provide an accurate marker of the position of the aortic root.

Aortic reference: Alternatively a pigtail catheter can be placed retrogradely in the aortic root via a femoral artery puncture. However, care must be taken to ensure the catheter is advanced fully into the aortic root.

The procedure

- Anatomical reference markers are placed according to the operator's preference.
- Access is gained to the right femoral vein and a wire is advanced to the SVC under fluoroscopy (Fig. 5.1).
- The trans-septal sheath with its dilator is advanced over the guidewire into the SVC. (Some operators prefer to pre-dilate the groin with a short sheath before passing the trans-septal sheath.)
- The guidewire is withdrawn from the sheath and dilator.
- The needle is advanced within the dilator under fluoroscopy to a position where the tip of the needle lies just inside the dilator. The inner guidewire is then removed and pressure monitoring attached (note: many operators remove the guidewire and attach pressure monitoring before advancing the needle into the sheath and dilator). It is often helpful to practise this outside the body so that you are aware of how far the needle needs to be inserted before its tip extends beyond the end of the sheath. As the needle is inserted into the body it should be allowed to rotate freely within the sheath, as otherwise there is often some resistance as the needle passes under the inguinal ligament.
- The entire trans-septal apparatus (needle, sheath, and dilator) is fixed together with one hand and rotated so that the curve of the needle and sheath points posteromedially to between 4 and 5 o'clock on an imaginary clockface, where the patient's chest is 12 o'clock, left arm is 3 o'clock, and back is 6 o'clock.
- The entire trans-septal apparatus is then withdrawn slowly from the SVC into the right atrium, normally during continuous fluoroscopic screening in the LAO projection (although some operators do this in the PA projection).
- As the needle enters the right atrium it will appear to jump to the left of the body (right of the screen) twice. The first (often very small) jump happens as it comes around the indentation in the SVC caused by the knuckle of the ascending aorta, and the second (usually larger) jump happens as it crosses the upper limbus of the fossa ovale and falls into the fossa itself.
- Whilst in the right atrium, a right atrial pressure trace will be recorded. The trans-septal apparatus should then be advanced slightly into the fossa ovale. At this point the fossa ovale will become tented and the pressure trace from the trans-septal needle will become 'flat' as the needle tip abuts against tissue. The trans-septal needle itself will usually be felt to pulsate with the cardiac motion.
- The position of the trans-septal needle should be checked in both RAO and LAO projections. It should lie behind (to the left of) the aortic markers in the RAO projection and will often pass completely behind the aortic marker in the LAO projection.
- With the left hand holding the trans-septal sheath and dilator in position tenting the fossa ovale, the operator's right hand should advance the trans-septal needle out of the end of the sheath. A pop may be felt as the needle passes through the fossa into the left atrium (Fig. 5.2).

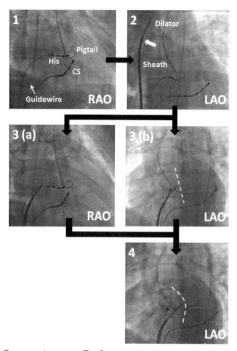

Fig. 5.1 Trans-septal puncture. The fluoroscopic projection is shown in the bottom right of each corner (RAO – right anterior oblique; LAO – left anterior oblique). 1. The guidewire is passed through the IVC, right atrium, and into the SVC. Catheters showing the location of the aortic root (Pigtail), the His bundle, and the coronary sinus (CS) are marked. 2. The trans-septal sheath and dilator have been advanced over the guidewire into the SVC. 3(a) & (b). The sheath and dilator have been withdrawn and have fallen towards the His catheter and the fossa. In the RAO view the tip is to the left or (posterior to) all catheters. In the LAO view it is to the right of (septal to) the His and aortic catheters (septum marked with dashed white line). 4. If pressure is applied gently on the sheath and dilator assembly the septum will tent (dashed white line). If a PFO or ASD is present, the dilator (± sheath) may slip through without requiring advancement of the needle.

- **CONFIRM POSITION OF THE NEEDLE TIP IN THE LEFT ATRIUM**:
  - A left atrial pressure trace will be seen – there should be two positive deflections of the pressure trace for each heart beat (if the patient is in sinus rhythm). The pressure measurement should also be significantly lower than arterial pressure, although this can be misleading in patients with significant MR. **Note: an atrial pressure trace can sometimes be seen with the needle in the pericardial space**.
  - It should be possible to withdraw bright red blood from the trans-septal needle. Arterial blood can also be withdrawn from the aorta but this will have a very different pressure trace. If the needle is in the pericardium no blood can be withdrawn. If it is still in the RA or in the PA, deoxygenated blood will be drawn back.
- If there is any doubt, the needle should be withdrawn and the process restarted. Otherwise the trans-septal sheath can be advanced into the left atrium. This can be done in one of two ways:
  - The trans-septal needle is fixed in position with the right hand whilst the dilator is advanced a few millimetres with the left hand. The needle and dilator are then fixed in position with the right hand whilst the sheath itself is advanced into the left atrium.
  - Alternatively the trans-septal needle can slowly be withdrawn completely and replaced with a guidewire, which is then advanced with fluoroscopic guidance into a pulmonary vein (usually on the left). The dilator and sheath can then be advanced over the wire into the left atrium without risk of perforating the atrial wall. This is particularly useful in patients with a tough interatrial septum, for example a patient who has previously had a trans-septal puncture performed. If the septum is really tough it is sometimes easier to advance the sheath if the wire is manipulated into a right-sided pulmonary vein.
- Dilator (and wire) are then withdrawn (Fig. 5.2). The sheath will appear to move down slightly into the LA as this happens.
- Before putting any catheters into the sheath, blood should be aspirated from it until no air is withdrawn (otherwise it is possible to get air introduced into the atrium). The line is then flushed (ideally with heparinized saline).
- The patient is then heparinized – the amount given and the desired ACT vary between operators and depend upon the case itself. Some operators will give the heparin before the puncture itself because of a fear of thrombus formation on the needle tip acutely.

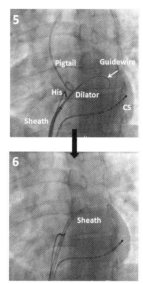

Fig. 5.2 Continuation of trans-septal puncture (Fig. 5.1). The fluoroscopic projection is left anterior oblique. 5. The guidewire is passed through the sheath and dilator into the left atrium. The dilator and sheath can then be advanced into the left atrium, and as long as neither goes past the tip of the guidewire there is no risk of perforation. 6. Once both sheath and dilator are in the left atrium, the dilator is removed and the sheath aspirated and flushed, ready for use.

Other technical variations

- *Contrast staining of the septum* – small quantities of contrast are injected through the trans-septal needle when it is against the septum. If it is within the fossa ovale the dye infiltrates the septum and can be seen to 'stain' the tissue. The needle will tent the septum when in the correct position (Fig. 5.1) and the needle is then advanced as described previously.
- *Echocardiographic guidance* – the puncture may be performed whilst using intracardiac echocardiography (which requires an extra venous sheath and an intracardiac echo catheter) or using transoesophageal echocardiography (which is possible under conscious sedation but is more straightforward under general anaesthesia).
- *Patent foramen ovale (PFO)* – in some patients a PFO may have already been identified (on a previous echocardiographic study, for example). The trans-septal needle may not need to be advanced if the sheath can be advanced through the PFO with gentle pressure on the sheath alone. Even if a PFO is not known about already, pressure should be gently applied before the trans-septal needle is advanced out of the sheath in case a PFO is present.
- *Double trans-septal puncture* – with the increase in procedures to ablate atrial fibrillation, there is an increase in the number of cases where access is needed for more than one catheter in the left atrium at the same time (📖 Chapter 20). Various techniques exist for gaining 'double trans-septal' access. The most straightforward is for two separate trans-septal punctures to be performed with two sheaths. In this case it is important to ensure the second sheath is not held away from the septum by the first sheath. It is sometimes necessary to rotate the second sheath 360° clockwise or anti-clockwise to make sure the sheath falls towards the septum – this will be seen as a drop towards the septum, as with any other trans-septal puncture. Alternatively a single trans-septal puncture is performed and after the sheath is advanced into the LA a guidewire is passed through the sheath into the LA and placed in a stable position (often the left upper pulmonary vein). The sheath can then be withdrawn into the right atrium (and advanced to and fro through the septum to ensure a hole is present). With the first sheath in the RA, a catheter (usually a steerable ablation catheter) is passed through the second trans-septal sheath, used to locate the initial puncture site and hole, and advanced into the LA. Once the catheter is across the septum it is deflected maximally to ensure it will not perforate the LA and the sheath is advanced through. The first sheath can now be advanced back through the puncture using the guidewire so two sheaths are in the LA.

Approach to the difficult trans-septal puncture

Where a previous trans-septal puncture has been performed and was noted to be difficult it is possible to prepare for the second time, but difficulty is encountered without any warning in some cases. Some difficulties that are encountered include:

- *A more anterior fossa than usual* – this is an anatomical variation and means that the sheath may only need to be in a 3 o'clock position rather than the usual 4–5 o'clock position. The concern is that there is a risk of puncturing the aorta if the needle is too anterior and so this may be best performed either with transoesophageal or intracardiac echocardiographic guidance.

- *A tough septum/fossa* – this may be because the muscular septum was punctured rather than the membranous part. If the whole fossa is thick then some other types of trans-septal needles may provide more support without the risk of pushing too hard, e.g. a two-part Endrys needle consisting of not only the inner sharp needle but also an outer metal dilator that goes inside both a specific trans-septal sheath and its own dilator.

- *The sheath does not 'catch' in the fossa but slides up and down the septum freely* – if the septum is entirely smooth then the sheath does not engage the fossa. Again, echocardiographic guidance can be helpful. Some operators will position the sheath just below (0.5 cm) where the fossa should be anatomically (using the standard references that they have in place, e.g. the aortic and CS catheters) and then advance the needle out of the sheath. This tends to straighten up the position slightly, lifting the needle to the correct position and the whole apparatus is then advanced. With the needle out of the sheath it now catches on the septum and punctures at this level. If it too slides freely then **STOP** and consider using imaging to help.

- *The sheath does not seem to fall across to the fossa* – particularly where there is right atrial dilatation, the standard curve on the trans-septal needle may not be enough to reach across to the fossa. There are specific needles designed with sharper curves as described previously (📖 p. 89), but it is possible to simply reshape the standard needle outside of the body with a sharper curve and then re-insert it into the sheath. Care needs to be taken when doing this not to damage the inner lumen of the needle, and with the sharper curve the needle tends to catch more as it is inserted into the sheath, especially as it goes under the inguinal ligament.

Management of trans-septal sheaths

- Once the trans-septal sheath is in the left atrium and has been flushed (📖 p. 90) catheters can be inserted. These should be inserted and withdrawn slowly as it is possible to create a negative pressure effect at the haemostatic valve (particularly on removing the catheter) and introduce air into the sheath.
- Whenever a catheter is removed from the sheath, before another catheter is inserted the sheath should be aspirated so that blood is flowing freely with no evidence of air, and then flushed with (heparinized) saline to avoid the risk of air embolism.
- Where trans-septal sheaths are going to be in the left atrium for longer periods of time (e.g. a number of hours for AF ablation procedures), many operators will continuously infuse saline or heparinized saline through the side arm (at rates of 30 ml/hr or more).

3-D cardiac mapping

Overview

Mapping refers to the process of integrating electrical information with cardiac anatomy. It is an essential step that allows the understanding of arrhythmia substrate needed to target ablation therapy.

Recent advances in technology have enabled mapping systems to:
• Display three-dimensional representation of cardiac chambers.
• Provide a visual display of the arrhythmia activation sequence.
• Display the arrhythmia substrate, e.g. scars, areas of conduction block.
• Non-fluoroscopically navigate catheters in real-time.
• Annotate sites of ablation lesions.

The systems that are most commonly used in clinical practice include sequential site mapping using magnetic field (CARTO) or electrical field (NavX) guidance, and simultaneous multisite non-contact reconstruction of endocardial electrical signals (Ensite Array).

The increasing complexity of ablation procedures, especially in the field of atrial fibrillation ablation, has led to the development of image integration techniques in an attempt to improve the accuracy and safety of ablation delivery. Detailed CT or MRI of the left atrium can be segmented from the original images and imported into mapping systems using the Merge software for CARTO and Fusion for NavX.

Three-dimensional electroanatomical mapping also provides an opportunity to elucidate the substrate of an arrhythmia. Mapping of electrogram voltage and local excitability helps to delineate areas of interest including potential scar or channels of conduction in re-entry circuits.

It is likely that cardiac mapping technology will continue to improve and refine to provide increasingly realistic anatomical representations and accurate guidance for ablation. Such developments have contributed not only in the clinical context but also in research into mechanisms of arrhythmia.

CARTO mapping

System overview

The CARTO system uses ultra-low magnetic fields to localize a specialized ablation catheter that contains a magnetic sensor at the distal electrode (Navistar). These magnetic fields are generated by three coils mounted under the examination table. The three-dimensional position and orientation (pitch, roll, and yaw) of the catheter tip can be determined. An external reference electrode patch placed on the patient's back is also required to compensate for patient movement.

Electrical data are collected sequentially by the Navistar from one or more cardiac chambers of interest. The system constructs a 3-D geometric 'shell' representing the shape and size of the chamber. Electroanatomic data can be shown in a number of ways:

- *Local activation time (LAT) map (Fig. 6.1)*. The timing of each individual recorded signal relative to a chosen reference is allocated a specific colour from the rainbow spectrum (earliest in red, latest in purple). The activation sequence and path of an arrhythmia are displayed in 3-D. Multiple chamber mapping can be performed.
- *Isochronal map (Fig. 6.1)*. Similar to the LAT map, but each colour is allocated a specific duration (e.g. 5 ms) so that conduction velocity is better appreciated.
- *Propagation map (Fig. 6.2)*. This is an animated version of the LAT map. The spread of wavefront propagation is projected in two colours as a running movie.
- *Voltage map*. The recorded signal amplitudes are allocated colours and the scale is manually adjusted to highlight abnormal myocardium (usually areas of low amplitude) in red. Sites with no electrograms or no capture consistent with scar can be tagged in grey.
- *Mesh map*. The chamber shell is shown as a transparent mesh so that annotated areas (e.g. ablation sites) from the whole chamber can be seen from one view.
- *CFAE (Complex fractionated atrial electrograms) map*. This is used in persistent atrial fibrillation ablation to display in red colour atrial sites with predefined local high frequency electrograms or fractionation (e.g. cycle length <120 ms).

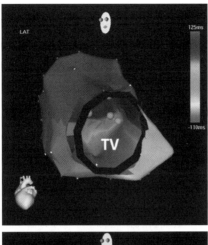

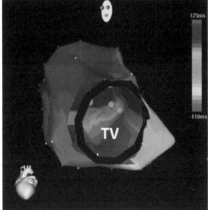

Fig. 6.1 CARTO local activation timing (LAT) map (top) and isochronal map (bottom) of the right atrium in LAO view. The activation sequence demonstrates a typical (counter-clockwise) right atrial flutter. TV – tricuspid valve annulus (black ring). The blue balls on the posterolateral wall (seen through the TV, red arrow) show the location of the crista terminalis. (☐ Plate 3 for colour version.)

Technical considerations
- Resolution: <1 mm for catheter position; <1 degree for orientation.
- Data sampling rate: 60 Hz.
- Bipolar and unipolar contact electrograms recorded by the Navistar catheter can be used for mapping.
- Combination with current-based localization technology can allow simultaneous display of a multi-polar mapping catheter.
- The reference patch should be placed close to the chamber of interest and checked by fluoroscopy. The patch position relative to the location pad is confirmed in the reference location dialogue box.

Advantages
- Geometry construction and annotation of sites of interest are accurate and intuitive.
- Electrical data and anatomic locations are collected and displayed by the system simultaneously during construction of the chamber geometry.
- Respiratory motion artefacts are relatively limited.
- LAT maps can be superimposed on a substrate map (e.g. scar).
- The CARTO algorithm is suitable for generating endocardial and epicardial anatomic maps.

Limitations
- Sequential site mapping can be time-consuming.
- Mapping of non-sustained tachycardia may be very difficult.
- Arrhythmias that are not well tolerated haemodynamically are usually not mappable.
- A change in tachycardia cycle length or morphology requires new mapping of the chamber.
- Only the Navistar catheter location can be shown (in earlier software versions).

When to use CARTO
- Sustained atrial or ventricular arrhythmias.
- Macroreentry atrial tachycardia in the setting of previous cardiac surgery and when atrial scarring is anticipated.
- Atrial tachycardia after atrial fibrillation ablation.
- Atrial fibrillation ablation.
- Endocardial and epicardial ablation of scar-mediated ventricular tachycardia.
- Substrate mapping for ablation of unmappable ventricular tachycardia.

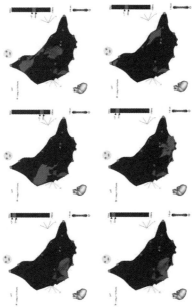

Fig. 6.2 CARTO propagation map of the right atrial flutter from Fig. 6.1. (📖 Plate 4 for colour version.)

NavX mapping

System overview

The Ensite NavX system generates a transthoracic electrical field by three pairs of orthogonal cutaneous patches. Catheter locations can be determined by measuring the local voltage gradient along each axis with respect to a reference electrode. Sequential positioning of a conventional catheter along the endocardial surface defines the geometry of a cardiac chamber. Separate geometries can be constructed for vessels attached to the chamber. The mapping catheter then collects electrical data and the system sequentially displays the information onto the geometry.

- *Diagnostic landmarking tool (Fig. 6.3)*. Activation timings relative to a chosen reference electrogram are shown on the geometry in a colour isochronal map (earliest in white, latest in purple).
- *Voltage mapping*. Electrogram amplitudes can be displayed in colour on the geometry using the diagnostic landmarking tool. Low amplitude electrograms below a specified threshold may be allocated a grey colour to represent areas of potential scar. High-voltage areas are labelled purple.
- *CFAE mapping*. The system computes a colour-coded map of atrial electrogram cycle lengths based on an algorithm that measures peak-to-peak electrogram intervals over a specified duration (e.g. 6 seconds). A fractionated index is calculated as mean or standard deviation of local electrogram intervals.

Technical considerations

- Resolution: <1 mm for catheter position.
- Data sampling rate: 1.2 kHz.
- Three pairs of cutaneous electrodes are applied to form the orthogonal axes of X, Y, and Z (left to right lateral, and neck to left leg, anterior to posterior).
- A 5.6 kHz low-level current is delivered alternately between these pairs of patches.
- Catheter locations are updated 93 times per second for up to 64 electrodes.
- A stable reference catheter is essential for the geometry, e.g. the coronary sinus catheter, a quadripolar catheter in the aorta, or an active-fixation catheter in the right atrium or ventricle.
- A respiratory compensation algorithm corrects for respiratory changes in thoracic impedance during the ablation procedure.
- A Field scaling algorithm may be applied after geometry construction to correct for impedance non-linearity that can distort the anatomical shape of the chamber.

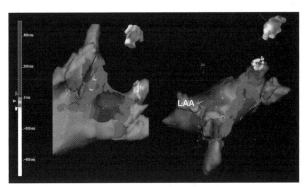

Fig. 6.3 Diagnostic landmarking of the left atrium during left atrial appendage (LAA) pacing to demonstrate a line of block on the atrial roof. The left infero-posterior view is shown on the left image; the superior view is shown on the right image. The colour scale refers to timing relative to a CS reference. Caudal to cranial activation of the posterior left atrium is demonstrated on the left image. (📖 Plate 5 for colour version.)

- Multi-polar catheters may be used to simultaneously collect electroanatomical data from multiple sites at the same time.
- Catheter navigation is fast and responsive.
- Any conventional mapping catheter may be used, thus reducing costs.
- Any energy source may be used for ablation.
- Multiple chamber mapping can be performed.

Limitations

- Chamber surface interpolations ('false space' without collected points) can occur in complex geometries.
- Catheter navigation accuracy can be affected by changes in respiratory patterns in a conscious patient.
- Mapping of non-sustained or poorly tolerated tachycardia may be difficult.
- A change in tachycardia cycle length or morphology requires repeat sequential mapping of the tachycardia circuit.

When to use NavX

- Sustained atrial or ventricular arrhythmias.
- Atrial fibrillation ablation.
- Atrial tachycardia after atrial fibrillation ablation.
- Endocardial ablation of ventricular tachycardia.
- Desire to perform multiple chamber mapping in conjunction with non-contact mapping (e.g. multiple tachycardia morphologies or non-sustained tachycardia).
- Conventional EPS/catheter ablation procedures with zero or minimal fluoroscopy.

Non-contact mapping

System overview

The Ensite multi-electrode array (MEA) is a specialized catheter designed to provide global, simultaneous electrical mapping of any cardiac chamber. It is positioned within the chamber of interest without direct contact with the endocardium. A conventional catheter is used to define the chamber geometry by sequentially mapping the endocardial border relative to the MEA (Fig. 6.4). Intracavity unipolar signals are then acquired by the MEA, amplified, and processed using inverse mathematics to reconstruct 'virtual' unipolar electrograms on the geometry.

- *Isopotential mapping*. In the review mode, the workstation can play back dynamic isopotential maps for any chosen heart beats. Filter settings and voltage thresholds may be manually specified to focus on local unipolar depolarization and to eliminate far-field potentials and repolarization changes. Depolarized regions are shown in white with the electrically silent background in purple. The entire arrhythmia circuit may be examined using adjustable playback speed and sequence.
- *Isochronal mapping*. A static map. It provides a colour representation of arrhythmia activation on the geometry for any chosen single beat. The earliest activation is displayed in white, and the latest in purple.
- *Dynamic substrate mapping*. This is a unipolar voltage map constructed from a selected cardiac cycle during sinus rhythm or pacing. The algorithm facilitates identification of low-voltage areas based on a percentage of the peak maximum unipolar voltage within the chamber. The system displays lines on the geometry encircling areas with the selected percentage voltage threshold.
- *Combined contact and non-contact mapping*. It is now possible to combine MEA-recorded unipolar signals with contact electrograms from a mapping catheter on the same geometry to enhance the display of substrate mapping.

Technical considerations

- The MEA consists of a 64-electrode mesh surrounding a 7.5 ml ellipsoid balloon that is mounted on a 9 Fr catheter.
- Resolution: <1 mm for mapping catheter position. A low-level current is passed at 5.68 kHz from the roving catheter to two ring electrodes of the MEA to allow determination of its location.
- Data sampling rate: 1.2 kHz.
- The system can generate 3360 virtual electrograms over the geometry at any one time.
- The reference electrode for the MEA is located in its shaft 16 cm proximal to the balloon.

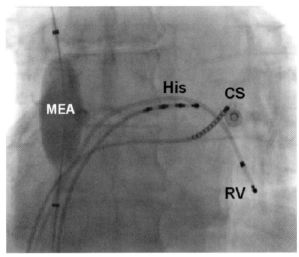

Fig. 6.4 Ensite multi-electrode array (MEA) in a right atrial electrophysiological study (AP view). Also shown are a quadripolar mapping catheter in the His region (His), a decapolar catheter in the coronary sinus (CS), and a bipolar catheter in the right ventricle (RV).

Advantages
- Ability to map non-sustained arrhythmias.
- Ability to quickly map multiple or changing arrhythmia circuits.
- Ability to map arrhythmias that cause haemodynamic instability.
- An entire arrhythmia circuit can be mapped in a single heart beat.
- Non-contact maps can be combined with contact data (NavX) using the same geometry.

Limitations
- Less suitable in larger cardiac chambers (accuracy reduced at distances >40 mm from the MEA).
- Low amplitude signals (e.g. fractionation, diastolic pathways) are not always detected by the MEA.
- Geometry construction can be distorted by false spaces.
- Isopotential maps are highly dependent on manual adjustment of filter settings and voltage thresholds.
- Inadvertent contact of the MEA with the endocardium or ablation catheter may cause artefacts or data saturation.

When to use non-contact mapping
- Ablation of non-sustained atrial or ventricular arrhythmias.
- Unifocal or multifocal right atrial tachycardia ablation.
- Atypical right atrial flutter ablation.
- Ablation of ventricular tachycardia with multiple morphologies.
- Ablation of ventricular tachycardia associated with haemodynamic instability.

Image integration

Image integration involves combining two representations of the same cardiac chamber that are created by two different modalities. In clinical practice, it most commonly refers to importing CT or MRI images of the left atrium into NavX (Figs. 6.5 and 6.6) and CARTO (Fig. 6.7) mapping systems for guidance of atrial fibrillation ablation. The accuracy of these techniques has been validated in animal and clinical studies. It is also valuable as a learning tool in complex anatomical ablation.

There are three fundamental processes involved in image integration:
• Image acquisition: The original rendering of cardiac anatomy using CT, MRI, intracardiac echocardiography (ICE), or rotational angiography.
• Segmentation: The isolation of an image of a cardiac chamber from neighbouring structures.
• Registration: The alignment and incorporation of the segmented chamber image with an electroanatomic map.

Different modalities of imaging techniques can be integrated with current mapping and navigational technologies, for example:
• CT/MRI with 3-D electroanatomical mapping.
• CT/MRI with 2-D fluoroscopy.
• Intracardiac echocardiography with 3-D electroanatomical mapping.
• 3-D electroanatomical mapping (± CT/MRI) with remote navigational systems (magnetic or robotic).
• Rotational angiography with 2-D fluoroscopy.

Image acquisition

Radiological modalities using CT or MRI can provide realistic images representing the actual anatomy of cardiac chambers. The qualities of CT or MRI images are similar, although CT carries a significant radiation dose. The choice is usually dependent on local expertise.

A number of factors may affect the quality and applicability of the images:
• *Rate and rhythm*. Images acquired during atrial fibrillation or tachycardia may be suboptimal.
• *Volume status.* Differences in volume loading during image acquisition and ablation may affect the size of the left atrium.
• *Respiratory phase.* CT/MRI performed during end-inspiration, whereas electroanatomical maps constructed in end-expiration. Errors are more likely to involve pulmonary vein branches than the left atrial body.
• *Timing prior to ablation*. Imaging should be performed as close as possible to the ablation procedure. Real-time imaging with ICE avoids this problem.

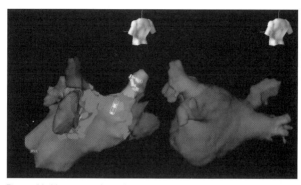

Fig. 6.5 NavX geometry of the left atrium and its DIFF image segmented from a cardiac MRI. It is possible to simultaneously display the circular mapping catheter in the right upper pulmonary vein (yellow). The tip of the ablation catheter is shown in green. Ablation lesions around the pulmonary veins and a roof line are shown as red dots. (📖 Plate 6 for colour version.)

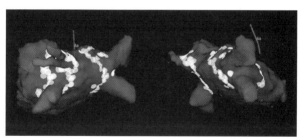

Fig. 6.6 An Ensite Fusion case of atrial fibrillation ablation. An MRI of the left atrium has been fused with the NavX geometry. The fused image provides accurate anatomical guidance for targeting ablation therapy (white dots). Note that a reference catheter has been positioned in the ascending aorta. (📖 Plate 7 for colour version.)

Segmentation

Electroanatomical mapping systems provide specific software tools to segment cardiac chambers of interest. Typically, segmentation involves the following:

- Select the thoracic level of interest.
- Adjust the blood pool density to highlight the cardiac chamber.
- Label, then segment the chamber from surrounding structures.
- Manual tailoring of inaccuracies in the final image.

Registration

For left atrial registration, it is recommended that pulmonary vein angiography is performed before registration to define the anatomy of the venous ostia.

CARTO merge

- Landmark registration is usually performed first. Three to four specific landmarks (usually at the ostia) are identified and labelled at matching locations on both the segmented image and the real-time electroanatomical map.
- Navistar catheter locations on fluoroscopy are matched with respective locations on the CT/MRI image.
- The two images are then superimposed.
- Surface registration is performed with the Navistar catheter by collecting location points along the endocardial surface of the chamber. The system automatically aligns the contour of the CT/MRI image to these points.
- An alternative strategy is to perform surface registration before landmark registration. Only a single landmark is required.
- Aim for a mean registration error of <3 mm.

NavX Fusion

- A NavX geometry is created first using an ablation or circular mapping catheter.
- A Field scaling algorithm is applied.
- Fiducial pairs of points on CT/MRI and NavX geometries are matched side-by-side (primary fusion).
- The two images are superimposed.
- Supplemental fiducial points are placed at respective sites on the two images to improve registration. The size and rotation of the NavX geometry may be optimized to fit the radiological anatomy (secondary fusion).

After completion of registration, the electroanatomical map can be hidden. Visualization of the mapping catheter and annotation of ablation sites can then be made directly on the CT/MRI image.

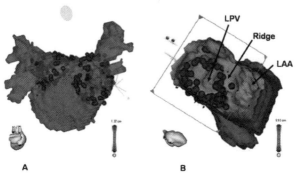

A   **B**

Fig. 6.7 A CARTO merge case of atrial fibrillation ablation. An MRI of the left atrium has been merged with the CARTO shell. Panel A shows a PA view of the left atrium. Circumferential ablation lesions (red dots) have been delivered around the left and right pulmonary veins in pairs. In panel B, the image has been clipped to allow direct endocardial visualization of the left pulmonary venous ostia (LPV) and left atrial appendage (LAA). The LAA ridge can be demonstrated between the LAA and the left pulmonary veins. (📖 Plate 9 for colour version.)

Potential pitfalls of image integration and solutions

- Volume loading may alter chamber size. Perform CT/MRI close to day of ablation.
- Tenting of the left atrial roof or anterior wall during surface registration or secondary fusion may distort the electroanatomic map. Manually delete these points.
- Significant rotational registration error may occur in the sagittal plane if only pulmonary venous ostia are used as landmarks. Use landmarks at the mitral annulus or appendage.
- Registration can be affected by movement artefacts. Consider using general anaesthesia.

Geometry construction

A mapping catheter is positioned sequentially along the endocardium or epicardium of a cardiac chamber. These locations are then registered by the system to create an anatomical representation of the chamber. Different algorithms are used to construct this geometry:

- *CARTO* creates an impression of a shell based on the 3-D locations of the acquired points.
- *NavX* and *Ensite Array* calculate and update the outermost locations of the mapping catheter and define the geometry border relative to a centre point.
- Before constructing an Ensite Array geometry, attempt to position the centre of the MEA close to the site of presumed earliest activation.

Practical tips

- Ensure adequate catheter contact before accepting its location.
- Acquire at least 30–40 well-distributed locations around the chamber.
- Label the anatomical relations of the chamber, e.g. for the right atrium, label the locations of the tricuspid annulus, caval veins, and coronary sinus.
- Attempt to acquire points at the same phase of respiration, and discard points acquired during sudden changes of respiratory pattern.
- Delete location points acquired when the chamber shape has been distorted, e.g. tenting of the left atrial roof by the catheter tip.
- For NavX and Ensite Array geometries, the algorithm occasionally generates false spaces – create separate geometries, e.g. for atrial body, pulmonary veins, and appendage.

Analysis of arrhythmia activation

Contact mapping

- Reference signal: A stable and consistent signal is required. This may be chosen from a temporary screw-in lead or the coronary sinus catheter. Select a CS signal with a large-amplitude atrial electrogram and minimal ventricular electrogram. For ventricular arrhythmias the surface ECG QRS complex may be used as a timing reference.
- Data resolution: At least 50–100 points are usually required to accurately define arrhythmia mechanisms. Ten to twenty points should be focused on the areas of earliest activation or slow conduction.
- Window of interest/diagnostic landmarking (Fig. 6.8): This creates a window of sensing to determine electrogram timing (early or late) relative to the reference. If mapping is performed during pacing, the window should be manipulated to blank out 10 ms after the pacing spike. If re-entrant tachycardia is suspected, the window duration should be selected to cover 90–100% of tachycardia cycle length. Sequentially map the whole chamber and generate a 3-D activation map.
- In focal tachycardia, there is a centrifugal pattern of activation from a discrete site of earliest activation. Usually <50% of tachycardia cycle length can be mapped within the chamber.
- In re-entrant tachycardia, >90% of tachycardia cycle length can be mapped. The circuit may involve several segments of the chamber (macroreentry), or less commonly occurs within a small segment (microreentry).
- In CARTO, the 'early-meets-late' algorithm highlights in purple the progression from adjacent late to early sites to prevent colour interpolation.

Practical tips

- The left margin of the sensing window should be placed before the onset of the earliest activation on the surface ECG to capture diastolic activity.
- For fractionated potentials, label activation timing at the onset of the electrograms.
- For double potentials, choose local timing at the larger of the two electrograms.
- Clearly annotate areas of scar to minimize colour interpolation between adjacent sites with differences in activation times.
- Re-map is necessary if the tachycardia cycle length or morphology has changed. Collect new points on the same chamber shell.

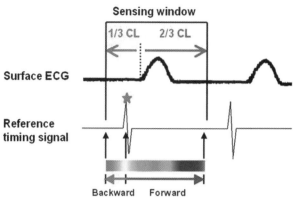

Fig. 6.8 Sensing window calculation: forward and backward timing durations are measured relative to a reference timing signal. The onset of the window is taken before tachycardia onset from the surface ECG (approximately 1/3 of the tachycardia cycle length) to include potential diastolic activity in a re-entry circuit. In this example, the sensing window covers 100% of the tachycardia cycle length. (☐ Plate 10 for colour version.)

Non-contact mapping

- The Ensite system reconstructs 3360 virtual unipolar electrograms over the entire geometry surface. The user may manually select electrogram waveforms from the geometry for display and examination.
- Electrogram data can be recorded as desired by the operator during sinus rhythm or arrhythmia. Theoretically, only a single beat is needed to establish the activation pattern of an arrhythmia. In practice, it is essential to analyse a number of beats of the same tachycardia to ensure consistency of the reconstructed data.
- To define the tachycardia mechanism using isopotential mapping, review the activation sequence in a slow playback speed (e.g. 1:50) over several beats (Fig. 6.9). Manually adjust the voltage scale to trace the earliest activation sites.
- Stretch out the virtual electrogram waveforms by displaying at fast-sweep speed (e.g. 400 mm/s).
- The earliest QS complex denotes the earliest site of activation.
- An initial R wave may suggest activation from a neighbouring site or chamber.
- Once an area of potential ablation target has been identified on the geometry, label it and confirm electrogram characteristics using a contact mapping catheter.

Practical tips

- Select high-pass filter at >4 Hz initially to minimize repolarization artefacts.
- When examining areas of slow conduction or possible diastolic pathways, select high-pass filter at 1 Hz and ensure the autofocus function is switched off.
- Differences in direction of activation or timing (> 40 ms) over adjacent areas may suggest a line of conduction block.
- If initial attempts at ablation are not successful, record and review the arrhythmia again to exclude changes in the tachycardia circuit.

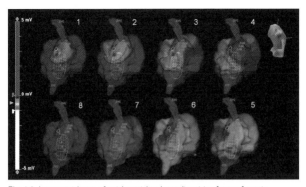

Fig. 6.9 Isopotential map of a right atrial tachycardia arising from a focus in the superior crista terminalis adjacent to the sinus mode. The sequence of depolarization is marked in order of from image 1 to 8. The green SAN labels mark the sinus node. The green numbers 6–10 mark the crista terminalis. Activation begins inferior and posterior to the sinus node (1) and spreads inferiorly and to the septum but is blocked by the crista terminalis (2–4) before passing through a gap (green number 10, 5) and spreading anteriority (6–8). (📖 Plate 11 for colour version.)

Substrate mapping

This is particularly important in scar-related ventricular tachycardias or incisional tachycardias in which tachycardias are haemodynamically poorly tolerated, non-inducible, or non-sustained at the time of the ablation procedure.

Contact voltage mapping in the ventricle (Fig. 6.10)

- Bipolar amplitude <1.5 mV is considered abnormal.
- Bipolar amplitude <0.5 mV has been referred to as 'dense scar'.
- Bipolar amplitude <1.0 mV and contact unipolar amplitude <5.8 mV have been validated with delay enhancement MRI as scar consisting of critical areas of post-infarction ventricular tachycardia.
- Failure to locally capture at >10 mA at 2 ms pulse width within a low voltage area may identify electrically unexcitable scars that form the border of re-entrant circuits.

Contact voltage mapping in the atrium

- Contact voltage mapping to define scarring in the atrium is less well validated.
- Bipolar amplitude <0.5 mV is probably abnormal.
- Bipolar amplitude <0.05–0.1 mV is likely to represent scar.
- Label electrically silent areas, double potentials, and fractionation on a voltage map to define the potential re-entry circuits.

Non-contact substrate mapping

- The dynamic substrate mapping (DSM) algorithm uses a percentage of the peak negative voltage of a chamber.
- DSM can be performed in sinus rhythm or constant pacing.
- It does not use an absolute cut-off value because MEA reconstructed voltages can be affected by differences in chamber size and mass.
- High-low pass filter settings: 2–150 Hz.
- During sinus rhythm, peak negative voltage <34% using DSM correlates with MRI and experimental ventricular scar.
- During ventricular pacing, the peak negative voltage cut-off is adjusted to <20%.
- DSM of the atrium is less well defined. The peak negative voltage is likely to be much lower than in the ventricle.

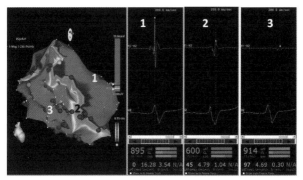

Fig. 6.10 CARTO bipolar voltage map of the left ventricle in sinus rhythm (modified RAO view). This patient has a prior inferior infarction with a large scar in the infero-posterior left ventricle. Representative sites from different regions are selected for display. 1 – normal myocardium (3.54 mV); 2 – probable border zone (1.04 mV); 3 – likely scar (0.30 mV). (📖 Plate 12 for colour version.)

Part 2

Electrophysiological testing for specific indications

Narrow complex tachycardia

Introduction

Intracardiac EPS is most commonly performed for patients with recurrent episodes of regular narrow complex tachycardia or 'supraventricular tachycardia' (SVT). The primary goal is to identify the mechanism of the tachycardia as an essential prelude to curative catheter ablation.

- In the past, purely diagnostic EPS could be conducted in exhaustive detail without time constraints. However, now that combined diagnostic/ablation procedures have become the norm, there is pressure to determine the arrhythmia mechanism as quickly as possible and proceed to therapeutic intervention with minimal delay.
- In most cases, the mechanism is easily identified through simple pattern recognition. Nevertheless, the operator needs to follow a systematic approach with basic checklists to avoid diagnostic pitfalls that could lead to potentially disastrous misclassification of an arrhythmia and inappropriate ablation therapy.
- Unpredictable/unusual findings are relatively common and operators must be alert to any divergences from the standard patterns and be prepared to adjust their routine protocols to fully investigate and account for such discrepancies *before* attempting ablation. The commonest explanation is the co-existence of more than one SVT mechanism in an individual patient (5–10% cases).

Differential diagnosis

Awareness of the differential diagnosis of narrow complex tachycardia and the relative frequency of the arrhythmia mechanisms (Table 7.1) is essential.

- The two commonest conditions, typical AVNRT and accessory pathway-mediated AVRT, account for around 80% of cases.
- Atypical forms of AVNRT, focal atrial tachycardias including sinus node re-entrant tachycardia (SNRT), and macroreentrant atrial tachycardias (atrial flutter) make up most of the remainder.
- Although MRAT/atrial flutter is a relatively common arrhythmia in clinical practice, most cases are diagnosed on the basis of ECG alone. Therefore it is an infrequent cause of undiagnosed regular narrow complex tachycardia coming to EPS.

Table 7.1 Differential diagnosis of narrow complex tachycardia

Mechanism	Frequency	📖
Typical AVNRT	50–60%	p. 236
AVRT (± WPW syndrome)	30%	p. 250
Atypical AVNRT	5–10%	p. 242
Focal atrial tachycardia including SNRT	10%	p. 290
Typical atrial flutter Other macroreentrant atrial tachycardia	5–10%	pp. 292–294
Automatic atrial tachycardia Junctional ectopic tachycardia	<5%	p. 290

Four-step diagnostic approach to regular narrow complex tachycardias

A systematic approach should always be followed although the steps may not always be performed in the standard order (for example if catheter placement provokes SVT before antegrade/retrograde curves can be performed).

Step 1: Clues from existing ECG data

Careful *pre-operative* review of available non-invasive data often provides valuable clues to guide EPS:

- 12-lead ECG during sinus rhythm ± result of adenosine testing.
- Examination of 12-lead ECGs during narrow complex tachycardia (wherever possible).
- ECG rhythm strips showing initiation/termination.
- Response of tachycardia to vagal manoeuvres and/or adenosine.
- Occasional diagnostic ECG findings.

Step 2: Identification of arrhythmia substrate(s)

Analysis of antegrade and retrograde conduction to identify potential SVT substrates (AV nodal duality, accessory pathways etc.) using:

- Basic intervals.
- Assessment of retrograde conduction.
- Assessment of antegrade conduction.
- Parahisian pacing.

Step 3: Induction and analysis of tachycardia

Induction and analysis of clinical tachycardia, particularly:

- Mode of initiation and termination.
- AV relationship during tachycardia.
- VA time and atrial activation sequence (midline vs. eccentric).
- Effect of cycle length variation.
- Effect of bundle branch block aberration.

Step 4: Pacing manoeuvres during tachycardia

Specific pacing manoeuvres to assess tachycardia mechanism:

- Response to ventricular entrainment.
- Diastolic scanning with ventricular extrastimuli including His-synchronous VPC.
- Response to atrial overdrive pacing or extrastimuli (rarely).
- Response to adenosine or other anti-arrhythmic agents.

Step 1: Clues from existing ECG data

Every effort should be made to obtain ECG documentation of narrow complex tachycardia prior to EPS, ideally a full 12-lead ECG. Also ambulance rhythm strips, Holter or transtelephonic ECG recordings, particularly any showing initiation/termination, variable AV block, or onset/offset of bundle branch block. Details of tachycardia response to IV adenosine or vagal manoeuvres should be checked, including the ECG rhythm strips if obtainable.

12-lead ECG in sinus rhythm

- Pre-excitation indicates an antegradely conducting accessory pathway and favours diagnosis of AVRT (Fig 7.1).
- The absence of a delta wave does not exclude AVRT:
  - Latent pre-excitation (📖 p. 248): i.e. it takes so long for atrial activity to reach accessory pathways located in a left free wall that the ventricles have already been normally activated via the His-Purkinje system. Delta wave can be revealed by IV adenosine to block AV nodal conduction.
  - Intermittent pre-excitation (📖 p. 257): suggests a relatively long antegrade pathway ERP.
  - Concealed accessory pathways: these only conduct in a retrograde direction from ventricle to atria so do not give rise to a delta wave but can sustain orthodromic AVRT.
- The presence of a delta wave is not diagnostic of AVRT. In around 10% of patients with a pre-excited ECG, the accessory pathway is a bystander and the underlying mechanism of SVT is AVNRT.

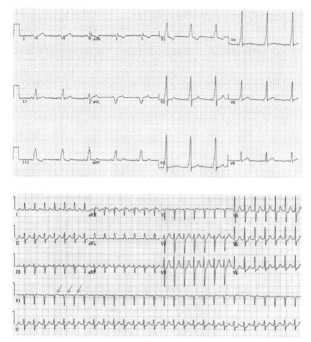

Fig. 7.1 ECG showing sinus rhythm and pre-excitation consistent with a left lateral accessory pathway (top). ECG showing orthodromic AVRT in the same patient (bottom). The arrows indicate the retrograde P waves.

12-lead ECG during tachycardia

The key is to identify the P waves (atrial activity) and their relationship to the QRS complexes (AV relationship). Interpretation may be facilitated by comparison with the 12-lead ECG in sinus rhythm (ideally recorded with the same leads/ECG machine), particularly when the P waves are inscribed over the QRS complexes.

- >1:1 AV ratio is highly suggestive of an atrial tachyarrhythmia (either focal or macroreentrant).
  - May be transient.
  - May be difficult to identify due to fusion of atrial activity/T waves.
  - Rarely, AVNRT is conducted with infranodal AV block (usually 2:1).
- No isoelectric baseline suggests macroreentrant tachycardia (flutter).
  - Typical sawtooth baseline is seen with counter-clockwise cavotricuspid isthmus-dependent ('common') atrial flutter.
  - Common atrial flutter is often associated with a ventricular rate around 150 bpm but **most cases of narrow complex SVT at around 150 bpm are due to junctional mechanisms** (AVNRT or AVRT).
- In typical AVNRT, the retrograde P waves are inscribed over the QRS complexes (Fig. 11.3).
  - Easier to identify by comparison with sinus rhythm ECG.
  - Pseudo R' in lead V1 or pseudo S in lead II result from P wave superimposed on the terminal portion of the QRS and are highly suggestive of AVNRT.
  - Rarely seen with focal atrial tachycardia and PR interval similar to tachycardia cycle length, and never with AVRT.
  - Commonest explanation for **narrow complex tachycardia with no discernible P waves**.
- Visible P waves after the QRS complexes are commonly seen in AVRT (Fig. 7.1).
  - May also occur in intermediate AVNRT and atrial tachycardia.
  - In AVRT and atypical AVNRT the P waves will usually be inverted in the inferior leads.
  - QRS alternans during tachycardia (variation in the beat-to-beat QRS amplitude by >1 mm) is commoner in AVRT than AVNRT.
  - Repolarization abnormalities (T wave inversion or ST depression) are also commoner in AVRT than AVNRT.

Response of tachycardia to IV adenosine (Fig. 7.2)

Bolus IV adenosine blocks the AV node, unmasking atrial arrhythmias and terminating junctional tachyarrhythmias dependent on AV node conduction (*NB failure to achieve termination or transient AV block suggests too low a dose of adenosine has been used – this may require >12 mg*).

Table 7.2 Response of tachycardia to IV adenosine

Arrhythmia	Effect of adenosine during tachycardia
AVRT	Terminates tachycardia
AVNRT (typical and atypical)	Terminates tachycardia
Focal atrial tachycardia	Transiently blocks AV conduction revealing rapid atrial activity; rarely terminates tachycardia
Sinus node re-entrant tachycardia	Terminates tachycardia
Atrial flutter (MRAT)	Transiently blocks AV conduction to reveal continuous underlying atrial activity

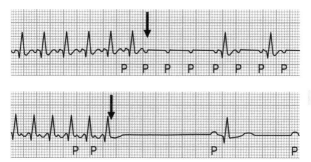

Fig. 7.2 Figure showing the effects of adenosine administration (arrow) on SVT. The upper strip shows ongoing fast atrial activity (unchanged) during AV block and then as AV conduction starts to recover, indicating **atrial tachycardia** (AV node is bystander). In the lower strip, SVT terminates with adenosine administration, consistent with a tachycardia that is dependent on the AV node for its maintenance, i.e. **AVNRT** or **AVRT**.

Other diagnostic ECG clues

A number of uncommon but characteristic ECG appearances can suggest or identify the likely mechanism of tachycardia, as outlined below. These are usually obtained from Holter ECG recordings or ward telemetry ECG monitors.

- Onset or offset of bundle branch block (BBB) during tachycardia (usually due to repetitive concealed penetration of the bundle):
  - Development of BBB during the tachycardia associated with **increase** in the cycle length (i.e. **slowing**) is diagnostic of AVRT utilizing an accessory pathway on the **same** side as the BBB (prolongs conduction time in the ventricle) (Fig. 7.13).
  - BBB with **no change** in cycle length is consistent with any SVT mechanism including AVRT (pathway and BBB on different sides).
  - Only applies if narrow QRS tachycardia and BBB are observed within the same episode of tachycardia.
  - Rate-related BBB is relatively uncommon with SVT but may be associated with **acceleration** at onset of BBB.
- Observations at initiation of tachycardia:
  - Initiation with sudden jump in PR interval, often following an APB, is suggestive of typical AVNRT (Fig. 7.3).
  - Initiation by VPB is unusual in typical AVNRT or atrial tachycardia and suggests AVRT.
  - Focal atrial tachycardia due to automaticity may exhibit 'warm-up' at initiation (Fig. 7.10).
- Observations at termination of tachycardia:
  - Typical AVNRT and AVRT usually terminate with antegrade block in the AV node such that the final beat of tachycardia has a P wave not followed by a QRS complex.
  - Atrial tachycardias are independent of the AV node, so the final beat of tachycardia consists of a P wave that is followed by a conducted QRS complex.
  - Atypical forms of AVNRT or AVRT (long RP tachycardia) often terminate retrogradely in the AV node, mimicking atrial tachycardia.
  - Termination by a VPB is unusual with typical AVNRT or atrial tachycardia and is suggestive of AVRT.
- Miscellaneous:
  - Sinus node re-entrant tachycardia (SNRT) produces a sudden change in heart rate at onset/offset with no change in P wave morphology (📖 p. 297).
  - Narrow complex tachycardia with AV ratio <1:1, i.e. VA block (usually 2:1), is diagnostic of AVNRT.
  - Atrial tachyarrhythmias with 2:1 block may be transiently accelerated to 1:1 conduction and sudden doubling of the heart rate.

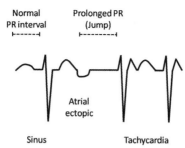

Fig. 7.3 Typical initiation of AVNRT with a critically timed atrial premature beat. The PR interval prolongs with the premature atrial ectopic (the ECG demonstration of decremental conduction and an AH jump demonstrated with intracardiac electrograms in Fig. 7.6.

Step 2: Identification of possible arrhythmia substrates

Introduction

Following placement of catheters, a search is made for evidence of the two commonest arrhythmic substrates – AV nodal duality supporting AVNRT and accessory pathways supporting AVRT. This is based on:

- Basic intervals.
- Assessment of retrograde conduction.
- Assessment of antegrade conduction.
- Parahisian pacing in specific cases if indicated.

(NB Some electrophysiologists prefer to assess antegrade conduction before retrograde but either approach is acceptable.)

It is important to note that:

- Identified arrhythmia substrates often predict the mechanism of SVT but may be bystanders (especially AV nodal duality) – definitive proof requires induction of tachycardia.
- More than one substrate and/or SVT mechanism is present in a significant minority of cases.

Therefore, a complete evaluation for potential arrhythmia substrates should be performed in all cases, even if the process is interrupted by induction of tachycardia and Steps 3 and 4 (see below).

Basic intervals

- Is there manifest pre-excitation with short or negative HV?
- Is there latent pre-excitation with early local V activation in the distal CS poles?

Assessment of retrograde conduction (Figs. 7.4 and 7.5)

Some electrophysiologists routinely start with assessment of antegrade conduction, but initial assessment of retrograde conduction has several advantages and is our preferred approach:

- Enables early identification of accessory pathway.
- If VA Wenckebach or block, accessory pathway/AVRT very unlikely.
- If VA Wenckebach, AVNRT is most likely diagnosis but will need autonomic manipulation (isoprenaline ± atropine) to induce sustained tachycardia.
- Complete VA block despite autonomic manipulation makes AVNRT or AVRT very unlikely; the probable diagnosis is an atrial tachyarrhythmia.

Normal retrograde conduction patterns (⊞ Retrograde curve, p. 72)

- No VA conduction or VA Wenckebach conduction.
- Decremental, midline conduction.
- Extra ventricular beats ('V4R') following the extrastimulus (S2) due to bundle branch re-entry or ventricular echo.
- Gap phenomena.

Evidence of retrograde accessory pathway (AP) conduction (⊞ p. 246)

- Non-decremental conduction.
- Eccentric activation for right and left free wall APs with earliest atrial activation at HRA and distal CS respectively.
- Midline activation for septal APs with non-decremental VA conduction down to pathway ERP followed by:
  - 'jump' in VA interval with subsequent decremental conduction due to switch to AV node conduction
  - VA block if retrograde AV nodal ERP is > retrograde AP ERP.

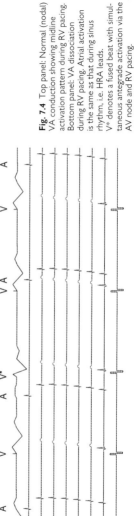

Fig. 7.4 Top panel: Normal (nodal) VA conduction showing midline activation pattern during RV pacing. Bottom panel: VA dissociation during RV pacing. Atrial activation is the same as that during sinus rhythm, i.e. HRA leads. V* denotes a fused beat with simultaneous antegrade activation via the AV node and RV pacing.

Difficulties with interpretation of retrograde curve

- AV nodal fusion and retrograde latency (Fig. 7.5):
  - Retrograde AP conduction is masked as the atria are activated by retrograde conduction via the AV node ('fusion') before the impulse reaches the AP.
  - Such 'retrograde latency' is most often seen with left-sided APs.
  - Usually unmasked during retrograde curve as the extrastimulus decrements in the AV node, delaying nodal activation compared to non-decremental activation via the AP. With left-sided APs, this results in shift from midline to eccentric CS activation.
  - Latent retrograde AP conduction may also be unmasked by:
    (i) pacing at shorter cycle lengths; (ii) LV pacing for left-sided APs (i.e. closer to AP insertion); (iii) IV adenosine to transiently block retrograde AV nodal conduction.
- Septal AP and AV nodes have similar retrograde conduction times at AP ERP – no VA 'jump' or change in midline activation as conduction switches from AP to AV node, so presence of AP may be missed:
  - AP should be suspected if IV adenosine fails to produce VA block.
  - Confirm/refute presence of AP by parahisian pacing (📖 p. 150).
  - Presence of AP may also be confirmed if SVT is inducible and His-synchronous VPC advances atrial activation (📖 p. 166).
- Retrograde AV nodal conduction is exclusively via fast pathway with minimal decrement followed by VA block at coupling intervals < AV node ERP – resembles septal AP conduction:
  - AP is unlikely if IV adenosine produces VA block.
  - Presence of AP can be refuted by parahisian pacing.
  - AP is unlikely if SVT is inducible but His-synchronous VPC fails to advance atrial activation.

Key questions to answer when assessing retrograde conduction

- Is there is VA conduction? If not, AVRT is very unlikely.
- Is VA conduction normal, i.e. midline atrial activation and decremental? If not, then there may be retrogradely conducting AP.
- Location of AP, i.e. where is the earliest retrograde A?
- What is the ERP of AP?
- Can the AP support re-entry, i.e. AVRT?

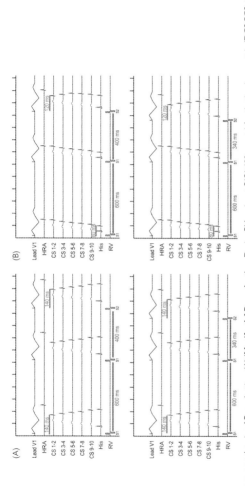

Fig. 7.5 Retrograde curves showing AP conduction. (A) **'Manifest' AP conduction**: During RV pacing at S1S1 600 ms, atrial activation is eccentric (DCS-PCS, then His and HRA). No decrement in VA interval (140 ms) following extrastimulus at S1S2 400 ms (upper panel), vs. S1S2 340 ms (lower panel). LA is being activated entirely via left lateral AP conduction – *no fusion* with retrograde AV nodal conduction. (B) **'Latent' AP conduction**: Retrograde AV node conduction activates the LA from the septum, before the paced impulses reach the insertion of the left lateral AP. Thus, during RV pacing at S1S1 600 ms, activation is midline (His, then PCS-DCS). An extrastimulus at S1S2 400 ms (upper panel) delays AV nodal activation due to decremental conduction but has no effect on AP conduction, resulting in fusion of the two wavefronts and a 'reverse chevron' pattern (earliest DCS and His, later at mid-CS). S1S2 340 ms (lower panel) further delays AV nodal conduction but not AP conduction (VA interval at DCS unchanged at 120 ms), resulting in LA activation entirely via the AP and the eccentric DCS-PCS pattern.

Assessment of antegrade conduction (Figs. 7.6 and 7.7)

The main aim is to check for dual AV nodal pathways as a potential substrate for AVNRT but occasionally the assessment unmasks 'latent pre-excitation' indicating an antegradely conducting accessory pathway.

- Based primarily on extrastimulus technique/antegrade curve (📖 p. 68).
- If normal or indeterminate, can try:
  - Different drive/pacing cycle length.
  - Double atrial extrastimuli.
  - Incremental atrial pacing.
  - Some or all of the above after autonomic manipulation (isoprenaline ± atropine, rarely β-blocker).

(NB If sustained tachycardia is initiated during this stage, assessment of antegrade conduction can be completed after Steps 3 and 4).

Normal antegrade conduction
- Smoothly decremental AV and AH conduction.
- Clear His electrogram with normal constant HV interval.

Is there evidence of antegrade accessory pathway conduction?
- Decremental AH conduction but non-decremental AV conduction.
- HV interval becomes progressively more negative and His electrogram may be lost in the ventricular electrogram.
- Pre-excitation becomes progressively more manifest.
- Latent pre-excitation unmasked.
- Pacing near the site of AP will increase pre-excitation and reduce the P to delta interval (usually CS pacing for left free wall pathways).
- Antegrade pathway conduction blocks when S1S2 is < AP ERP – if AVN ERP is < AP ERP, antegrade AV nodal conduction resumes with normalization of HV and disappearance of delta wave.

Is dual AV nodal physiology demonstrable? (Figs. 4.13, 4.14, 7.6)
- In typical cases, faster conducting route ('fast pathway') has longer ERP than slower conducting route ('slow pathway').
- Decremental AV and AH conduction down fast pathway until ERP of fast pathway is reached, then conduction switches to slow pathway with sudden increase in A2H2 interval – the AH 'jump' (📖 p. 238).
- AH jump is defined as increase of A2H2 or H1H2 interval of ≥50 ms with a 10 ms decrease of A1A2 (or S1S2) coupling interval.
- Produces discontinuity of the antegrade curve.
- Occasionally observe more than one jump in antegrade curve.

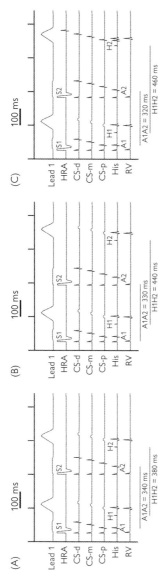

Fig. 7.6 Antegrade curve showing evidence of dual AV nodal physiology. (A) Atrial pacing from HRA. Normal decremental antegrade conduction with atrial extrastimulus results in A1A2 of 340 ms conducted with H1H2 of 380 ms. (B) Shortening extrastimulus by 10 ms results in A1A2 of 330 ms and a 'jump' in H1H2 by 60 ms to 440 ms, reflecting antegrade block in the fast pathway and switch to slow pathway conduction. However, the impulse terminates in the ventricle with no echo beat back to the atria. (C) Shortening the coupling interval further results in A1A2 of 320 ms and delays H1H2 to 460 ms, sufficient for fast pathway refractoriness to recover and conduct an echo beat back to the atria with midline activation sequence 'jump + echo'. These findings in a patient with documented narrow complex tachycardia are highly suggestive of AVNRT but it is still essential to induce sustained tachycardia to confirm the diagnosis.

Potential difficulties in detecting AV nodal duality

- Conduction times of fast and slow pathways are similar at coupling intervals near to fast pathway ERP, so that the 'jump' is <50 ms:
  - Repeat antegrade curve with faster drive cycle length.
  - Repeat antegrade curve with autonomic manipulation (isoprenaline ± atropine, rarely β-blocker).
- Fast pathway ERP is not reached due to progressive intra-atrial conduction delay (i.e. A1A2 > S1S2) at short coupling intervals:
  - Try double atrial extrastimuli.
  - Try incremental atrial pacing to check if Kay's sign (Fig. 4.17).
  - Pacing from a different site, e.g. PCS.
- Fast pathway ERP < slow pathway ERP:
  - Repeat antegrade curve with autonomic manipulation.
  - Repeat antegrade curve with a slower drive cycle.

Are there atrial echo beats (Fig. 7.6 and Fig. 7.7)?

- AV nodal duality may be incidental (detectable in 30% of population) and its presence does **not** prove AVNRT.
- An atrial echo beat occurs when an extrastimulus is conducted antegradely down the SP and then retrogradely via the FP to the atria:
  - Timing of typical echo beat is similar to ventricular activation (impulses travel down His-Purkinje system and up FP simultaneously).
  - If SP has recovered by the time the impulse travels up FP, it can re-conduct antegradely and potentially support AV nodal re-entry.
- Atrial echo beats must be differentiated from intra-atrial re-entry beats:
  - True nodal echoes exhibit midline activation.
  - Caudo-cranial activation (His/PCS precedes HRA).
  - Consistent VA timing over a range of coupling intervals.
- Intra-atrial re-entry suggested if:
  - Abnormal atrial activation pattern (HRA before low RA/PCS or eccentric CS pattern) (Fig. 7.7).
  - Inconsistent VA interval with repeated testing over range of coupling intervals.
- Presence of atrial echo beats makes AVNRT very likely (>90%) but definitive proof still requires induction of tachycardia (Steps 3 and 4).

Key observations during assessment of antegrade conduction

- Is there manifest pre-excitation on ECG? If yes:
  - Determine AP location, i.e. where is the earliest V activation?
  - Determine AP antegrade conduction properties, i.e. AP ERP and minimum pre-excited RR interval during AF and/or incremental atrial pacing.
  - Does AP support tachycardia, i.e. AVRT?
- Is there latent pre-excitation?
  - Early V activation in distal CS poles.
  - Non-decremental AV conduction with unmasking of pre-excitation at shorter coupled extrastimuli.
  - Alternatively use adenosine, pacing at short cycle lengths, or pacing near AP atrial insertion site to unmask pre-excitation.
- If AV conduction is decremental, check for dual AV node physiology:
  - Is there an AH jump on the antegrade curve?
  - Are there one or more atrial echoes?
  - Does the AV node support AVNRT?

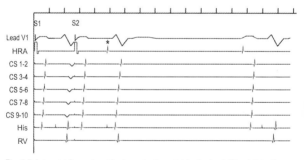

Fig. 7.7 Intra-atrial re-entrant beat – not a true atrial echo beat. The atrial activation is cranio-caudal (HRA precedes His and PCS, *) – an AV nodal echo beat exhibits caudo-cranial activation (His and PCS precede HRA).

Parahisian pacing (Figs. 7.8 and 7.9)

This elegant technique is invaluable to distinguish retrograde AV node conduction from septal accessory pathway (AP) conduction, particularly as it does not depend on inducibility of sustained tachycardia, unlike the use of His-synchronous VPCs (see Step 3). Ideally parahisian pacing should also be performed in all patients with septal APs prior to ablation for pre-/post-comparison to confirm abolition of AP conduction.

Technique

- Can use a customized octapolar catheter for RV septal pacing with simultaneous recording at His bundle region, but parahisian pacing is more commonly performed with standard diagnostic catheters by repositioning the His catheter.
  - Pacing is delivered at the RV septum close to the His bundle and the right bundle branch.
  - Catheters should be positioned for clear recording of retrograde His and atrial activation to enable beat-to-beat monitoring of S1A1 and H1A1 intervals.
- High output pacing (e.g. 20 mA at 2.0 ms pulse width) captures **both** the His bundle (central fibrous body) and septal RV myocardium:
  - The impulse is retrogradely conducted through the AV node.
  - If a septal AP is present, retrograde atrial activation also takes place directly via the RV septum and AP.
  - QRS complexes are relatively narrow because ventricular activation is partly via antegrade conduction through the His-Purkinje system.
- As pacing output is gradually reduced, septal myocardium is still captured but there is loss of capture of His bundle (central fibrous body), manifesting as sudden QRS broadening to LBBB morphology.

Interpretation

- With exclusive AV nodal conduction and no AP (**'nodal response'**), activation now spreads to the RV apex, then up RBB and AV node to the atria, rather than directly via His bundle and AV node. Therefore:
  - S1A1 increases, typically by >50 ms (delayed His activation via RV).
  - H1A1 remains constant (atria still activated via His → AV node).
- In presence of septal AP, retrograde atrial activation via the RV septum and AP is maintained (**'extranodal response'**). Therefore:
  - S1A1 is unchanged or increases by <40-s.
  - H1A2 shortens (delayed His activation via RV with constant S1A1).

Possible confounding factors

- Difficulty achieving His bundle capture:
  - Reposition catheter.
  - His capture may only be intermittent at maximum output, varying with respiratory swings.
- Local atrial capture.

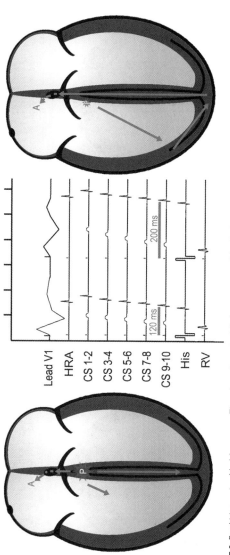

Fig. 7.8 Parahisian pacing. Nodal response. The schematic on the left shows capture of the His bundle with antegrade activation of the His–Purkinje system and retrograde activation of the atrium via the AV node. This results in a narrow QRS complex (first beat of the electrogram panel) with a stimulus to atrium time of 120 ms. The schematic on the right shows loss of capture of the His (as the pacing output is reduced) and now activation of the ventricle is through the myocardial tissue alone before retrogradely activating the His–Purkinje system and then the atrium. This creates a delay in the signal recorded in the atrium as shown in the second beat of the electrogram panel – the QRS is now broad and the stimulus to atrial time is 200 ms, i.e. >50 ms more than with the narrow QRS complex beat, suggesting that retrograde conduction is AV nodal.

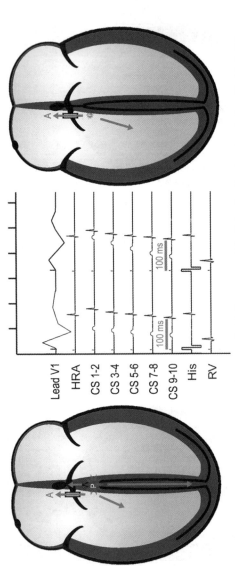

Fig. 7.9 Parahisian pacing. Extranodal response. The schematic on the left shows capture of the His bundle with antegrade activation of the His-Purkinje system and retrograde activation of the atrium via the AV node and a septal accessory pathway. This results in a narrow QRS complex (first beat of the electrogram panel) with a stimulus to atrium time of 100 ms. The schematic on the right shows loss of capture of the His (as the pacing output is reduced) and now activation of the ventricle is through the myocardial tissue alone. Retrograde activation, however, is still through the septal accessory pathway of the atrium. There is no change in the signal recorded in the atrium as shown in the second beat of the electrogram panel – the QRS is now broad but the stimulus to atrial time is still 100 ms, i.e. no more than with the narrow QRS complex beat, suggesting that retrograde conduction is extranodal.

Step 3: Induction and analysis of tachycardia

Initiation of sustained SVT is an absolute pre-requisite for definitive characterization of narrow complex tachycardia prior to catheter ablation. The only exceptions to this rule (i.e. ablation performed despite non-inducibility) are:

- Suspected AVRT in WPW when ablation of the pathway is mandated on prognostic grounds (📖 p. 257).
- Clear evidence of concealed AP with clinical ECG suggestive of AVRT.
- Clinical ECG highly suggestive of common atrial flutter.
- (Occasionally) AV nodal duality ± echo beats and clinical ECG highly suggestive of typical AVNRT.

Inducibility of tachycardia at EPS is variable even after withdrawal of anti-arrhythmic agents and may be more difficult under GA or with deep 'conscious' sedation. Steps 3 and 4 should be undertaken as soon as sustained tachycardia is observed. This may occur:

- At baseline, i.e. spontaneous or incessant SVT.
- Following introduction of catheters.
- During retrograde or antegrade curves (± double extrastimuli) or incremental atrial pacing (📖 p. 74).
- During isoprenaline infusion ± atropine plus programmed stimulation.
- Rarely with β-blocker ± atropine plus programmed stimulation.
- Other programmed stimulation techniques (rapid burst pacing, multiple extrastimuli, alternate pacing sites such as CS or LV, etc.).

Comparison of ECG to clinical tachycardia

Having induced tachycardia, 12-lead ECG of the tachycardia should be compared to any 12-lead ECGs of the clinical tachycardia to ensure that the induced tachycardia is clinically relevant. Ideally the ECG of the tachycardia induced in the lab will be identical to that seen during symptomatic episodes (apart from subtle differences reflecting the altered autonomic state and supine posture of the patient in the EP lab).

P waves

The P wave axis and relationship of P waves to the QRS complexes are the most important features. Any overt difference (e.g. long RP vs. short RP interval) may suggest that the induced tachycardia has a different mechanism to the clinical SVT.

QRS complexes

Patients commonly develop constant 'traumatic' RBBB during EPS precluding direct comparison with the clinical tachycardia. Other cases of BBB during tachycardia represent 'functional aberration' due to repetitive concealed conduction of a bundle. Unlike traumatic RBBB, in functional aberration the BBB resolves on restoration of sinus rhythm or may be abolished during ongoing tachycardia by critically timed extrastimuli (📖 p. 164).

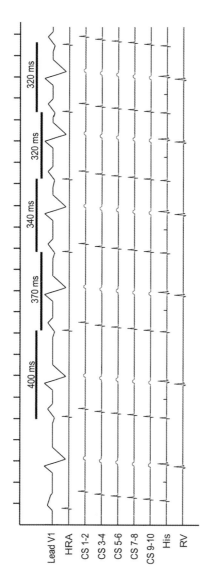

Fig. 7.10 Initiation of atrial tachycardia with 'warm up'. Spontaneous onset of automatic right atrial tachycardia (second beat) accompanied by a subtle change in P wave morphology and atrial activation sequence compared to sinus rhythm (first beat). This is followed by acceleration of the tachycardia cycle length from 400 ms to 320 ms within a few beats.

Analysis of initiation and termination

Valuable clues as to the nature of the tachycardia can be gained by analysing electrograms at the start and end of the tachycardia.

Initiation

- **AVNRT**: Usually initiated by atrial extrastimuli or incremental atrial pacing close to Wenckebach cycle length, with induction dependent on a critical AH interval to enable recovery of FP excitability and retrograde conduction of the atrial echo beat (📖 p. 236). Often the requisite AH delay occurs at the 'jump' from FP to SP conduction (Fig. 7.6). In practice, typical AVNRT is seldom inducible reliably by ventricular extrastimuli or pacing.
- **AVRT**: Often can be initiated by either atrial or ventricular extrastimuli/pacing. In WPW syndrome the classical pattern is that AVRT starts with an atrial extrastimulus shorter than the antegrade ERP of the accessory pathway and is conducted decrementally via the AV node (producing a non-pre-excited QRS complex) with sufficient delay to enable conduction retrogradely to the atria via the pathway initiating tachycardia. The other common pattern is initiation by a ventricular extrastimulus (particularly in patients with concealed pathways), which blocks retrogradely in the AV node but is conducted via the pathway.
- **Atrial tachycardia**: These are usually less dependent on the occurrence of a critically timed ectopic beat. In contrast to AVNRT, AVRT, and re-entrant atrial tachycardias, focal tachycardias often show a warm up phenomenon with the rate increasing gradually over a few beats (Fig. 7.10).

Termination

- **AVNRT**: Usually terminates with antegrade block in slow pathway, i.e. final electrogram recorded is atrial (may be difficult to see on ECG as P wave is buried at the end of QRS complex).
- **AVRT**: Also commonly terminates with antegrade block in the AV node producing a final atrial electrogram.
- **Atrial tachycardia**: Atrial tachycardias are not dependent on the AV node, so the last beat of atrial tachycardia will be conducted to the ventricle. Atrial tachycardias usually terminate with ventricular electrograms – if a tachycardia consistently terminates with an atrial electrogram, it is unlikely to be intra-atrial in origin.

A:V relationship during tachycardia

The commonest finding is an A:V relationship = 1:1 (A = V) and this can be found in AVNRT, AVRT, and atrial tachycardia. A:V relationship >1:1 (A > V) usually indicates an atrial tachyarrhythmia, the only common exception being AVNRT with 2:1 infranodal block. A:V relationship <1:1 (V > A) with narrow complex tachycardia is rare but the causes are shown below (📖 exceptions box).

Exceptions

AVNRT with 2:1 AV block

Occasionally infranodal block in AVNRT produces a tachycardia with A:V relationship 2:1. If the block is at infra-His level, careful examination shows that each atrial electrogram is preceded by a His electrogram.

AVNRT with complete AV block

Rarely, during attempted slow pathway ablation for AVNRT, inadvertent interruption of AV conduction below the level of the lower turnaround results in complete AV dissociation with ongoing AVNRT.

Narrow complex tachycardia with V > A

This can be seen in several situations, all very rare:

Junctional ectopic tachycardia (JET). VA dissociation is a common finding with each ventricular electrogram preceded by His electrograms; however, around 90% of patients do show some VA conduction.

AVNRT with VA block. Strictly HA block, usually with Wenckebach periodicity but occasionally 2:1 VA block may be seen.

Nodofascicular pathway. With antegrade conduction down the His-Purkinje system and retrograde conduction over the nodofascicular pathway.

1:2 tachycardia. Sinus beats conducted via dual AV nodal pathways resulting in two conducted ventricular electrograms for each atrial electrogram.

Atrial activation pattern (Fig. 7.11)

Activation of the atria during a tachycardia is usually described as:

- **Midline** (referred to inappropriately as 'concentric') – i.e. the earliest atrial electrograms at His or PCS, with activation spreading from PCS → DCS, and HRA later than His or PCS (caudo-cranial activation).
- **Eccentric** – atrial activation not spreading in classical midline pattern, usually DCS → PCS, still with caudo-cranial activation of HRA.
- **Cranio-caudal** – atrial electrograms in HRA precede earliest atrial activity in His or PCS.

Midline atrial activation

Typical of AVNRT, but also seen in orthodromic AVRT with septal or postero-septal APs, or in atrial tachycardia arising from the septum.

'Eccentric' atrial activation patterns

This usually excludes AVNRT but may be seen in both atrial tachycardias and AVRT. The pattern of atrial activation provides useful clues as to the location of the pathway or the focus of the tachycardia:

- **DCS → PCS**: AVRT via a left lateral AP; the distal CS is activated earliest with spread of the atrial electrograms proximally. Rarely atrial tachycardia originating in the lateral left atrium will produce an identical DCS → PCS pattern during tachycardia but with normal decremental midline activation during the retrograde curve.
- **CS chevron pattern**: With left-sided pathways located posteriorly on the mitral valve annulus, the mid-CS electrodes are activated first producing a 'chevron' pattern of atrial activation in the CS.
- **HRA earliest**: In the presence of a right lateral pathway, CS activation will be from proximal to distal, but the HRA electrograms may be simultaneous with or even precede atrial activation in the His and PCS. A similar pattern can also be seen with right atrial tachycardias including SNRT – differentiation may require careful scrutiny of the retrograde curve as well as pacing manoeuvres (📖 p. 172).

Pitfalls

- CS catheter not positioned fully within the coronary sinus, resulting in a false chevron CS pattern rather than midline atrial activation.
- CS catheter too deeply engaged, resulting in reverse chevron CS pattern (DCS, PCS earlier than mid-CS due to LA activation from both anterior and posterior septum) rather than midline activation.
- AVNRT with left-sided connection of retrograde fast pathway fibres resulting in chevron pattern of CS activation (requires differentiation by parahisian pacing and His-synchronous VPCs, 📖 pp. 150, 166).
- Misplacement of His catheter resulting in inaccurate timings of atrial activation.
- Failure to use a HRA catheter (may miss right free wall pathway).

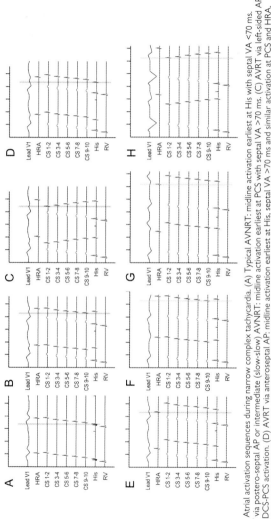

Fig. 7.11 Atrial activation sequences during narrow complex tachycardia. (A) Typical AVNRT: midline activation earliest at His with septal VA <70 ms. (B) AVRT via postero-septal AP or intermediate (slow-slow) AVNRT: midline activation earliest at PCS with septal VA >70 ms. (C) AVRT via left-sided AP: eccentric DCS-PCS activation. (D) AVRT via anteroseptal AP: midline activation earliest at His, septal VA >70 ms and similar activation at PCS and HRA. (E) AVRT via right lateral AP or right atrial tachycardia: cranio-caudal activation, HRA precedes His and PCS. (F) Atypical (fast-slow) AVNRT: long RP tachycardia with midline activation earliest at PCS and septal VA >150 ms. (G) High RA tachycardia (including SNRT): cranio-caudal activation earliest at HRA. (H) Left atrial tachycardia: eccentric DCS-PCS activation and long VA interval.

Septal VA interval with midline atrial activation (Fig. 7.11)

The temporal relationship of ventricular and atrial electrograms in the septal region can be useful in diagnosing **narrow complex tachycardia with midline atrial activation sequence**.

- In AVRT the ventricles and atria are activated sequentially. It takes at least 70 ms for electrical activity to pass from the ventricles to the atria via an accessory pathway. V activation always precedes A.
- In typical AVNRT both the ventricles and the atria are activated simultaneously or A activation may be slightly before or after V.
- In atrial tachycardia (low RA origin) A always precedes V activation, but often with slightly varying conduction delay through the bystander AV node resulting in an 'unstable' VA interval.

How to do it

Measure the interval between the earliest ventricular activation in the His or PCS and the earliest atrial activation in the same channels.

What does the VA time mean?

- **VA time <70 ms**: This is classically seen in typical AVNRT where atrial and ventricular activity occur almost simultaneously. It excludes AVRT as a mechanism. A short VA time may also be seen in an atrial tachycardia, where the AV delay is nearly identical to the cycle length of the tachycardia but may fluctuate slightly beat-to-beat due to variable AV nodal conduction.
- **VA time >70 ms**: This is seen in AVRT and in intermediate AVNRT where electrical activity is conducted back to the atria via a relatively slow 'fast pathway' ('slow-slow AVNRT'), thus atrial activation occurs well after ventricular activation. It is also seen in atrial tachycardias where the AV delay is shorter than the cycle length of the tachycardia.
- **Long RP tachycardia** (📖 p. 182) is effectively narrow complex tachycardia with VA time >50% of tachycardia cycle length.

Cycle length variation (Fig. 7.12)

Small variations in cycle length are sometimes observed during 'regular' narrow complex tachycardia. They are more common in atrial tachycardia but are also seen in both AVRT and AVNRT. Careful measurement of the AA and HH intervals during tachycardia can identify where the variations in cycle length are occurring and thus the underlying mechanism of the tachycardia.

How to do it

Measure the intervals between a series of consecutive atrial electrograms in a single atrial channel (HRA or CS), taking care to measure between identical points on each electrogram (AA intervals). Next measure the intervals between the His depolarizations of the same portion of the tachycardia (HH intervals). Are changes in the tachycardia cycle length seen first in the HH intervals and mirrored in the subsequent AA intervals, or vice versa?

What does it mean?

- **HH intervals precede or 'lead' AA intervals**: This is seen in tachycardias that that are dependent on the AV node, usually AVNRT or AVRT. Electrical conduction in the AV node is highly dependent on autonomic tone and varies slightly beat-to-beat. In contrast conduction within the atria, ventricles, and retrogradely conduction via the fast pathway or accessory pathways is very stable. Thus most variation in cycle length occurs during antegrade AV nodal conduction (i.e. A → H). Therefore, the HH interval will almost always change before the AA interval.

- **AA intervals precede or 'lead' HH intervals**: Atrial tachycardias do not depend on the AV node. Thus changes in AV node conduction have little effect on the AA intervals. In contrast the HH intervals are dependent on the preceding AA interval.

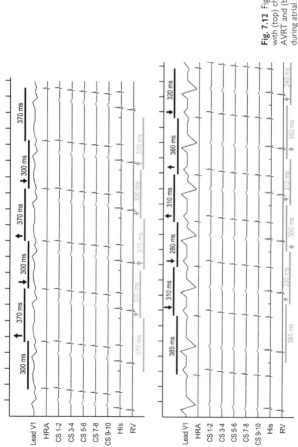

Fig. 7.12 Figure of HH and AA relationship with (top) change in HH leading AA during AVRT and (bottom) change in AA leading HH during atrial tachycardia.

Development of bundle branch block during tachycardia (Fig. 7.13)

Change in cycle length may occur if a bundle branch block (BBB) develops during tachycardia, either due to spontaneous VPBs or programmed ventricular extrastimuli causing functional aberration due to repetitive concealed penetration of the bundle.

- Development of BBB has little effect on the cycle length of either AVNRT or an atrial tachycardia, as neither is dependent on ventricular myocardium.
- Ventricular myocardium is an important part of the re-entrant circuit in AVRT. Ipsilateral BBB (**i.e. accessory pathway is on the same side of the ventricle as the BBB**) lengthens the re-entrant circuit because impulses must travel via the opposite bundle and ventricle and across the IVS to reach the V insertion of the accessory pathway. This increases VA interval and tachycardia cycle length.
- LBBB will increase the cycle length of an AVRT via a left-sided pathway but will have no effect on an AVRT dependent on a right-sided pathway. RBBB has the opposite effect.
- A positive finding is an increase in VA interval and TCL >20 ms with onset of BBB.
- Development of LBBB *per se* is highly suggestive of AVRT and only rarely seen in AVNRT.

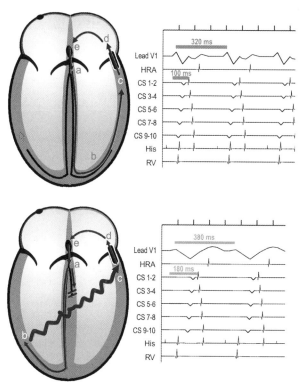

Fig. 7.13 Effect of bundle branch block on tachycardia cycle length. The upper panel shows AVRT via a left-sided accessory pathway with eccentric DCS-PCS atrial activation. TCL is 320 ms (representing A.B.C.D.E.) with ventriculo-atrial (VA) conduction interval 100 ms (representing A.B.C.). Following onset of ipsilateral bundle branch block (i.e. LBBB), the circuit is extended with impulses having to reach the LV via the right bundle and septum (A.B.C.), resulting in an increase in VA interval to 180 ms and TCL to 380 ms but no change in intra-atrial conduction (D.E.) from pathway insertion to AV junction, or in AV conduction time (E.A.).

Step 4: Pacing manoeuvres during tachycardia

Pacing manoeuvres during tachycardia are key to identifying/confirming the mechanism of a narrow complex tachycardia, particularly if doubts remain after Steps 1–3. Pacing the ventricles is of much greater diagnostic value in SVT than atrial pacing manoeuvres and ideally should be performed routinely for confirmation even if the operator is reasonably confident about the mechanism of tachycardia.

Diastolic scan with ventricular extrastimulus

This involves scanning of diastole with single ventricular premature beats induced by pacing the RV catheter. It can provide useful diagnostic information in two ways:
• Response to His-synchronous VPB.
• Induction of bundle branch block.

His-synchronous ventricular premature beat (VPB) (Figs. 7.14, 7.15, and 7.16)

This is used to identify the presence of a retrogradely conducting septal accessory pathway.
• Following activation of the bundle of His it becomes refractory.
• Thus a critically timed VPB coincident with His activation cannot be transmitted retrogradely to the atria via the AV node. It can only activate the atria via an accessory pathway.
• If a His synchronous VPB advances the next atrial beat it confirms the presence of an accessory pathway.

How to do it
• Programme the stimulator to pace and sense from the RV catheter.
• During tachycardia, measure the time from the peak electrograms in the RV catheter to the His electrograms in the His catheter.
• Add around 20 ms to this value.
• Deliver a single pacing stimulus via the RV catheter exactly this length of time after the last RV electrograms. Repeat a number of times, each time reducing the delay by 10 ms increments.

What to measure
• Choose the VPB that is timed closest to the predicted time of the His electrograms. Confirm that the VPB is His-synchronous.
• Measure the interval between the two atrial electrograms (PCS and/or His catheters) of the beat immediately preceding the His-synchronous VPB and the beat immediately afterwards.
• If this second interval is shorter than the first then the **atria have been advanced by the His-synchronous VPB (Fig. 7.14)**.
• Next measure the interval between the two atrial electrograms following the His-synchronous VPB. If this interval is the same as the cycle length of the tachycardia this means that the **tachycardia circuit has been advanced by the His-synchronous VPB**.

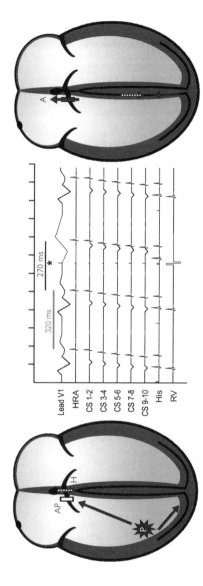

Fig. 7.14 Role of the His-synchronous VPB (see also Fig. 7.15). Intracardiac signals show narrow complex tachycardia at CL 320 ms with midline atrial activation but VA interval >70 ms, consistent with either AVRT via septal accessory pathway or intermediate AVNRT. A ventricular extrastimulus (P in the left-hand panel) is delivered immediately prior to the His deflection but nevertheless is conducted retrogradely advancing atrial activation by 50 ms to 270 ms (shown in red). As the AV junction below the His bundle is refractory, this confirms the presence of a separate septal accessory pathway (AP) allowing atrial reset (A in the right-hand panel) to occur.

Interpretation
- Atrial advancement by a His-synchronous VPB confirms the presence of an accessory pathway.
- No atrial advancement suggests that **either** there is no accessory pathway **or** a left **or** right free wall pathway remote from the pacing site, such that the conduction time to the bypass tract's ventricular insertion is too long for there to be any atrial pre-excitation.
- No atrial advancement by His-synchronous VPB makes a midline or septal accessory pathway unlikely, and AVNRT likely (Fig. 7.15).
- Atrial **and** tachycardia advancement by His-synchronous VPB normally suggests that the accessory pathway is part of the re-entrant circuit rather than a bystander, i.e. diagnosis is AVRT, **but** …
- Because of the decremental conduction properties of the AV node, atrial pre-excitation by the VPB often results in a compensatory delay. Thus even when the pathway is part of the circuit, atrial reset is not always accompanied by advancement of the tachycardia.
- Conversely, when the accessory pathway is a bystander to an AVNRT, the advanced atrial beat may be able to enter the slow pathway early and advance the tachycardia.

Caveats
- Atrial advancement by a His-synchronous VPB only confirms the presence of an accessory pathway, not that it is playing a role in the tachycardia. It may simply be acting as a bystander in either an atrial tachycardia or AVNRT.
- Failure to advance the atria does not rule out the presence of an accessory pathway (Fig. 7.16).
- Cycle length variation or alternans makes the His-synchronous VPB uninterpretable.

Other useful observations
- Tachycardia termination by a His synchronous VPB that is **not** conducted to the atria confirms that the ventricle is part of the re-entrant circuit and the mechanism must be an AVRT.
- Atrial delay following a His synchronous VPB occurs very rarely but is diagnostic of an orthodromic AVRT in the unusual situation where the accessory pathway has decremental conduction properties. The VPB causes such delay in retrograde conduction in the accessory pathway that electrical activity reaches the atria later than it would have done during AVRT.

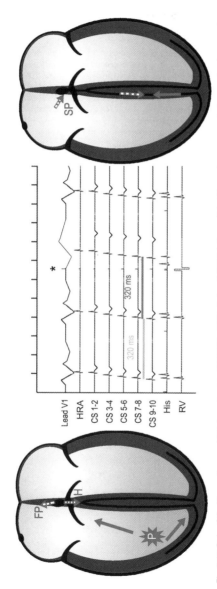

Fig. 7.15 Role of the His-synchronous VPB. In contrast to AVRT (Fig. 7.12), during AVNRT delivery of the His-synchronous ventricular stimulus does not alter or reset atrial activation because the AV junction and fast pathway (FP) are refractory.

Induction of bundle branch block

Diastolic ventricular pacing can induce (or abolish) bundle branch block during tachycardia due to repetitive concealed penetration. In a patient with an AVRT, development of a bundle branch block on the same side as the accessory pathway will lead to an increase in the ventricular portion of the re-entrant circuit and thus increase the cycle length of the tachycardia (📖 p. 164).

- Induction of bundle branch prolongs tachycardia cycle length: This confirms both the presence of an ipsilateral accessory pathway and that it participates in the tachycardia.
- BBB has no effect on tachycardia cycle length: This is seen in AVNRT or atrial tachycardia, but also in AVRT if the accessory pathway that is part of the re-entrant circuit is on the other side of the heart to the bundle that blocks.

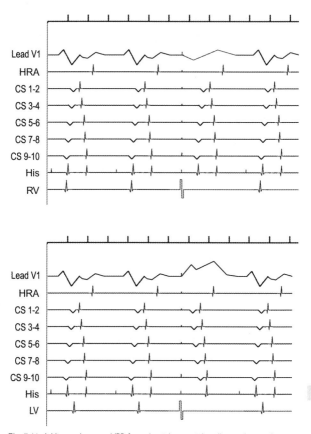

Fig. 7.16 A His-synchronous VPB from the right ventricle will not advance the atria in an AVRT secondary to a left lateral accessory pathway (top). In contrast, a His-synchronous VPB delivered in the left ventricle (nearer the accessory pathway) will cause atrial advancement (bottom). This is because the LV catheter is delivering an extrastimulus very close to or **within** the tachycardia circuit, whereas the RV catheter is outside the circuit.

Ventricular entrainment (Figs. 7.17, 7.18, and 7.19)

The response to RV pacing at a slightly faster rate than TCL provides important clues as to its underlying mechanism based on:
- Activation pattern and timing during pacing.
- Electrogram sequence upon discontinuation of pacing.
- Return cycle upon discontinuation of pacing (post-pacing interval).

In the majority of cases, **the electrogram sequence at offset of pacing provides the most important diagnostic information**, i.e. differentiating atrial tachycardia from AVRT and AVNRT.

How to do it

Overdrive RV pacing at cycle length 10–40 ms (usually 20 ms) shorter than the tachycardia cycle length. Once the atria are entrained to the faster pacing rate, pacing is stopped. **It is important to confirm acceleration of the atria to the ventricular pacing cycle length**.

Reasons for failure to entrain the atria:
- Termination of tachycardia during RV pacing – re-induce tachycardia and repeat manoeuvre.
- VA block at cycle length greater than tachycardia cycle length – manoeuvre not diagnostically useful.

Interpretation – VA interval and activation sequence during pacing
- Change in atrial activation sequence suggests atrial tachycardia due to activation retrogradely via AV node (Fig. 7.18). Sequence should be unchanged in AVNRT (Fig. 7.19) and in AVRT (Fig. 7.17), unless the PCL < retrograde AP ERP resulting in switch to nodal activation.
- Change in VA interval, measured in the lead with earliest atrial activation during tachycardia. In AVRT, VA time should be the same during ventricular pacing as in tachycardia. Increase in VA time by ≥85 ms during ventricular entrainment suggests atrial tachycardia or AVNRT.
- Further information can be gained by entraining from two sites. In AVNRT and atrial tachycardia, shortest VA time is seen with apical pacing (i.e. near insertion of right bundle) rather than basal pacing. With AVRT via septal AP, entrainment from the base (i.e. near pathway insertion) will produce a shorter VA time than from the apex.

Interpretation – electrogram sequence after termination of pacing

The sequence of electrograms seen immediately on cessation of ventricular pacing depends on the underlying mechanism. This is only relevant if the tachycardia continues after ventricular entrainment:
- V-A-V sequence is consistent with AVRT or AVNRT (Figs. 7.17 and 7.19).
- V-A-A-V sequence is indicative of atrial tachycardia (Fig. 7.18).

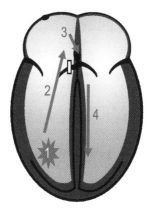

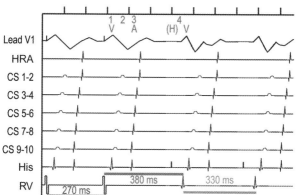

Fig. 7.17 Ventricular entrainment in AVRT. Narrow complex tachycardia at CL 330 ms with midline atrial activation and VA >70 ms. (1) The final beat of RV overdrive pacing (V) is conducted (2) via the accessory pathway (3) to the atria (A) and then (4) via the AV node and His (H) back to the ventricles (V), producing a V-A-H-V sequence ('V-A-V'). This excludes atrial tachycardia but could be consistent with either AVRT or AVNRT. Post-pacing interval (PPI) is 380 ms and (unadjusted) PPI – TCL = 50 ms, making AVRT very likely. This is because pacing is being delivered within the tachycardia circuit.

Explanation

- Following entrainment of AVRT the last paced beat (V electrogram) is conducted to the atria via the accessory pathway (A electrogram) and then back down via the AV node to continue the tachycardia (V electrogram), hence the V-A-V sequence or 'response'.
- During AVNRT, a similar pattern is seen to AVRT. The last entrained ventricular beat is conducted to the atrium via the AV nodal fast pathway and then down the slow pathway to continue the tachycardia, again producing a V-A-V response.
- Atrial tachycardia is suppressed by ventricular entrainment. Thus the last paced beat (V electrogram) is conducted to the atria (A electrogram) followed by resumption of the first beat of atrial tachycardia (A electrogram) conducted back to the ventricles via the AV node (V electrogram), hence the V-A-A-V sequence or response.

Interpretation – post-pacing interval (PPI) (see Figs. 7.17 and 7.19)

This is the time between the last pacing stimulus and the next ventricular electrograms in the RV catheter as the tachycardia resumes (return cycle). It is useful to distinguish between AVRT and AVNRT. However, ideally the PPI should be adjusted for the decremental properties of the AV node, which will tend to lengthen the apparent PPI:

$$\text{adjusted PPI} = \text{PPI} - (\text{AH}_{PPI} - \text{AH}_{tachycardia})$$

AH_{PPI} = first AH interval after the end of ventricular pacing
$\text{AH}_{tachycardia}$ = AH interval during tachycardia

- In AVRT the ventricle is part of the re-entrant circuit so the adjusted PPI is usually within 115 ms of the cycle length of the tachycardia.
- In AVNRT the ventricle is not part of the re-entrant circuit and the adjusted PPI is usually >115 ms longer than the tachycardia cycle length (last paced impulse travels retrogradely up the AV nodal fast pathway, then to sustain tachycardia re-enters the slow pathway before reaching the AV node and reactivating the ventricle).

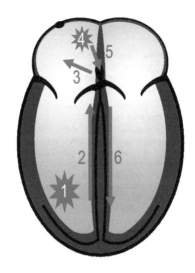

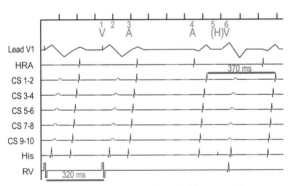

Fig. 7.18 Ventricular entrainment in atrial tachycardia. Narrow complex tachycardia at CL 370 ms with cranio-caudal atrial activation. (1) The final beat of RV overdrive pacing (**V**) is conducted retrogradely (2) via the AV node (3) to the atria (**A**), resulting in a change to midline caudo-cranial activation. Because the AV node is now refractory, unlike in AVNRT and AVRT, the last retrogradely conducted A is not conducted back antegradely to the ventricles. After a compensatory pause, the atrial tachycardia resumes (4) with cranio-caudal atrial depolarization (**A**) conducted antegradely (5) via the AV node and His (**H**) (6) back to the ventricles (**V**), producing a V-A-A-H-V sequence ('V-A-A-V'). This is indicative of atrial tachycardia and excludes AVRT or AVNRT.

Pitfalls in interpretation

Failure to entrain:

Misinterpretation can occur if the tachycardia is not entrained by the ventricular pacing, but carries on independently. It is essential to confirm the AA interval (i.e. between **atrial** electrograms) during ventricular pacing is the same as the pacing interval and thus shorter than the tachycardia cycle length.

Pseudo V-A-A-V response in AVNRT:

The VA time during entrainment of typical AVNRT is short and the last V of the V-A-V response often occurs almost simultaneously with the next atrial beat. If the VA time is negative during tachycardia this can even lead to an apparent V-A-A-V response to ventricular entrainment. The key is to look at the His electrogram. In typical AVNRT the first A of the V-A-V is conducted to the ventricle via the AV node and His bundle, producing a His electrogram (H) immediately prior to the simultaneous A and V electrograms. Thus a V-A-H-A-V pattern is seen. In contrast the first A of a V-A-A-V response in atrial tachycardia is not conducted down the AV node so there is no His electrogram between the two A electrograms (i.e. V-A-A-H-V).

Termination:

Occasionally RV pacing may terminate the tachycardia repeatedly, even using a pacing interval only slightly shorter than the tachycardia cycle length, and so precluding successful entrainment. Interpretation is then not possible with the exception that, if a tachycardia is consistently terminated by ventricular pacing **without capture of the atrium**, it is very unlikely to be an atrial tachycardia (Fig. 7.20).

Bystander pathways:

Patients may suffer from AVNRT, but also have a retrogradely conducting bystander accessory pathway. This can lead to confusion. The VA time may not prolong as much as expected, but the patient will still have a relatively long PPI and a VAV response to ventricular entrainment.

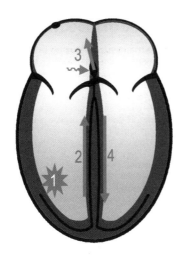

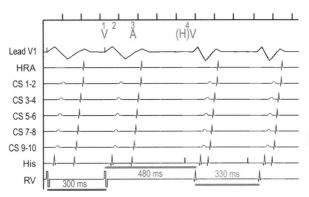

Fig. 7.19 Ventricular entrainment in AVNRT. Narrow complex tachycardia at CL 330 ms with midline atrial activation and VA <70 ms. (1) The final beat of RV overdrive pacing (**V**) is conducted (2) retrogradely via the AV nodal fast pathway (3) to the atria (**A**) and then (4) antegradely via the AV nodal slow pathway and His (**H**) back to the ventricles (**V**), producing a V-A-H-V sequence ('V-A-V'). This excludes atrial tachycardia but could be consistent with either AVRT or AVNRT. Post-pacing interval (PPI) is 480 ms and (unadjusted) PPI – TCL = 150 ms, making AVNRT very likely (see Fig. 7.17 for comparison). The relatively long PPI reflects the fact that pacing is being delivered outside the tachycardia circuit.

Other diagnostic manoeuvres

Role of atrial pacing manoeuvres during tachycardia

These are generally of much less value and only rarely used.

- **Transient overdrive atrial pacing** performed repeatedly:
  - At just faster than TCL but without terminating tachycardia. If VA interval of return cycle (discontinuation of pacing) is consistently within 10 ms of VA interval during tachycardia, AVRT or AVNRT are likely, whereas atrial tachycardia produces a variable VA timing.
  - At longest CL that resulted in AV block with analysis of last AH before cessation of pacing. If tachycardia termination is associated with relatively short AH intervals compared to AH intervals when tachycardia continues, termination is AH dependent, i.e. AVNRT or AVRT likely, atrial tachycardia unlikely.
- **Single atrial extrastimuli** during a narrow complex tachycardia with a short VA time may help to distinguish between typical AVNRT and a non-re-entrant junctional tachycardia.
  - His-synchronous atrial extrastimulus delivered when the AV node is refractory will have no effect in a non-re-entrant junctional tachycardia. In contrast, in typical AVNRT the slow pathway will not be refractory. This may either lead to advancement of the next His electrograms, or delay of the next His beat as a result of the decremental properties of the slow pathway. Either response is diagnostic of AVNRT rather than a non-re-entrant junctional tachycardia.
  - An atrial extrastimulus delivered significantly earlier than the His electrograms in a non-re-entrant junctional tachycardia will be able to penetrate the fast pathway and advance the His without terminating tachycardia. In contrast, in AVNRT, if an early APB does advance the His electrograms, it can only do this via the fast pathway, rendering it refractory and terminating the tachycardia. Thus advancement of the His by an early atrial premature beat without termination suggests a non-re-entrant junctional tachycardia rather than AVNRT.

Adenosine in tachycardia

Adenosine blocks the AV node conduction and can be useful to confirm the presence of an atrial tachycardia with persistent tachycardia despite ventricular dissociation. It is important to be aware that adenosine also terminates sinus node re-entrant tachycardias and a significant minority of atrial tachycardias. However, in atrial tachycardias it will usually block the AV node slightly before it terminates the tachycardia, leading to a small number of non-conducted beats of atrial tachycardia.

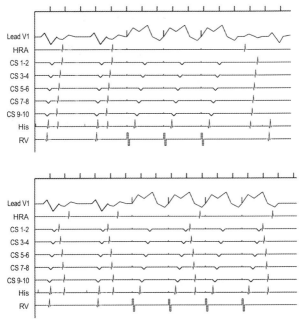

Fig. 7.20 Termination of AVNRT (upper panel) and AVRT via left lateral AP (lower panel) by ventricular overdrive pacing without capture or resetting of the atria excludes atrial tachycardia.

Two- or three-catheter studies

Traditionally four to five catheters are used in EP studies for narrow complex tachycardias: CS multi-polar catheter; quads for the RV, HRA, and His; ± additional roving catheter for mapping/ablation. However, it is possible to perform studies and ablations for supraventricular arrhythmias with only three or even two catheters.

Three-catheter studies

A diagnostic coronary sinus catheter is used to detect atrial and ventricular electrograms and to pace the atria. A His catheter is used to mark the AV node and map the His electrograms. In addition an ablation catheter is placed in the right ventricular apex and used to stimulate the ventricle during the electrophysiology study. Once the tachycardia has been induced the ablation catheter is withdrawn from the right ventricle and used to perform ablation.

Advantages
- Fewer diagnostic catheters used, saving money.
- Fewer venous sheaths required.

Disadvantages
- If no ablation is performed the more expensive mapping catheter is used unnecessarily. However, in most series this is outweighed by the use of fewer diagnostic catheters in patients who do undergo ablation.
- Fewer electrograms can make it more difficult to diagnose the mechanism underlying the tachycardia. This is particularly a problem for fellows learning electrophysiology, for whom it is very helpful to have as much information as possible. A particular difficulty can be in distinguishing intra-atrial re-entrant beats from echo beats in patients with AVNRT. Potentially this could lead to problems defining the endpoint to ablation in AVNRT. It is also difficult in patients with complex substrates such as multiple pathways, atypical arrhythmias, or multiple potential arrhythmia mechanisms. However, in experienced hands a three-wire study is just as safe and effective as a five-wire study for the vast majority of supraventricular tachycardias. If an atypical arrhythmia is encountered more catheters can be added.

Two-catheter studies

It is possible to perform an electrophysiological study for a narrow complex tachycardia with only two wires. A catheter is placed in the coronary sinus to map atrial and ventricular electrograms and pace the atria. The ablation catheter is then moved between the RV position and the His position to perform the EP study. However, it is much more difficult to perform and interpret pacing manoeuvres. It also means that the His position cannot be marked during ablation of the slow pathway, potentially increasing the risk of complete heart block.

Special situations

Long RP tachycardia

Long RP tachycardias are a special group of narrow complex tachycardias. They are characterized by a longer VA interval than AV interval during tachycardia. They are caused by the same arrhythmias as other narrow complex tachycardias:

- Atrial tachycardia – this is much more common as a cause of a long RP tachycardia than other narrow complex tachycardias.
- Atypical AVNRT.
- AVRT with a slow-conducting accessory pathway.

The basic approach to a long RP tachycardia should be the same as that used in other supraventricular tachycardias, whilst the pacing manoeuvres will be identical. However, there are special considerations:

Pseudo V-A-A-V response to ventricular entrainment

If the VA time is long, it may prolong further during ventricular entrainment, such that the VA time is longer than the pacing interval. This can lead to an apparent V-A-A-V response at the end of ventricular entrainment. The last paced beat is followed by two atrial electrograms; however, the first of these is dependent on the second-to-last pacing beat with the next atrial beat following on from the last ventricular electrogram. Thus the interval between these atrial electrograms will be the same as the pacing interval. If this is consistently the case then the first of the two atrial electrograms may be ignored.

Patients with abnormal anatomy/congenital heart disease

Patients with congenital heart disease often develop narrow complex tachycardias. Frequently these include atrial tachycardia and both typical and atypical flutter. However, they are also prone to more common arrhythmias such as AVNRT and even AVRT. Treatment of these patients requires a detailed understanding of the congenital abnormalities and any surgical correction that may have been performed in each individual patient. It may be awkward to correctly position catheters and ablation of even the more common arrhythmias may be difficult. Thus ablation should only be performed in these patients by operators and centres with extensive experience of congenital heart disease.

However, the basic electrophysiological testing and interpretation of electrograms at the initiation and termination of tachycardia and of manoeuvres such as ventricular entrainment and His-synchronous ventricular premature beats remains the same as in other patients.

Limited vascular access

Venous access to the right heart may be difficult in some patients because of their size (e.g. small children), previous operations and illnesses, or congenital anomalies. In these situations it is often necessary to perform the EP study with fewer catheters as described earlier.

A particular problem is seen in patients with an interrupted inferior vena cava, where it may not be possible to access the heart at all from a femoral route. In this situation a full electrophysiological study can be performed from a superior approach using subclavian and internal jugular venous access.

Non-inducibility

Many patients present to the lab with a history of arrhythmias, but no tachycardia can be easily induced in the lab. Initially, aggressive attempts should be made to induce arrhythmia using a combination of the following manoeuvres:

- Atrial pacing with one, two, or three extrastimuli, from multiple sites (coronary sinus and high right atrium).
- Burst pacing at short cycle lengths from multiple sites.
- Isoprenaline infusion.
- Atropine.
- Beta-blockers – in a small proportion of patients arrhythmias cannot be induced by pacing manoeuvres in the presence of either atropine or isoprenaline, but can be induced in the presence of intravenous beta-blockers.

If no arrhythmias can be induced despite these manoeuvres, the approach depends on what information has been elicited from the EP study and the clinical history.

Patients with dual AV node physiology

If a patient has clearly demonstrable dual AV node physiology with a jump and double echo beats during the antegrade curve, and with an ECG during clinical tachycardia that is suggestive of AVNRT, most electrophysiologists will attempt slow pathway modification. Some will also perform ablation in similar patients with a good history of a recurrent persistent tachycardia that terminates with vagal manoeuvres, even in the absence of ECG documentation, particularly if they have throbbing in their neck during tachycardia suggesting cannon waves.

The situation is more difficult in patients whose only evidence of AVNRT in the lab is single echo beats. A major problem is the lack of an endpoint during ablation if no tachycardia can be induced, as single echo beats are usually accepted as a satisfactory endpoint to a standard slow pathway modification. However, in patients with clear evidence of troublesome narrow complex tachycardia terminated with adenosine, who have a jump and single echo beats during the antegrade curve but no other abnormalities during EP study, many electrophysiologists will attempt a cautious slow pathway modification.

Patients with an accessory pathway

Most electrophysiologists will ablate antegradely conducting accessory pathways in patients with a pre-excited ECG or a good history of tachycardia even if no AVRT can be induced in the lab. This is particularly true if the pathway can be shown to conduct antegradely at a short cycle length (<250 ms on isoprenaline), suggesting they may be at risk of pre-excited AF. However, the position of the pathway is also critical: the closer the pathway is to the AV node, the more important it is to have a clear mandate for ablation. In the case of parahisian pathways, many electrophysiologists will want to stop the procedure and have a detailed discussion with the patient before proceeding to ablation.

The situation is also more difficult in patients with concealed accessory pathways that only conduct retrogradely. Again the position of the pathway is important, but even if the pathway is in a relatively straightforward position to ablate, many electrophysiologists will only perform an ablation if there is either ECG documentation of the arrhythmia or a clear history of tachycardias reliably terminated with vagal manoeuvres.

Recurrent atrial fibrillation during the EP study

Recurrent atrial fibrillation is the bane of the electrophysiologist performing EP studies for regular narrow complex tachycardias. It is a particular problem in patients with either incessant tachycardia that rapidly degenerates into AF or difficult-to-induce arrhythmias. Aggressive burst pacing of the atria, or drive trains with short coupled extrastimuli, can easily induce atrial fibrillation. Atrial fibrillation in this setting does not usually mean the patient suffers clinically from atrial fibrillation. However, it can make it difficult both to complete the diagnostic EP study and to carry out ablation. It can also make it impossible to confirm lines of atrial block such as a cavotricuspid isthmus block for typical atrial flutter.

Once atrial fibrillation has started it may terminate spontaneously, but often it persists. There are a number of possible management options:

- **Internal cardioversion**: An internal cardioversion catheter can be passed via a 7 Fr venous sheath into the right atrium, through the right ventricle and into a pulmonary artery (ideally the left). Once in position the patient can then be cardioverted with a small electrical shock (15–30 J). However, this either requires removing one of the diagnostic or ablation catheters or placing a new venous sheath. Placing the catheter in the pulmonary artery can also be time-consuming. External cardioversion is also possible but the patient requires much deeper sedation.
- **Flecainide**: Frequently once a patient has developed atrial fibrillation they can enter a downward spiral with increasingly frequent atrial fibrillation requiring repeated cardioversions. In this situation small doses of flecainide (typically 30 mg initially) can be used to try and maintain sinus rhythm long enough to complete the study and treat the patient. The downside is that even small doses of flecainide may make it difficult to induce tachycardia, and in particular may block accessory pathways.
- **Ablation in atrial fibrillation**: It is possible to ablate accessory pathways during pre-excited atrial fibrillation, although it can be more difficult to identify a perfect signal. In contrast it is usually not recommended to perform slow pathway modifications for AVNRT during atrial fibrillation. The presence of atrial fibrillation makes it difficult to assess the rate of any junctional rhythm induced during the burn and makes it impossible to detect VA block during the burn. Similar considerations apply to parahisian pathways.

How to recognize and avoid common pitfalls

Sub-optimal placement of catheters

Taking the time to correctly position the diagnostic catheters is critical to ensure that correct diagnoses are made. This is particularly important with the His and coronary sinus catheters.

Coronary sinus catheter

This sits in the coronary sinus and records electrograms from both the atrium and ventricle. In both two- and three-wire EP studies it is also used to pace the atrium. Misplacement can cause confusion in a number of ways:

Is atrial activation midline or eccentric?

Normally midline activation of the atria leads to proximal to distal activation of the coronary sinus catheter electrodes. However, in small patients or patients with a valve in the distal coronary sinus it can be difficult to place all the poles of the catheter within the coronary sinus and the proximal poles hang out in the RA. This can lead to atrial activation being earliest in the middle poles of the catheter, which if not recognized can give the false impression of a left posterior or postero-septal accessory pathway. This can also occur if the coronary sinus catheter slips back into the RA after being placed. The position of this catheter should always be checked with fluoroscopy before diagnosing such a pathway.

Atrial or ventricular capture?

If the coronary sinus catheter is used to pace the atrium, care should be taken to examine the surface ECG to confirm that it is indeed capturing the atrium. The distal poles of the coronary sinus catheter can become lodged in a left ventricular branch, leading to ventricular capture (with a broad QRS) during pacing.

His catheter

The His catheter marks the position of the bundle of His, slightly superior and anterior to the AV node. The position of this catheter is critically important to mark this structure in order to prevent inadvertent AV node ablation during slow pathway modification and ablation of septal pathways. It is also used as a marker of the aortic root when performing a trans-septal puncture. If the His catheter is in an incorrect position this can increase the chance of complications. A well-sited catheter will have three signals: atrial, ventricular, and a sharp His electrogram. If no atrial signal is seen it suggests that the catheter is pushed too far into the ventricle and is probably recording a right bundle potential.

Broad complex tachycardia

Introduction

Electrophysiology studies have been used extensively in patients with broad complex tachycardia. The primary goal is identification of arrhythmia mechanism(s) prior to planning therapy (this could be as a prelude to ICD implantation, curative catheter ablation, and/or pharmacological therapy).

- In the past, purely diagnostic EP studies were routinely conducted in patients with broad complex tachycardia as part of the diagnostic process. Now many of these arrhythmias, including ventricular tachycardia, can be definitively treated with catheter ablation, often at the same sitting. There is therefore pressure to determine the arrhythmia mechanism as quickly as possible and decide on the therapeutic strategy with minimal delay.

- In many cases, the mechanism is easily identified through simple pattern recognition. Nevertheless, the operator needs to follow a systematic approach with basic checklists to avoid diagnostic pitfalls that could lead to potentially disastrous misclassification of an arrhythmia and inappropriate therapy.

- Unpredictable/unusual findings may occur and operators must be alert to any divergences from the standard patterns and be prepared to adjust their routine protocols to fully investigate and account for such discrepancies *before* deciding the therapeutic strategy.

Differential diagnosis

Awareness of the differential diagnosis of broad complex tachycardia and the relative frequency of the arrhythmia mechanisms is essential.

- Ventricular tachycardia, SVT with aberrancy, and SVT with pre-excitation are the three differential diagnoses.

- The likelihood of a particular diagnosis is significantly affected by a number of factors including features of the ECG and the presence or absence of structural heart disease.

Four-step diagnostic approach to broad complex tachycardias

Like the approach to diagnosis of narrow complex tachycardias, a systematic approach should also always be followed for broad complex tachycardias. The steps may not always be performed in the order presented (for example if catheter placement provokes tachycardia before antegrade/retrograde curves can be performed), but a knowledge of each step will help to make the correct diagnosis.

Step 1: Clues from existing ECG data and clinical data

Careful *pre-operative* review of available non-invasive data often provides valuable clues to guide EP studies in patients with broad complex tachycardia:
- 12-lead ECG during sinus rhythm (may show pre-excitation).
- Examination of 12-lead ECGs during tachycardia (wherever possible).
- ECG rhythm strips showing initiation/termination.
- Response of tachycardia to vagal manoeuvres and/or adenosine.
- Review of Holter ECG or rhythm strips of tachycardia initiation/termination patterns.
- Cycle length changes with spontaneous episodes of BBB aberration.
- Impact of structural heart disease on likelihood of VT.
- Occasional diagnostic ECG findings.

Step 2: Identification of arrhythmia substrates

Analysis of antegrade and retrograde conduction to identify potential substrates:
- Latent pre-excitation, AH jumps, echo beats, and AV nodal duality.
- Presence or absence of VA conduction.
- Midline vs. eccentric atrial activation, decremental vs. non-decremental conduction.
- Gap phenomena, V4R, etc.
- Parahisian pacing.
- Recognition of SVT substrate as a bystander.

Step 3: Induction and analysis of tachycardia

Induction and analysis of clinical tachycardia, particularly:
- Mode of initiation and termination.
- AV relationship during tachycardia (1:1 or not).
- VA time and atrial activation sequence (midline vs. eccentric).
- Comparison of QRS morphology with clinical tachycardia.
- Effect of cycle length variation.
- Role of His recording and analysis of HV interval.
- Analysis of VH and VA relationship.
- Identification of bundle branch re-entry.

Step 4: Pacing manoeuvres during tachycardia

Specific pacing manoeuvres to assess tachycardia mechanism:

- Diastolic scanning with ventricular extrastimuli including His-synchronous VPC (what to look for).
- Response to ventricular entrainment.
- Role of atrial extrastimuli.
- Inducing or suppressing BBB aberration and cycle length changes.
- Patterns of tachycardia termination.
- Role of atrial extrastimuli and atrial pacing to dissociate atria and in His activation.
- Characterization of pre-excited tachycardias.

Step 1: Clues from existing ECG data and clinical data

Every effort should be made to obtain ECG documentation of the broad complex tachycardia prior to EP study. Ideally a full 12-lead ECG is most helpful but if not available ambulance rhythm strips, Holter or transtelephonic ECG recordings, or defibrillator recordings can provide valuable information. If drug challenges are performed, e.g. IV adenosine, then a rhythm strip must be recorded at the very least.

12-lead ECG in sinus rhythm

- Pre-excitation indicates an antegradely conducting accessory pathway and may suggest a diagnosis of SVT with pre-excitation (antidromic AVRT or pre-excited AF), but one needs to be aware that the pathway could be a bystander in terms of the broad complex tachycardia, i.e. not directly involved in maintaining tachycardia.
- QR (Coumel) complex – the presence of Q waves in a territory consistent with coronary artery disease may indicate myocardial infarction as a substrate for VT. The presence of identical QRS morphology during tachycardia is very suggestive of VT involving this area of scar.
- Bundle branch block during sinus rhythm may be reproduced identically during tachycardia. Also, minor conduction abnormalities during sinus rhythm should make one alert to the possibility of bundle branch re-entry (📖 p. 316).

Examination of 12-lead ECGs during tachycardia (wherever possible)

- Numerous electrocardiographic criteria have been described to differentiate between VT and SVT as the cause for a broad complex tachycardia (📖 Box: ECG features of broad complex tachycardia favouring VT).
- Most of these are not 100% specific or sensitive.
- In the clinical setting, it is often safest to assume a broad complex tachycardia is VT rather than SVT with aberrancy or pre-excitation.

Response of tachycardia to vagal manoeuvres and/or adenosine

- Response of SVT to vagal manoeuvres or adenosine is described on 📖 p. 137. With VT there is no response to adenosine. As with narrow complex tachycardia, adequate doses of adenosine must be given to block the AV node. However, unlike the narrow complex tachycardia scenario, eventually one has to accept that a lack of response to increasing doses of adenosine must indicate VT rather than an SVT mechanism.

ECG features of broad complex tachycardia favouring VT

- QRS complexes >140 ms for RBBB (a predominantly positive QRS complex in lead V1) and >160 ms for LBBB tachycardia (a predominantly negative deflection in lead V1). (NB In the absence of drugs that might affect QRS duration.)
- Superior frontal plane axis in RBBB and a right inferior axis in LBBB tachycardias.
- Evidence of AV dissociation.
- Capture/fusion beats.
- Negative/positive concordance.
- ECG lead morphology – leads V1–2 and V6:
  - RBBB: monophasic R, qR, Rr', and RS in V1 and RS ratio <1 in V6.
  - LBBB: initial r wave ≥40 ms or an interval of ≥70 ms from the QRS onset to the nadir of the S wave in V1–2 (Fig. 8.1), notching of the downstroke of the S wave in V1–2, or an initial q wave in V6.

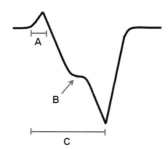

Fig. 8.1 Features of the QRS complex in V1–2 favouring VT. Time A ≥40 ms, slurring/notching at B, and time C ≥70 ms.

Review of Holter ECG or rhythm strips of tachycardia initiation/termination patterns

- A number of uncommon but characteristic ECG appearances can suggest or identify the likely mechanism of tachycardia (📖 p. 138).

Occasional diagnostic ECG findings

- If aberrant conduction during sinus rhythm is slower than during the broad complex tachycardia, i.e. the QRS complex during broad complex tachycardia is narrower than during sinus rhythm, the diagnosis is VT. It cannot be SVT with aberrant conduction because during tachycardia it would have a QRS duration at least as long as (if not longer than) sinus rhythm (Fig. 8.2).
- Broad complex tachycardia may be seen to spontaneously change to a narrow complex tachycardia (often with a critically timed ventricular extrastimulus – this can be reproduced in the EP lab as a diagnostic manoeuvre) and supports a diagnosis of SVT with aberrant conduction.

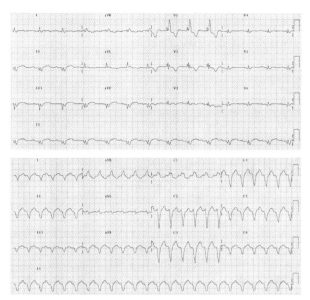

Fig. 8.2 12-lead ECGs showing a broad QRS (180 ms) during sinus rhythm (top), whilst during tachycardia (bottom) the QRS is narrower (140 ms), suggesting this must be VT rather than an SVT with aberrant conduction.

Step 2: Identification of possible arrhythmia substrates

Introduction

Following placement of catheters, a search is made for evidence of arrhythmic substrates. This is based on analysis of antegrade and retrograde conduction to identify potential substrates:

- Presence or absence of VA conduction.
- Midline vs. eccentric atrial activation, decremental vs. non-decremental conduction.
- Latent pre-excitation, AH jumps, echo beats, and AV nodal duality.
- Parahisian pacing.
- Recognition of SVT substrate as a bystander.

Presence or absence of VA conduction

- Assessment of retrograde conduction is described on 📖 p. 72.
- Absence of VA conduction (both with and without provocation using isoprenaline) makes AVNRT and AVRT very unlikely.
- Atrial tachycardia with aberrant conduction and VT remain possibilities.

Midline vs. eccentric atrial activation, decremental vs. non-decremental conduction, and other phenomena

- The variations in VA conduction and their implications are described on 📖 p. 72.
- Extra ventricular beats ('V4R') following the extrastimulus (S2) may be due to:
  - bundle branch re-entry (📖 p. 316), **or**
  - ventricular echo (📖 p. 238).
- Gap phenomena (📖 p. 72).
- These findings may still not identify the cause of the tachycardia and tachycardia itself needs to be induced.

Latent pre-excitation, AH jumps, echo beats, and AV nodal duality

- Assessment of antegrade conduction is described on 📖 p. 68.
- Is there manifest pre-excitation with short or negative HV or is there latent pre-excitation with early local V activation in the distal CS poles?
- Identification of AV nodal duality and echo beats raises the possibility of AVNRT.

Parahisian pacing

- Parahisian pacing and implications of the findings are outlined on 📖 p. 150.

Recognition of SVT substrate as a bystander

- Although the findings from the retrograde and antegrade curves may identify a substrate for an SVT mechanism, this does not mean that the broad complex tachycardia is an SVT and it is still essential to induce tachycardia, analyse the electrograms during it, and perform appropriate manoeuvres as described in the next two steps.

Step 3: Induction and analysis of tachycardia

Induction and analysis of clinical tachycardia is required to definitively identify the underlying mechanism, and hence guide effective therapy, particularly catheter ablation. There are some circumstances where a patient with BCT may be ablated without induction of tachycardia. These are:

- Suspected AVRT in WPW when ablation of the pathway is mandated on prognostic grounds (📖 p. 257).
- Mahaim pathway (📖 p. 376).
- Suspected fascicular VT (📖 p. 520).
- Ischaemic VT where substrate mapping and ablation is performed (📖 p. 502).

Inducibility of tachycardia at EPS is variable even after withdrawal of anti-arrhythmic agents and may be more difficult under GA or with deep 'conscious' sedation. Steps 3 and 4 should be undertaken as soon as sustained tachycardia is observed. This may occur:

- At baseline, i.e. spontaneous or incessant tachycardia.
- Following introduction of catheters.
- During retrograde or antegrade curves (± double extrastimuli) or incremental atrial/ventricular pacing (📖 p. 74).
- During isoprenaline infusion ± atropine plus programmed stimulation.
- Due to other programmed stimulation techniques (rapid burst pacing, multiple extrastimuli, alternate pacing sites such as CS or LV, etc.).

Comparison of ECG to clinical tachycardia

Having induced tachycardia, 12-lead ECG of the tachycardia should be compared to any 12-lead ECGs of the clinical tachycardia to ensure that the induced tachycardia is clinically relevant. Ideally the ECG of the tachycardia induced in the lab would be identical to that seen during symptomatic episodes (apart from subtle differences reflecting the altered autonomic state and supine posture of the patient in the EP lab).

P waves

The P wave axis and relationship of P waves to the QRS complexes are the important features. In particular the presence of dissociated P wave activity supports the diagnosis of VT.

QRS complexes

The axis of the QRS complexes and precordial transition should be compared to the clinical tachycardia and confirmed to be the same.

Analysis of initiation and termination

Valuable clues as to the nature of the tachycardia can be gained by analysing electrograms at the start and end of the tachycardia.

Initiation
- **AVNRT**: 📖 p. 156.
- **AVRT**: 📖 p. 156.
- **Atrial tachycardia**: 📖 p. 156.
- **VT**: Re-entrant VT will normally be induced by programmed electrical stimulation (PES) from the ventricle. It is not normally inducible with PES from the atrium, with the exception of fascicular VT (📖 p. 520). Other forms of VT that are automatic/triggered, e.g. RVOT VT, are more commonly initiated with burst pacing.

Termination
- **AVNRT**: 📖 p. 156.
- **AVRT**: 📖 p. 156.
- **Atrial tachycardia**: 📖 p. 156.
- **VT**: Where there is AV dissociation tachycardia will end with a ventricular electrogram and then resumption of the patient's normal underlying rhythm. If VA conduction is present then the final electrogram at tachycardia termination may be atrial.

A:V relationship during tachycardia

A 1:1 A:V relationship does not exclude VT as retrograde conduction through the AV node can give this pattern. A:V relationship >1:1 (A > V) indicates an SVT rather than VT, whilst an A:V relationship <1:1 (V > A) with a broad complex tachycardia will mostly occur in VT (📖 exceptions below).

Exceptions

The following exceptions are only likely to occur in the presence of bundle branch block during sinus rhythm (📖 p. 157 for details of each):

AVNRT with 2:1 AV block

AVNRT with complete AV block

Other SVTs with V > A:

Junctional ectopic tachycardia (JET)

AVNRT with VA block

1:2 tachycardia

Atrial activation pattern

Atrial activation patterns and their implications and pitfalls are described in detail in relation to narrow complex tachycardias (📖 p. 158). In a patient with BCT, the same rules and principles apply, particularly in terms of diagnosing an SVT mechanism as the cause. With VT there will either be VA dissociation (in which case the atrial activation pattern should be midline, i.e. normal antegrade conduction), or some degree of retrograde VA conduction (in which case atrial activation will also be midline, but retrograde).

Septal VA interval with midline atrial activation

The temporal relationship of ventricular and atrial electrograms in the septal region can be useful in diagnosis and is described in detail in relation to narrow complex tachycardia (📖 p. 160). During VT the VA time may be continuously varying, i.e. reflecting VA dissociation, or have a VA time that corresponds to the retrograde route of activation if VA conduction is present.

Cycle length variation

Variations in cycle length may be observed during broad complex tachycardia. They are more common in automatic triggered arrhythmia (atrial tachycardia, idiopathic VT) than in re-entrant arrhythmia (AVRT, AVNRT, macroreentrant VT). Unlike narrow complex tachycardias, measurements of the AA and HH intervals during tachycardia are only useful if there is an SVT mechanism (📖 p. 162). More helpful is measuring AA and VV intervals to identify which leads.

How to do it

Measure the intervals between a series of consecutive atrial electrograms in a single atrial channel (HRA or CS), taking care to measure between the identical points on each electrogram (AA intervals). Next measure the intervals between the ventricular electrograms (e.g. from the RV channel) of the same portion of the tachycardia (VV intervals). Are changes in the tachycardia cycle length seen first in the VV intervals and mirrored in the subsequent AA intervals, or vice versa?

What does it mean?

- **VV intervals precede or 'lead' AA intervals**: This is most commonly seen in VT (Fig. 8.3), although it is theoretically possible to see this during AVNRT or AVRT.
- **AA intervals precede or 'lead' VV intervals**: Seen with atrial tachycardias and not with VT.

Role of His recording and analysis of HV interval

A clear His recording may be important to make the diagnosis:
- In patients with VT the His may be absent or demonstrate variable block (the absence of a recorded His is presumably mostly because it is buried in the ventricular deflection).
- A shorter HV interval during broad complex tachycardia than during sinus rhythm (in the absence of pre-excitation) implies retrograde activation and suggests VT.

Analysis of VH and VA relationship

Measurement of VH and VA intervals are part of the diagnostic process for broad complex tachycardia. Commonly the VH and VA (or HA) times need to be measured during tachycardia and during pacing (at or near to the tachycardia cycle length):
- **AVNRT**: A shorter VH and VA time during tachycardia than pacing makes AVNRT a possibility.
- **AVRT**: 📖 p. 272.
- **Atrial tachycardia**: Similar VH and VA times during tachycardia and pacing support is a possible diagnosis of atrial tachycardia. There may be some degree of variation but less than with VT.
- **VT**: If retrograde 1:1 atrial activation is present, similar VA times are seen during tachycardia and pacing. If there is no clear VA/VH relationship then VT is likely. The VH interval may not be helpful in all patients – activation of the His-Purkinje system because of proximity of the VT circuit may mean the VH/HV time can be normal, short, or long.

Identification of bundle branch re-entry

📖 p. 316 for the mechanism of bundle branch re-entry.
- Every ventricular electrogram is preceded by a His electrogram with a stable HV interval.
- Variations in VV interval are preceded and predicted by variations in HH interval.
- Induction occurs with a critical delay in the VH interval (sometimes referred to as a VH jump).

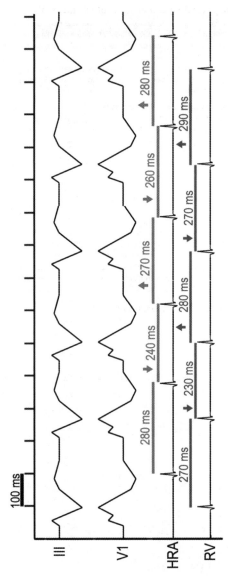

Fig. 8.3 Figure showing VV interval predicting AA interval during a broad complex tachycardia suggesting VT.

Step 4: Pacing manoeuvres during tachycardia

Pacing manoeuvres during tachycardia are key to identifying/confirming the mechanism of a broad complex tachycardia, particularly if doubts remain after Steps 1–3. Unlike narrow complex tachycardias, pacing the ventricles is of less diagnostic value, and atrial pacing manoeuvres may have an important role in differentiating VT from SVT mechanisms. These manoeuvres should be performed routinely for confirmation even if the operator is reasonably confident about the mechanism of tachycardia.

Diastolic scanning with ventricular extrastimuli including His-synchronous VPC and response to ventricular entrainment

📖 p. 172 for details of assessment in relation to SVT mechanisms. Ventricular entrainment may result in termination of the tachycardia irrespective of the mechanism, but other responses (V-A-V or V-A-A-V) suggest an SVT mechanism.

Role of atrial extrastimuli/pacing (Fig. 8.4)

The response to pacing the atrium at a slightly faster rate than the tachycardia cycle length or introducing atrial extrastimuli provides important clues as to the underlying mechanism.

How to do it

Overdrive pace the right atrium at a cycle length 10–40 ms (usually 20 ms) shorter than the tachycardia cycle length. Once the atria are entrained to the faster pacing rate pacing is stopped. It is important to confirm capture of the atria to the pacing cycle length before drawing any conclusions. Atrial extrastimuli can be added (either single or multiple) to attempt to dissociate the atrial from the ventricular activity and diagnose VT.

Reason for failure to entrain the atria:
• Termination of tachycardia during pacing – makes a diagnosis of VT very unlikely except for fascicular VT, which has other characteristic features anyway (📖 p. 322).

Interpretation

• The ability to dissociate the atria and continue tachycardia in the ventricles at the same cycle length effectively makes the diagnosis of VT (the only rare exception is with AVNRT where it may be possible to dissociate the A from V).
• If the atrium can be captured and the QRS changes to a sinus QRS (even for just a single beat) then the diagnosis is VT.
• Degeneration to AF at faster atrial pacing rates can also be useful as it may demonstrate dissociation, i.e. the tachycardia continues without any change in cycle length, or if the mechanism is SVT-dependent then the change may unmask narrow complexes or pre-excitation.

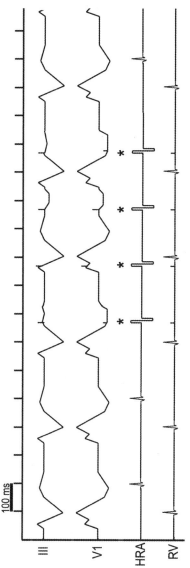

Fig. 8.4 Figure shows atrial pacing during a broad complex tachycardia that dissociates atrial activity from ventricular activity, which continues at the same cycle length as the original tachycardia, confirming VT.

Inducing or suppressing BBB aberration and cycle length changes

📖 p. 170 for methods for inducing BBB. A similar technique can be used to try to suppress BBB with a broad complex tachycardia and hence exclude a diagnosis of VT. With the change/suppression of BBB, analysis of cycle length can give important clues to the underlying diagnosis (📖 p. 272).

Electrophysiological testing for sudden cardiac death risk assessment

Programmed ventricular stimulation

Programmed electrical stimulation can be performed from anywhere within the heart that can be captured electrically. In the case of ventricular stimulation this can be from anywhere in either ventricle that can be captured.

Indications

- Evaluation of patients deemed to be at risk of VT, mainly to identify need for ICD implantation (including those with structural heart disease who have unexplained syncope/non-sustained VT).
- Evaluating the effect of anti-arrhythmic treatment on inducibility of VT.
- Induction of VT as a prelude to catheter ablation.

For a complete description of how to perform programmed ventricular stimulation 🕮 p. 80.

Interpretation of programmed ventricular stimulation: sensitivity vs. specificity

If pacing is performed aggressively enough (triple or quadruple extrastimuli with short coupling intervals), polymorphic VT or ventricular fibrillation will eventually be induced in almost every individual, particularly those with structural heart disease. This is therefore not routinely accepted as a specific endpoint (i.e. clinically relevant) for ventricular arrhythmia risk assessment in most patients – the only exception may be in channelopathy patients, e.g. those with Brugada syndrome (🕮 p. 212). There is probably increased specificity of polymorphic VT/VF induced with only single or double extrastimuli but this is still not as specific as induction of sustained monomorphic VT, which is considered as specific however it is induced. Therefore more aggressive protocols increase the sensitivity (or pick-up rate of VT) but may decrease specificity (or the clinical relevance). Likewise induction from sites other than the RV apex, or with pharmacological stimulation, may not be deemed to be as specific in terms of risk assessment, but this may not be of importance when these strategies are employed (🕮 p. 82).

Practical note

during programmed ventricular stimulation it is common to get a single ventricular beat after the extrastimulus (or a short burst of 3–5 ventricular beats), which often have a similar morphology to the paced QRS. this is known as a 'repetitive ventricular response' and is probably caused by local re-entry within the adjacent myocardium or in the bundle branches. It is of **no** clinical significance.

Role of programmed stimulation in ICD patient selection

Patients with coronary artery disease and impaired LV function

Benefit from ICD therapy as primary prevention of sudden cardiac death. Although some studies demonstrate this benefit is independent of inducibility of VT at programmed stimulation (MADIT II),[3] others used inducibility of monomorphic VT as part of the selection criteria for implantation (MADIT)[1] and this has been incorporated into some national guidelines too (e.g. NICE in the UK).

Brugada syndrome

Initial descriptions of programmed ventricular stimulation in asymptomatic patients with Brugada syndrome suggested that it did have a role in predicting risk of future ventricular arrhythmias/sudden cardiac death, and therefore need for an ICD. However, more recent studies (including larger patient populations) and meta-analysis have reported mixed results, making its role less clear.

Further confusion arises from variation in the protocols used for stimulation and the definitions of inducibility (🕮 p. 210), e.g. some accept VF, PMVT, or monomorphic VT as a positive result, even if induced with aggressive stimulation protocols.

Syncope and family history of sudden cardiac death have been associated with risk of sudden cardiac death in Brugada patients (as well as previous sustained VT/VF arrest, of course) so current international guidelines (HRS for devices) recommend ICD implants only in patients who have these risk factors and suggest no role for programmed ventricular stimulation.

Other non-ischaemic cardiomyopathies

DCM

Programmed ventricular stimulation has not been shown to be predictive of SCD risk in patients with non-ischaemic DCM (PMVT can be induced in most DCM patients but is non-specific). Even in the absence of inducible sustained monomorphic VT, there is still a high risk of VT occurrence in these patients.

Heart muscle disease

In patients with HCM the predictive value of programmed stimulation is low. In patients with ARVC there is also limited benefit and it is not recommended. There has been some limited evidence for its use in patients with cardiac sarcoid but it is still not routinely recommended.

Table 9.1 Trials demonstrating efficacy of ICD therapy in reducing sudden cardiac death in patients with coronary artery disease

Eligibility criteria	MADIT[1]	MUSTT[2]	MADIT II[3]
Coronary artery disease	MI ≥3 weeks previously, NYHA I–III	MI, PCI, or CABG ≥96 hours previously	MI ≥30 days previously
LV ejection fraction (%)	≤35%	≤40%	≤30%
Documented VT	NSVT; inducible monomorphic VT	NSVT ≥96 hours post-MI, PCI, or CABG	None necessary
EP study	Yes	Yes	No

MI – myocardial infarction; NYHA – New York Heart Association; PCI – percutaneous coronary intervention; CABG – coronary artery bypass grafts; NSVT – non-sustained ventricular tachycardia.

References

1. Moss AJ, Hall WJ, Cannom DS, *et al.*, for the Multicenter Automatic Defibrillator Implantation Trial Investigators (1996) Improved survival with an implanted defibrillator in patients with coronary disease at high risk for ventricular arrhythmia. *N Engl J Med*, **335**: 1933–1940.
2. Buxton AE, Lee KL, Fisher JD, Josephson ME, Prystowsky EN, Hafley G, for the Multicenter Unsustained Tachycardia Trial Investigators (1999) A randomized study of the prevention of sudden death in patients with coronary artery disease. *N Engl J Med*, **341**: 1882–1890.
3. Moss AJ, Zareba W, Hall WJ, *et al.*, for the Multicenter Automatic Defibrillator Implantation Trial II Investigators (2002) Prophylactic implantation of a defibrillator in patients with myocardial infarction and reduced ejection fraction. *N Engl J Med*, **346**: 877–883.

Electropharmacological testing

In the past, programmed stimulation was used to test the efficacy of pharmacological agents in suppressing ventricular arrhythmias. This routine practice has now been generally discontinued.

Drugs are also used to risk-stratify patients in other circumstances, as described below.

Ajmaline challenge (📖 p. 217)

Brugada syndrome is a sodium channelopathy but the classical ECG changes may not be manifest all the time. The administration of an agent that blocks Na^+ channels will unmask the ECG changes. Ajmaline is a very short-acting Na^+-channel blocker that is administrated intravenously whilst the patient is monitored. Twelve-lead ECGs are recorded at given time intervals (📖 p. 215) to see if the ECG changes become apparent. To increase the sensitivity of the test, the precordial leads V1, V2, and V3 are placed one intercostal space higher than usual. Other drugs can be used, e.g. flecainide, procainamide, propafenone, or pilsicainide, but their longer half-lives mean the patient needs monitoring for longer than with ajmaline.

Adrenaline challenge (📖 p. 215)

This is used in patients suspected of having long QT syndrome but in whom the resting ECG does not show QT prolongation. It is important to note that:

• ~50% of LQT1 patients have a normal QT interval at rest when they arrive for the test.
• Paradoxical absolute QT-interval prolongation, defined as a ≥30 ms increase, can be applied as a diagnostic test for LQT1 or even in genetically proven (KCNQ1 mutation) LQT1 to assess whether the identified gene mutation can manifest physiologically.
• Diagnostic accuracy is sensitivity 92.5%, specificity 86%, positive predictive value 76%, and negative predictive value 96%.
• A β-blocker washout period is recommended prior to testing with inpatient monitoring if necessary (β-blockade reduces the diagnostic accuracy substantially). Stop β-blockers five days before.
• Unless complications occur during the test, the entire protocol should be followed and not stopped even if QT interval prolongs by at least 30 ms.

Adenosine challenge (📖 p. 218)

This may be performed in patients in whom it is unclear whether an antegradely conducting accessory pathway is present, e.g. where the PR interval is short but there is not an obvious delta wave. An EP study may provide a definitive answer but the administration of adenosine intravenously in a large enough dose (📖 p. 253) will either demonstrate manifest pre-excitation, or complete AV block (suggesting but not proving a lack of accessory pathway).

Adrenaline challenge protocol

Preparation:
- Consent appropriately (📖 side effects below).
- Check serum electrolytes and correct any imbalance before administration.
- Nil by mouth for four hours before administration.
- Ensure resuscitation equipment and drugs available.

Dose:
- Add 5 ml of 1:10 000 (= 0.5 mg) adrenaline (epinephrine) to 45 ml normal saline (50 ml in total) = 10 mcg/ml
- The infusion is given in ml/hour (multiply dose in ml/hour/kg by the body weight in kg)
- Stage 1: 0.025 mcg/kg/min = 0.15 ml/hour/kg for 10 minutes.
- Stage 2: 0.05 mcg/kg/min = 0.3 ml/hour/kg for 5 minutes.
- Stage 3: 0.1 mcg/kg/min = 0.6 ml/hour/kg for 5 minutes.
- Stage 4: 0.2 mcg/kg/min = 1.2 ml/hour/kg for 5 minutes.

Monitoring during administration:
- Continuous 12-lead ECG monitoring for duration of challenge and for at least one hour after or until the ECG normalizes or until adverse effects have resolved.
- 12-lead ECG recorded at baseline, 5 minutes after starting infusion, and 30 seconds before the end of each stage.
- Patient's BP and pulse monitored at 5 minute intervals.

Reasons for ceasing adrenaline:
- Ventricular arrhythmias, including ventricular premature complexes.
- Completion of entire protocol.

Side effects:
- The main potential complications are VT or VF.
- Dysrhythmias are more common with overdose or too rapid injection. In extreme overdose there may be severe tachycardia, flushing, headache, abdominal pain (and any other symptom attributable to vasoconstriction and ischaemia).
- Development of angina and heart failure.

Ajmaline challenge protocol

Preparation:
- As for adrenaline challenge.

Dose:
- 1 mg/kg is administered (up to a maximum of 80 mg in our institution) intravenously with 10 mg given over a minute, every 2 minutes.

Monitoring during administration:
- Continuous 12-lead ECG monitoring (with accurate/alternative high precordial lead positions) for duration of challenge and for at least one hour after or until the ECG normalizes or until adverse effects have resolved.
- Patient's BP and pulse monitored at 5 minute intervals.

Reasons for ceasing ajmaline:
- Test is positive (to minimize adverse effects).
- Target ajmaline dose reached.
- Ventricular arrhythmias, including ventricular premature complexes, or when QRS widening (≥30% of baseline) observed or onset of bradycardia or AV block (type II or III).

Side effects:
- The main potential complications are VT or VF but other pro-arrhythmic effects (similar to all class I anti-arrhythmics) include sinus bradycardia, sino-atrial block, AV block, and QRS widening.
- Dysrhythmias are more common with overdose or too rapid injection. In extreme overdose respiratory depression, hypotension, coma, or cardiac arrest may occur.
- Development of heart failure and angina.
- Sensation of heat, flushing, paraesthesia, and gastrointestinal disturbances.

Cautions:
- BBB, sick sinus syndrome, or first degree AV block.
- Non-arrhythmogenic hypotension (<90 mmHg).
- Cholestatic jaundice.
- AF and atrial flutter (ventricular rate may increase dramatically).

Contraindications:
- Arrhythmias including second and third degree AV block, existing intraventricular conduction disorder, widening of QRS or PR or QT prolongation, tachycardia due to cardiac decompensation, bradycardia, or digitalis toxicity.
- Hypertrophic cardiomyopathy.
- Ajmaline hypersensitivity.
- Heart failure with LVEF <35%.
- ACS within three months.
- Pregnancy.
- Myasthenia gravis.
- Bacterial endocarditis.
- Liver disease.

Interpretation:
- A positive test is characterized by the development of the typical ECG appearances of Brugada syndrome (Fig. 9.1).

NB Ajmaline is not licensed for this use in some countries, e.g. the UK, but can be used on a named patient basis.

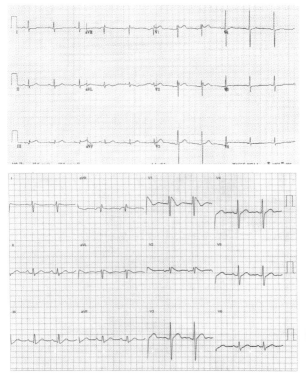

Fig. 9.1 ECG (top) at rest in a patient with syncope and a family history of Brugada syndrome. After administration of ajmaline (bottom) the typical ST elevation pattern of Brugada Type I is demonstrated in leads V1–2.

Adenosine challenge protocol

Preparation:
• As for adrenaline challenge.

Dose:
• 12 mg adenosine rapid bolus followed by 10–20 ml normal saline bolus into large gauge cannula in antecubital fossa.

Monitoring during administration:
• Continuous 12-lead (or at least multiple lead rhythm strip) ECG recording just before, during, and for 30–60 seconds after administration of adenosine.

Outcomes:
• Pre-excitation seen – diagnosis of accessory pathway made.
• AV block or PR prolongation with no delta – diagnosis of no accessory pathway.
• Neither of the above – need to give higher dose of adenosine; try 24 mg then 36 mg to try to achieve one of the first two outcomes.

Reasons for ceasing adenosine:
• None as very short acting.

Side effects:
• Sensation of chest tightness and lightheadedness ('impending doom'), which is very transient.
• Rebound tachycardia briefly.
• Theoretically VF if AV node blocked, patient goes into AF, and accessory pathway conducts rapidly.

Cautions:
• Asthma (even patients with asthma can be given high doses of adenosine – only need to avoid in those with very severe asthma, e.g. if they previously required intensive care treatment for asthma).

Electrophysiological testing for bradycardia

Assessment of sinus node function

Sinus node recovery time (SNRT)

The SNRT is the time taken for sinus rhythm to resume after a period of overdrive atrial pacing. If abnormal it suggests disease in the sinus node itself. The normal range varies between different electrophysiologists but a guideline is that the maximum SNRT should be less than 1500 ms.

Since the SNRT also varies with sinus rate, the SNRT can be corrected for this. The sinus rhythm cycle length immediately prior to the pacing is deducted from the SNRT to give the corrected SNRT. The normal maximum value is less than 550 ms. This is probably the most useful measure of sinus node function but may not be accurate if the sinus rate is very variable.

How to measure SNRT and corrected SNRT

- Pacing is performed from a quadripolar catheter in the high right atrium.
- Continuous pacing at a cycle length of 800 ms for 30 seconds and then stop pacing.
- Measurement of the SNRT and corrected SNRT is then done (Fig. 10.1).
- This is repeated with pacing at 700, 600, 500, 450, 400, 350, and possibly 300 ms.

Practical note

If the sinus rhythm cycle length is shorter than 800 ms then the initial pacing rate is reduced accordingly. The number of different pacing cycle lengths used for testing varies between electrophysiologists and many will only test at 600, 500, 400, and 350 ms, for example. Also, it does not matter if Wenckebach/AV block occurs at shorter cycle lengths as long as there is atrial capture at the pacing rate – it is the sinus node that is being tested, not the AV node. There is an overestimation in the time recorded compared to the actual time taken for sinus node tissue to recover. This is because time is taken for a paced impulse to invade the sinus node and for subsequent sinus node impulses to escape.

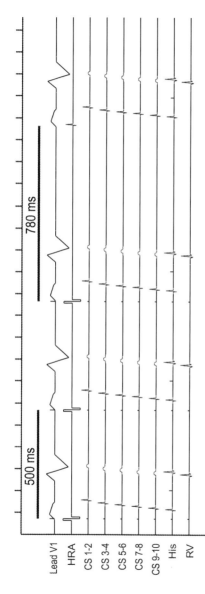

Fig. 10.1 Figure showing single ECG lead (V1), high right atrial (HRA), coronary sinus (CS), His, and right ventricular (RV) intracardiac recordings. The sinus rhythm (SR) cycle length (CL) is 600 ms (not shown). To measure sinus node recovery time (SNRT) in this case, pacing is performed from HRA at CL 500 ms for 30 seconds and then stopped d. The last three paced beats are shown followed by the subsequent first sinus beat. The SNRT is measured as 780 ms. The corrected SNRT is therefore 780 − 500 = 280 ms. Both of these values are normal.

Sino-atrial conduction time (SACT)

The SACT is a measurement of conduction between the sinus node and adjacent atrial tissue. Its measurement is dependent upon resetting the sinus node with high right atrial extrastimuli and examining the effect this has on the subsequent recorded response. There are four possible responses:

Blocked sinus impulse – a late atrial extrastimulus after a sinus beat collides with the next sinus impulse outside the node and blocks it. This does not affect the timing of the subsequent sinus impulse or its transmission. There is therefore a pause of twice the sinus CL between the two conducted sinus beats. It is said that there is no 'reset'.

Local re-entry – a very early coupled atrial extrastimulus may give rise to a very early beat, premature of that expected with the sinus impulse, because of a re-entrant phenomenon within the high right atrial/sinus node tissue.

Interpolated extrastimulus/reset – if the coupled atrial extrastimulus is not early enough to cause local re-entry, but not late enough to block the sinus impulse, one of two things may occur:

- Conduction of the impulse into the sinus node is blocked, the node is not affected, and the next impulse is conducted on time. The extrastimulus is said to be **'interpolated'** and has had no (or in reality little) effect on the sinus beat.
- An extrastimulus that is slightly later than the interpolated one but is earlier than a blocked one will be able to invade the sinus node and **'reset'** it. The next sinus beat is conducted to the atrium but delayed by the time it took for the extrastimulus to invade the sinus node (the SACT) and the time it takes for the next sinus impulse to escape the node and conduct to the atrium (the sinus CL + SACT). The time from the extrastimulus to the next recorded sinus impulse in the atrium (time x) is therefore the sinus CL + 2 × SACT. This will occur over a range of coupling intervals for the extrastimulus (the '*zone of reset*') and it is this zone and the corresponding time x that needs to be identified.

How to measure SACT

- Sinus rhythm CL is measured.
- Coupled atrial extrastimuli are added at SCL – 100 ms and decreased in decrements of 20 ms with at least ten beats of sinus rhythm between each extrastimulus.
- Time x is measured and the zone of reset identified where time x is minimally variable (remember, at coupling intervals longer than those in the zone of reset, the sinus node impulse is blocked so time x = 2 × SCL, and at shorter coupling intervals than the zone of reset the extrastimulus is either interpolated or creates local re-entry).

Normal values for SACT range from 50–115 ms. Reproducibility of the SACT measurement is difficult to achieve so SNRT and corrected SNRT are more commonly used. These measurements are made infrequently in current clinical practice. This is because sinus node dysfunction, and specifically the need for pacing as a result, is assessed through ambulatory monitoring or exercise testing. These measurements would only be performed if an EP study is otherwise indicated, as an adjunct to these non-invasive tests.

Assessment of AV conduction disorders

AH and HV intervals

AH interval

- The AH interval is the time taken for a cardiac impulse to travel through the AV node – this is measured as the time from the atrial signal arriving at the node to the time to activate the His bundle (Fig. 10.2). The AH interval is affected by autonomic tone and by pharmacological agents, e.g. sedation or beta-blockers will prolong AH interval whilst anxiety, atropine, or isoprenaline will shorten it.
- Recorded on the His catheter.
- Measurement started at the first high frequency component of the atrial electrogram (the 'intrinsic deflection', which represents onset of local activity rather than lower amplitude far-field activity – Fig. 10.2).
- Measured to the onset of the His electrogram (as this represents time of arrival of the impulse at the His bundle).
- Normal values: 55 to 125 ms.

HV interval

- The HV interval is the time taken for conduction through the His-Purkinje system to the ventricle.
- Recorded on the His catheter and commonly the surface QRS.
- Measurement from the onset of the His electrogram (as this represents time of arrival of the impulse at the His bundle).
- Measured to the earliest ventricular activation recorded, which is commonly onset of the surface ECG QRS (NB look for the earliest lead).
- Normal values: 35 to 55 ms.
- Note that the HV interval may be a negative value in patients with pre-excitation (📖 p. 262).

Prolongation of either of these intervals indicates AV nodal conduction delay. However, both intervals, but particularly the AH interval, are affected by a number of factors including autonomic tone (📖 p. 230).

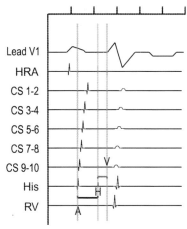

Fig. 10.2 Measurement of AH and HV intervals. A single ECG lead (V1), high right atrial (HRA), coronary sinus (CS), His, and right ventricular (RV) intracardiac recordings are shown.

Conduction curves and incremental pacing

- 📖 pp. 68–76 for how to perform these manoeuvres.
- The retrograde conduction curve adds no information to bradycardia assessment.
- The antegrade curve is used to measure the AVN ERP (📖 p. 66). Although this is subject to significant variation depending upon autonomic tone or drug provocation (📖 p. 230), information on the site of conduction block can be obtained (see below). Normal values: <400–450 ms.
- Incremental atrial pacing is used to determine the Wenckebach cycle length (📖 p. 75). This will also help determine the site of conduction block (see below).

Determination of the site of conduction block

Different responses during the antegrade curve have been described to indicate the site of conduction block (Figs. 10.3, 10.4, and 10.5).

Type I response

- Most common and represents block in the node itself.
- Progressive delay in the AV node with no change in infranodal conduction, characterized by prolongation in the AH interval (this may be smooth or with a jump – 📖 p. 238) but little/no change in the HV interval until loss of conduction at the level of the AV node (atrial electrogram but no His or V).

Type II response

- Less common.
- Delay in the AV node initially (prolongation of the AH interval as in type I) but at shorter coupling intervals during the antegrade curve gradual HV interval prolongation (representing delayed conduction in the His-Purkinje system). This is manifest as aberrant conduction on the 12-lead ECG. As the coupling interval is further decreased block may then occur either in the atrium itself (loss of any atrial capture), in the node (with AH block), or in the His-Purkinje system (an atrial and His electrogram are recorded but no ventricular electrogram or capture occurs).

Type III response

- Least common.
- Initially the same as type I but then a sudden increase in HV is seen. In this case subsequent conduction block is invariably seen first in the His-Purkinje system.

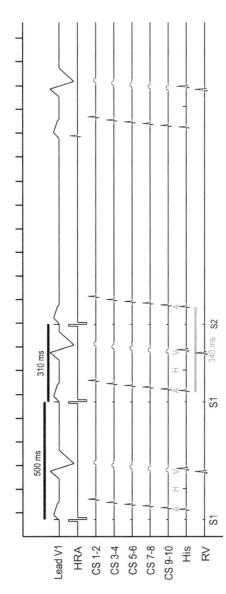

Fig. 10.3 Figure showing single ECG lead (V1), high right atrial (HRA), coronary sinus (CS), His, and right ventricular (RV) intracardiac recordings. The most common type of block with programmed electrical stimulation from the atrium is block in the AV node. The drive train CL is 500 ms. The last two paced beats of the drive train (S1) are shown followed by an atrial extrastimulus (S2) with a coupling interval of 310 ms. The atrium is captured 340 ms later but there is no conduction through the AV node (no His deflection). If a coupling interval of 320 ms is conducted through the AV node then 310 ms is the AV node effective refractory period (AVN ERP).

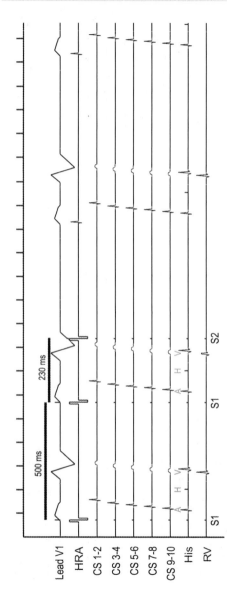

Fig. 10.4 Figure showing single ECG lead (V1), high right atrial (HRA), coronary sinus (CS), His, and right ventricular (RV) intracardiac recordings. The block with programmed electrical stimulation from the atrium is in the atrium itself in this example. The drive train CL is 500 ms. The last two paced beats of the drive train (S1) are shown followed by an atrial extrastimulus with a coupling interval of 230 ms. The atrium is not captured. If a coupling interval of 240 ms captures the atrium (as in Fig. 10.3) then the atrial effective refractory period (AERP) is 230 ms.

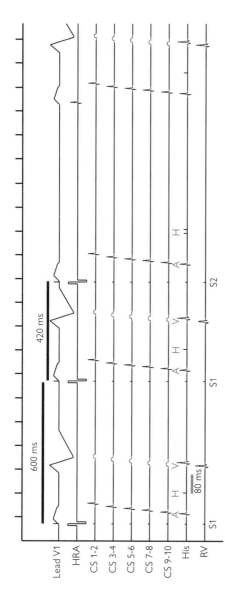

Fig. 10.5 Figure showing single ECG lead (V1), high right atrial (HRA), coronary sinus (CS), His, and right ventricular (RV) intracardiac recordings. The block with programmed electrical stimulation from the atrium is below the AV node and in the His-Purkinje system (infrahisian block) in this example. The drive train CL is 500 ms. The last two paced beats of the drive train (S1) are shown followed by an atrial extrastimulus with a coupling interval of 420 ms. The atrium and AV node are captured (an A and H signal are seen) but the ventricle is not captured. The actual level at which block occurs within the His-Purkinje system cannot be determined from these recordings.

Role of autonomic influence

AV nodal conduction is most susceptible to influence by autonomic tone, which makes definition of normal values for the refractory periods difficult (📖 p. 66). Atrial, ventricular, and His-Purkinje conduction are relatively less susceptible to autonomic tone changes, but still not completely independent. It is possible to control for this with autonomic blockade, e.g. using atropine, but this is not routinely done or necessary.

Role of drug provocation

As described on 📖 p. 224, various drugs may be used in testing AV nodal conduction.

Part 3

Mechanisms, ECGs, and electrophysiological features of the main cardiac arrhythmias

Atrio-ventricular nodal re-entrant tachycardia (AVNRT)

AVNRT

Atrio-ventricular nodal re-entrant tachycardia is common, occurring in 50–60% of patients presenting with regular narrow complex tachycardia. It is characterized by the presence of a re-entrant electrical circuit in or around the atrio-ventricular node itself.

AVNRT occurs more frequently in women than men (2:1) and may first present with recurrent palpitations at any age, although most commonly between 30 and 50 years.

Development of AVNRT is dependent on the presence of two function-ally discrete electrical pathways into the AV node, most commonly a fast and a slow one (Figs. 11.1 and 11.2). Dual AV nodal physiology such as this can be found in a significant proportion of the population, but only a small proportion go on to develop clinical tachycardia.

Fast pathway
- Located at the site just anteroseptal to the compact AV node.
- Rapid conduction of electrical impulse into the AV node.
- Long refractory period.
- Ablation of the fast pathway was initially used to treat AVNRT, but was associated with a high incidence of both complete heart block and subsequent development of incessant atypical AVNRT.

Slow pathway
- Enters the AV node from below. Most commonly it involves tissue lying between the anterior border of the coronary sinus orifice and the tricuspid valve posterior and inferior to the compact AV node. In some patients it also incorporates tissue in the roof of the coronary sinus and the left atrium.
- Slow pathway potentials may be identified in this area with a mapping catheter, which are discrete from both local atrial activation and the His potential.
- Slow conduction into the AV node.
- Shorter refractory period.
- May be multiple.

In sinus rhythm electrical activity normally enters the AV node through a fast pathway. AVNRT develops as a result of re-entry involving two pathways into the node.

Typical or atypical AVNRT
A number of different types of AVNRT exist, which are classified according to the precise nature of the re-entrant pathway.
- Typical AVNRT:
  - Slow pathway antegrade/fast pathway retrograde (slow-fast).
- Atypical AVNRT:
  - Fast/slow or slow/slow.

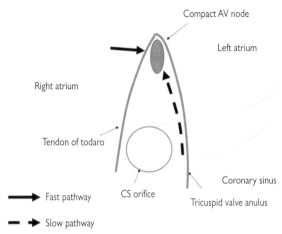

Fig. 11.1 Anatomy of the triangle of Koch as seen in a right anterior oblique view, showing the normal location of the fast and slow pathways.

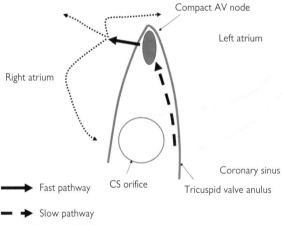

Fig. 11.2 Typical AVNRT. Electrical activity enters the compact AV node via the slow pathway, returns to the atria via the fast pathway, then re-enters the slow pathway to create a re-entrant loop.v

Typical or slow-fast AVNRT

The re-entrant circuit comprises antegrade conduction down the slow pathway into the compact AV node with retrograde conduction to the atria via the fast pathway.

Initiation

Typical AVNRT is usually initiated by an atrial ectopic beat that reaches the fast pathway when it is still refractory following the previous sinus beat. The activity is thus conducted antegradely down the slow pathway to the AV node. When the impulse reaches the AV node the fast pathway has now recovered, allowing rapid retrograde conduction back up to the right atrium, setting up the typical slow-fast re-entrant pathway and allowing the tachycardia to propagate.

Termination

The tachycardia is terminated by any manoeuvre that slows or blocks AV node conduction, including vagal manoeuvres, calcium channel blockers, beta-blockers, adenosine, or pacing manoeuvres (📖 p. 30).

Termination usually occurs in the slow pathway resulting in tachycardia ending with an atrial electrogram.

ECG

This typically shows a narrow complex tachycardia with a rate of 150–200 bpm (usually 180–200 in adults). The P waves are usually buried within the QRS complexes, although small deflections representing the P waves may be seen in the terminal portion of the QRS complex producing a 'pseudo r prime' appearance in V1 and a 'pseudo s prime' appearance inferiorly (Fig. 11.3).

AVNRT with 2:1 conduction: Occasionally AVNRT can occur with conduction block below the AV node with two atrial electrograms for each ventricular electrogram. This is characterized on the ECG by the presence of inverted P waves, midway between the QRS complexes.

Differential diagnosis

• Atrial tachycardia.
• Atrio-ventricular re-entrant tachycardia.

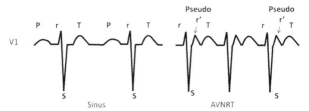

Fig. 11.3 Appearance of ECG in V1 in sinus rhythm and during AVNRT showing the presence of a pseudo r' wave at the end of the QRS complex, reflecting retrograde atrial activation.

Anatomical basis of AV node duality

There has been much debate about the precise anatomical structure and physiology of the AV node and how this relates to the development of AVNRT. The normal AV node is not clearly demarcated but is located within the triangle of Koch, an area bordered inferiorly by the attachment of the septal leaflet of the tricuspid valve, posteriorly by the coronary sinus os and superiorly by the Tendon of Todaro. The node itself consists of specialized AV nodal cells forming the compact AV node, the penetrating AV bundle (the bundle of His), and transitional cells that connect the AV node to the rest of the atrial tissue. In the normal heart these transitional cells are located in two main groups: the anterior (superior) input, which merges with the AV node near the apex of the triangle of Koch, and a posterior (inferior) input that connects the atrial tissue at the coronary sinus os to the AV node. A third middle group of transitional cells has also been identified connecting the AV node to the left atrium and septum. These provide an anatomical basis for dual AV node physiology.

Thus electrical activity enters the AV node from several directions: posteriorly from the crista terminalis; anteriorly via the septum along the fossa ovalis; and also via a broad mid-septal route across the tendon of Todaro. During sinus rhythm the predominant input is via the short anteroseptal approach with a relatively short conduction delay – the fast pathway. However, when the atria are paced at a fast rate (short coupling intervals) the anterior inputs are blocked and electrical activity enters the AV node via the longer posterior inputs – the slow pathway. The presence of dual pathway into the AV node is thus a characteristic of normal AV node physiology and does inevitably lead to AVNRT. However, features of 'dual AV nodal physiology' during standard electrophysiological testing, such as a jump in the antegrade curve and AV nodal echo beats, are seen in a significant proportion of normal subjects (25–40%). Only in a much smaller number of patients are the electrophysiological characteristics of the various inputs to the AV node sufficient to support AVNRT.

EP characteristics: sinus rhythm

Antegrade curve

- *Demonstration of dual AV node physiology*: Pacing from the right atrium demonstrates initially smooth midline decrementation of A-H conduction. However, as the refractory period of the fast pathway is reached, it will block causing a sudden prolongation of the A-H interval, as the AV node is activated through the slow pathway. This is described as a 'jump'. A jump is regarded as significant if a 10 ms reduction between S1 and S2 leads to a greater than 50 ms increase in the AH interval. The slow pathway then shows normal decremental properties (Fig. 11.4).
- *ECHO beats*: During the antegrade curve, once the fast pathway has blocked antegradely, conduction in the slow pathway may be delayed sufficiently for the fast pathway to have recovered by the time activity has reached the AV node. This allows retrograde conduction back into the atria, producing simultaneous atrial and ventricular activation. This is referred to as an atrial 'echo' and confirms both the presence of AV nodal duality and that the fast pathway is capable of retrograde conduction (Fig. 11.5). If the activation is again conducted down the slow pathway then a second cycle may be completed. If this persists then tachycardia is initiated (📖 p. 240).

Retrograde curve

- Concentric/midline CS activation or VA block (very unusual to have VA block in the presence of dual AV nodal physiology and if present at baseline then may develop VA conduction with isoprenaline).
- May demonstrate a jump retrogradely also.
- Occasionally induces tachycardia.

Tips for a reliable antegrade curve

- Ensure atrial capture – failure of S2 to capture the atria will result in apparent loss of AV nodal conduction.
- Intra-atrial delay – as the S2 is brought earlier, conduction delay within the atria will increase. Thus A1A2 should always be measured in the catheter nearest to the AV node (the His catheter). In extreme cases this may lead to an increase in A1A2 despite a decrease in S1S2. This can be reduced by decreasing the cycle length of the drive train (S1).

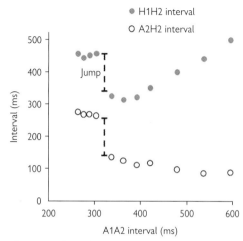

Fig. 11.4 Appearance of dual AV nodal physiology on an antegrade curve. At long A1A2 intervals conduction is solely down the fast pathway (grey circles). As the A1A2 interval is shortened further, the fast pathway becomes refractory and blocks and conduction is down the slow pathway (white circles) causing an abrupt increase in both the A2H2 and H1H2 intervals.

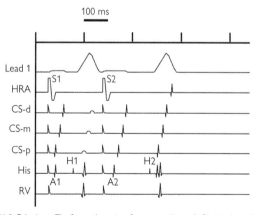

Fig. 11.5 Echo beat. The fast pathway is refractory to the early S2 stimulus, which is instead conducted down the slow pathway. By the time it reaches the AV node the fast pathway has recovered allowing the electrical activity to be conducted back up to the atria, leading to simultaneous activation of the atria and ventricle.

Note: (1) The HRA catheter is activated after His and CS-proximal, confirming an echo beat rather than a non-conducted atrial beat. (2) Because of intra-atrial delay, A1A2 is longer than S1S2. For this reason A1A2 should always be measured in the His catheter.

EP characteristics: tachycardia

Tachycardia is commonly initiated during the antegrade curve, usually in association with a jump. Much less commonly it may be induced during the retrograde activation curves. If no tachycardia can be initiated by these means, extrastimuli may be introduced to the antegrade curve or atrial burst pacing may be attempted. However, often the tachycardia can only be induced and sustained when these procedures are repeated in the presence of an isoprenaline infusion.

Basic characteristics (Fig. 11.6)

Typical AVNRT is characterized by:

- Short VA interval (usually less than 70 ms), often with simultaneous atrial and ventricular activation.
- Long AH interval.
- Concentric/midline coronary sinus activation.
- Earliest atrial activation is usually in the anterior septum detected by the His catheter, but less commonly the atria are activated via the posterior septum resulting in an earliest atrial signal in the proximal CS catheter.

Pacing manoeuvres

Ventricular entrainment (Fig. 11.7):
AVNRT is associated with a V-A-V response to ventricular entrainment.

His synchronous ventricular premature beat
The atrial activation is not advanced by a His-synchronous ventricular premature beat.

Effect of bundle branch block

Left or right bundle branch block may occur during tachycardia, or be present at rest. However, in contrast to atrio-ventricular tachycardias, development of bundle branch block has no effect on the tachycardia cycle length.

Ablation strategies

The safest approach to ablation of AVNRT is to abolish/modify the slow pathway by ablating between the anterior edge of the CS os and the tricuspid annulus. Occasionally further ablation is required within the roof of the CS or rarely within the left atrium (Chapter 17).

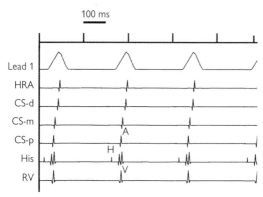

Fig. 11.6 AVNRT. There is a cycle length of 300 ms. Note simultaneous activation of atria and ventricles, with atrial activity earliest in His and proximal CS, but latest in HRA.

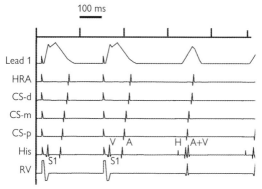

Fig. 11.7 AVNRT. Response to ventricular entrainment. The AVNRT is paced from the RV (S1) at a cycle length of 280 ms. When pacing stops the atria are then activated retrogradely via the fast pathway. Activity then goes down the slow pathway to activate the atria, producing a V-A-V response and excluding atrial tachycardia as a diagnosis. Note that in typical AVNRT the atria are then activated simultaneously with the ventricle. However, this can be distinguished from a V-A-A-V response because the second atrial beat occurs **after** the His signal in the His catheter.

Atypical AVNRT

Fast-slow AVNRT

Here electrical activity is carried into the compact AV node by the fast pathway and returns to the atria via the slow pathway.

Tachycardia characteristics

Fast-slow AVNRT is characterized by:

- Long HA interval.
- Shorter AH interval.
- Concentric coronary sinus activation.
- Earliest atrial activation in the triangle of Koch or coronary sinus.

ECG

This is a cause of a long RP tachycardia with discrete P waves separate from the QRS complexes (📖 p. 182).

Slow-slow AVNRT

This utilizes slow pathways for both limbs of the re-entrant circuit.

Tachycardia characteristics

Slow-slow AVNRT is characterized by:

- Long HA interval.
- AH interval longer than the HA interval.
- Concentric coronary sinus activation.
- Earliest atrial activation in the inferior triangle of Koch or coronary sinus.

Differential diagnosis

Atypical AVNRT is more difficult to distinguish from either an atrial tachycardia or an AVRT with a postero-septal accessory pathway than typical AVNRT.

Response to pacing manoeuvres

This is identical to typical AVNRT.

Practical tip: It is particularly important to ensure that ventricular entrainment is associated with atrial capture, otherwise atypical AVNRT may be misdiagnosed as an atrial tachycardia.

Table 11.1 How to distinguish AVNRT from orthodromic tachycardia via a septal accessory pathway

Feature		AVNRT	Septal pathway (orthodromic AVRT)
His synchronous VPB during tachycardia	Tachycardia continues	No atrial advancement	Atrial advancement
	Terminates tachycardia	Terminates with atrial electrogram	Terminates without atrial electrogram
Ventricular entrainment during tachycardia	Electrogram	V-A-V	V-A-V
	Post-pacing interval	>115 ms longer than cycle length	<115 ms longer than cycle length
VA time during ventricular pacing at tachycardia cycle length		Greater than 85 ms	Less than 85 ms
VA time with differential pacing from apex and base of RV		Shorter at apex	Shorter at base
Parahisian pacing – effect of loss of His capture		Increased stimulus to A time (>50 ms)	No change in stimulus to A time (<50 ms)

Accessory pathways and atrio-ventricular re-entrant tachycardia (AVRT)

Epidemiology and anatomy

- Defined as an additional electrical connection between the atrium and ventricle, across the AV groove.
- Prevalence ~0.1–0.4% of the general population. Risk is four times higher if a first-degree relative is affected.
- Remnant strand of electrically active tissue, typically with properties similar to atrial myocardium and spanning the AV groove that separates the atria from the ventricles.
- May occur anywhere at the mitral or tricuspid annuli and very rarely at the aorto-mitral continuity (Fig. 12.1). Some authorities have proposed discarding traditional terminology in favour of attitudinally-correct terms (Fig. 12.2).
- Most commonly single, but may be multiple pathways in 5% of patients.
- 75% are left-sided.
- May run straight or oblique course – significant separation between atrial and ventricular insertions may be present.
- CS musculature is also a potential site for AP. They may occur at the site of a coronary sinus diverticulum.
- May be endocardial or epicardial.

Importance
- Cause of paroxysmal SVT.
- Risk of sudden death from rapid antegrade conduction of AF, resulting in VF.

Important anatomical considerations
Left-sided pathways
- Require trans-septal puncture or retrograde aortic approach, thus increasing the procedural risk.
- The angulated, distinct mitral annulus permits stable catheter placement and greater success during ablation.

Right free wall pathways
- Lower procedural risk as requires venous access only and no trans-septal puncture.
- The flatter tricuspid annulus creates greater catheter instability, thus reducing the acute procedural success and increasing recurrence rates.

Postero-septal pathways
- Complex anatomy with proximity to AV nodal branch of RCA resulting in risk of heart block from arterial spasm/occlusion during ablation.
- Oblique orientation may result in earliest atrial and ventricular signals being recorded on opposite sides of the IAS.
- AP may lie at a depth requiring irrigated tip ablation.

Antero/mid-septal pathways
- Proximity to conduction system increases risk of iatrogenic complete heart block.
- A clear His potential may be recorded at successful final ablation site.

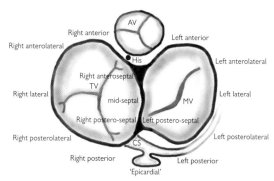

Fig. 12.1 Traditional AP localization terminology.

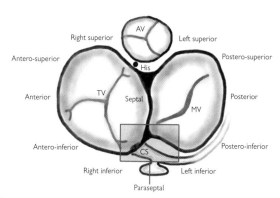

Fig. 12.2 Attitudinally-correct AP localization terminology.

Pathophysiology

The majority of APs demonstrate non-decremental conduction properties similar to those of atrial myocardium. Approximately 8% have decremental conduction.

Pre-excitation

APs may conduct in only one direction or may conduct in both directions. If they have antegrade conduction from atrium to ventricle they are capable of ventricular pre-excitation. If this is visible on the resting 12-lead ECG (a delta wave and short PR interval), the AP is said to show **manifest** pre-excitation. In some cases, particularly left free wall accessory pathways, by the time atrial depolarization has travelled all the way across both atria from the sinus node to the AP, depolarization has already passed through the AV node and His-Purkinje system and ventricular depolarization takes place through the normal route giving a narrow QRS and no ECG signs of pre-excitation. This is said to be **latent** pre-excitation. Both forms of ventricular pre-excitation are capable of producing antidromic AV reciprocating tachycardia and pre-excited atrial fibrillation. Most antegradely conducting APs also conduct retrogradely and can give rise to orthodromic AVRT.

The most common form of AP, however, is the **concealed** AP, which can only conduct from ventricle to atrium. As there is no antegrade conduction there is no pre-excitation on the resting ECG. Orthodromic SVT results from retrograde conduction. Pre-excited atrial fibrillation cannot occur.

APs create a substrate for re-entrant arrhythmias. They exhibit different conduction velocity and refractoriness from AV nodal tissue. The mitral and tricuspid valves otherwise act as an area of conduction block around which a re-entrant circuit may revolve. Critically-timed atrial or ventricular premature beats may reach the AV node and AP when one 'limb' is refractory and the other fully recovered and able to conduct. Depolarization therefore spreads from atrium to ventricle (or ventricle to atrium) down one rather than two routes. If by the time depolarization reaches the distal end of the previously refractory limb it has recovered, depolarization then conducts back to the original chamber in the opposite direction, completing a re-entrant loop. If the initial limb has recovered, a re-entrant circuit is established and tachycardia can perpetuate. Tachycardia may initiate with block in either the AV node or the AP and may result from block in antegrade or retrograde directions with atrial or ventricular premature beats, depending upon the particular conduction properties of the AP and AV node.

Definition

Wolff-Parkinson-White syndrome

Ventricular pre-excitation due to an accessory pathway AND symptomatic tachycardia (AV re-entrant tachycardia and/or atrial fibrillation).

Arrhythmia mechanisms

- AV re-entry:
  - Orthodromic AVRT.
  - Antidromic AVRT.
- Pathway-to-pathway AVRT.
- Pre-excited AF.
- Bystander pathway.

AV re-entry: orthodromic AVRT

- Antegrade conduction occurs via AV node, with retrograde atrial activation via AP (Fig. 12.3).
- Narrow complex (unless BBB), regular tachycardia with retrograde P waves inscribed in ST segment (usual VA time >70 ms, 📖 p. 272).
- Accounts for 95% of AP-mediated re-entrant arrhythmias.

AV re-entry: antidromic AVRT

- Antegrade conduction occurs via AP, with retrograde atrial activation via AV node (Fig. 12.4).
- Broad complex, regular tachycardia with delta wave morphology allowing localization of ventricular insertion site of AP (📖 p. 254).
- Retrograde atrial activation via AV node recognized by P wave morphology (📖 p. 254).
- Occurs in 5–10% of patients with WPW syndrome.

Pathway-to-pathway AVRT

- Both antegrade and retrograde activation occur via two separate APs.
- Broad complex, regular tachycardia with delta wave morphology allowing localization of ventricular insertion site of AP (📖 p. 254).
- Retrograde atrial activation via AP and atrial insertion site recognized by P wave morphology (📖 p. 254).
- Very rare.

Pre-excited AF

- Classic arrhythmia is fast, broad, and irregular ('FBI').
- Delta wave morphology and ventricular insertion of AP best identified from maximally pre-excited complexes. QRS morphology varies beat-to-beat depending upon degree of ventricular pre-excitation.
- Minimum pre-excited RR interval determined by AP antegrade effective refractory period.
- RR intervals <250 ms indicate risk of degeneration to VF and sudden death (📖 p. 257).
- One third of WPW patients have AF.

Bystander pathway

- Broad complex tachycardia with delta wave morphology allowing localization of ventricular insertion site of AP (📖 p. 254).
- AP activation occurs as a bystander to another underlying tachycardia mechanism (e.g. atrial tachycardia or AVNRT).
- Uncommon.

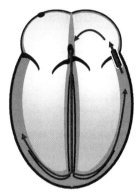

Fig. 12.3 Orthodromic AVRT.

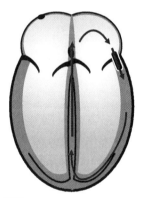

Fig. 12.4 Antidromic AVRT.

Clinical presentation and investigations

Clinical presentation

- Commonest presentation is with paroxysmal supraventricular tachycardia (PSVT).
- Symptoms may be present since childhood. SVT can even occur in the foetus.
- Instantaneous onset and offset.
- APBs/VPBs establish AV re-entry and are often noticed by the patient at onset.
- Rapid, regular palpitations often too fast for the patient to count.
- May be associated with dyspnoea, chest pain, presyncope, and syncope.
- Valsalva-type manoeuvres may terminate the arrhythmia.
- Atrial fibrillation.
- May be pre-excited with a rapid irregular ventricular rate, causing dyspnoea, chest pain, presyncope, and syncope.
- May also result from degeneration of orthodromic SVT in young patients with concealed APs.
- Aborted sudden death (pre-excited AF resulting in VF).
- Asymptomatic – incidental finding on ECG.

Investigations

Electrocardiogram

- In the baseline state, may permit localization of AP ventricular insertion site when antegrade conduction apparent as delta wave (manifest pre-excitation) (📖 p. 254).
- During tachycardia to confirm mechanism and involvement of AP.

24-hour Holter monitor

- May be of use if paroxysms occur relatively frequently, i.e. > once a week.
- Principally reserved for patients without manifest pre-excitation in whom the arrhythmia has not yet been captured on a 12-lead ECG.
- Often difficult to determine precise SVT mechanism, but allows distinction from benign palpitations, sinus tachycardia, atrial fibrillation or flutter, and ventricular arrhythmias.

TTE

- To exclude relevant structural heart disease, principally:
  - Ebstein's anomaly – associated with right-sided APs that are often multiple.
  - Aortic valve disease – may prohibit retro-aortic approach to left-sided APs (📖 p. 364).

IV adenosine

- Useful in cases of suspected subtle or latent baseline pre-excitation.
- When administered during sinus rhythm, adenosine delays or blocks AV node conduction.
- If an AP with antegrade conduction properties is present, a delta wave appears and manifest pre-excitation is briefly present.
- If there is no AP with antegrade conduction the normal response is PR prolongation with no delta wave, or complete AV block, depending upon the dose administered (Fig. 12.5).
- It is important to give an adequate dose (12–18 mg) so that either complete heart block occurs or there is manifest pre-excitation.
- Rarely, APs may be adenosine sensitive and also block during administration.

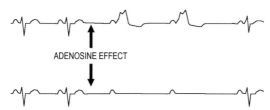

Fig. 12.5 IV adenosine response in a case of latent pre-excitation: (top) pre-ablation; (bottom) post-ablation.

ECG localization of accessory pathways

For those patients with manifest pre-excitation in the baseline state, numerous algorithms based on the delta wave and QRS morphology have been developed to permit localization of the ventricular insertion site of the AP. However, all have limitations, particularly in the accurate localization of mid- and anteroseptal accessory pathways. Close inspection of an ECG during orthodromic AVRT may reveal important clues regarding the atrial insertion site of an AP.

Delta wave and QRS morphology

- Basic principle of localization derives from knowledge that activation towards an ECG lead results in positive deflection and vice versa.
- Arruda *et al.* (1998) derived a method based on inspection of morphology of first 20 ms of delta wave (Fig. 12.6).
- QRS morphology and transition (from overall negative to R > S deflection) is also useful.

'Rules of thumb'

- Left free wall: −ve delta in lead I and aVL, V1 R > S.
- Right free wall: +ve delta in V1 but QRS transition R > S at V5.
- Septal: V1 isoelectric or −ve, R > S transition typically at V2.

Refining the position

- For free wall APs: +ve delta in aVF suggests anterior AP and −ve suggests posterior AP.
- For septal APs: −ve delta in aVF suggests postero-septal AP (−ve delta V1 right postero-septal and +ve delta left postero-septal). +ve delta aVL suggests AP closer to His; R > S in lead III suggests anteroseptal, else mid-septal position.

Retrograde P wave morphology

- Same general rules apply (see above).
- May be difficult to identify in some leads, due to morphology of ST segment and difficulty differentiating ST segment from P wave.
- Identifying atrial insertion point may suggest the presence of more than one AP (pre-excitation consistent with right free wall AP, but retrograde P wave morphology from left free wall AP).

'Rules of thumb'

- Left free wall: −ve P waves aVL/lead I.
- Right free wall: −ve P V1, +ve P aVL/lead I.
- Septal: more difficult – identify by exclusion.

Refining the position

- For all P wave morphologies, +ve P aVF suggests anterior, while −ve P aVF suggests posterior atrial insertion point.

Reference

1. Arruda MS, McClelland JH, Wang X, *et al.* (1998) Development and validation of an ECG algorithm for identifying accessory pathway ablation site in Wolff-Parkinson-White syndrome. *J Cardiovasc Electrophysiol*, 1998; **9**(1): 2–12.

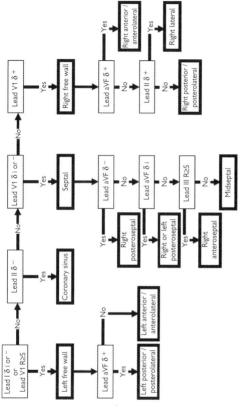

Fig. 12.6 Algorithm for AP localization (see text for details).

Prognosis

Atrial fibrillation (AF) in the patient with ventricular pre-excitation has the potential to be life-threatening by causing ventricular fibrillation. The mechanism by which this occurs is the extremely rapid conduction of depolarization over the AP in addition to the normal conduction system. A normal heart is protected during fibrillation by the decremental conduction properties of the AV node. APs, however, behave in a similar fashion to atrial myocardium and the His-Purkinje system, i.e. their refractory periods shorten the more rapidly they are stimulated. The shorter the AP refractory period, the more frequently irregular fibrillatory impulses can be conducted over the pathway, potentially resulting in ventricular rates in excess of 300 bpm.

AF appears to be more common in patients with ventricular pre-excitation. The two possible mechanisms are:
• AF results from the degeneration of AVRT.
• The AP is a source of focal automatic tachycardia that degenerates into fibrillation.

Pre-excited AF has a typical ECG appearance of a very rapid, irregular ventricular rate with broad QRS complexes with subtle differences in their morphology due to varying degrees of ventricular pre-excitation, possibly with the occasional narrow complex QRS complex.

Although hard to estimate, the risk of sudden cardiac death in asymptomatic patients with ventricular pre-excitation is estimated to be 0.1–0.2% per annum. The presence of additional risk factors may increase the annual risk of sudden cardiac death to as much as 0.3–0.6%.

Important points
• AF is only dangerous if the AP conducts antegradely, i.e. there is ventricular pre-excitation. Concealed accessory pathways do not pose a risk.
• Latent pre-excitation is just as potentially dangerous as manifest pre-excitation (the latent AP may still have a dangerously short refractory period during AF even if it is not manifest during sinus rhythm).
• It is the refractory period (recovery time), not the conduction velocity, that determines the ventricular rate during AF.
• AF with a rapid ventricular rate and narrow QRS complexes is not pre-excited – if narrow complex only, the normal conduction system is in use.

Risk stratification

Non-invasive
- Occasionally it is possible to identify low-risk APs by non-invasive means.
- Intermittent pre-excitation during sinus rhythm: Some QRS complexes are pre-excited and are followed by others that are not. This indicates that the AP has a very long refractory period.
- Sudden block in the AP during exercise: If pre-excitation disappears suddenly as the sinus rate increases during exercise, this indicates the AP has a long refractory period. There should also be a sudden return of pre-excitation during recovery. This must be distinguished from gradual loss of pre-excitation resulting from increases in adrenergic tone improving conduction through the AV node relative to the AP.
- Loss of pre-excitation during sinus rhythm following administration of a Class 1C drug or procainamide indicates a long refractory period.

Invasive
- Invasive assessment requires an electrophysiological study. This is usually performed with transvenous catheters but may also be performed with a transoesophageal pacing electrode in small children and infants.
- Direct assessment of the AP refractory period using programmed stimulation: High-risk pathways have antegrade refractory periods <260–270 ms. A sedated or anaesthetized patient, however, may have an AP that appears safe at rest but the refractory period may subsequently shorten to dangerous levels with adrenergic stimulation, e.g. exercise or stress.
- Inducibility of AVRT: If SVT is inducible the pathway is potentially higher risk but it also means a previously asymptomatic patient has the potential to develop AVRT. Non-inducibility may indicate a lower risk.
- Ventricular rate during AF: AF is induced with burst pacing and the shortest R-R interval measured. Isoprenaline may be infused to counter the effects of anaesthesia or sedation. Pre-excited R-R intervals of <200–220 ms are deemed to indicate high risk.

Table 12.1 Risk stratification

Low risk	High risk
Intermittent pre-excitation	aERP <270 ms
Sudden AP block on exercise	Shortest pre-excited R-R <200 ms during AF
AP block with Class 1C drug	Male gender
No arrhythmias and >35 years old	AF during a high adrenergic state
Shortest pre-excited R-R >300 ms during AF	Multiple APs
	Septal APs
	Symptomatic or inducible AVRT

Asymptomatic pre-excitation

The dilemma of whether or not to ablate asymptomatic accessory pathways

While there is little argument that radiofrequency ablation is an appropriate treatment for most patients with symptomatic AVRT or pre-excited AF, there is much debate for and against assessing and ablating asymptomatic APs. If no low-risk non-invasive markers are present, should asymptomatic patients undergo invasive assessment, with or without ablation?

The case for invasive assessment:
- The AP refractory period can be measured.
- Inducibility can be assessed.
- The anatomical site can be determined (will help define risk of heart block etc. with ablation and possible increased sudden death risk with septal APs).
- The presence of multiple APs can be determined (may increase risk of sudden death).
- A diagnostic EP study is extremely low risk.

The case for ablation:
- If the catheters are in place for diagnostic studies it is only a small step to go on and ablate.
- Many asymptomatic patients turn out to have potential high-risk feature on invasive testing.
- Ablation of the AP removes all risk of sudden death from pre-excited AF and the possibility of the future development of AVRT.
- Ablation is a low-risk procedure (📖 p. 260).

The argument against invasive assessment and empiric ablation:
- Ablation carries a risk (📖 p. 260).
- Asymptomatic patients, particularly those >35 years, are probably low-risk.

Practically speaking, every patient needs to be assessed on an individual basis, taking into account their age (particularly young children), their symptoms, the location of the AP based on the 12-lead ECG, and non-invasive assessment of the AP refractory period.

Approach to diagnostic EPS with accessory pathways

Purpose of EPS
- Confirm AP presence.
- Define role of AP in clinical arrhythmia.
- Determine conduction properties (and therefore risk) if ventricular pre-excitation.

Consent
- Acute procedural success rates 85–95%, depending upon AP location:
  - Right lateral, average 90%.
  - Left lateral, 96%.
  - Postero-septal 93–98%.
  - Mid/anteroseptal, 95%.
- 5–10% recurrence rate.
- Overall success after one or more procedures >95%.
- Complications:
  - RF application: AV block (0.17–1%, depending upon proximity to AVN); cardiac tamponade (0.13–1.1%); coronary artery spasm/occlusion ~0.06%.
  - Catheter manipulation: Vascular damage; microemboli; CS perforation; coronary artery dissection (all rare).
  - Vascular access: 1:100 pneumothorax, if subclavian access used; haematoma; DVT; AV fistula; arterial perforation (~0.25%, possibly under-reported).
  - Case fatality rate 0.08–0.13% (higher with left-sided AP due to risk of TSP/transaortic approach); CVA ~0.14%.
  - Overall complication rate 1.8–4.4%.

Patient preparation (📖 p. 36)
- Stop all anti-arrhythmic drugs at least five half-lives before EPS.
- Conscious sedation standard practice for most adult patients:
  - Midazolam (up to 0.2 mg/kg/hr), and
  - Fentanyl (up to 2 mg/kg/hr) IV.
- General anaesthesia for paediatric patients.

Choice of vascular access
- Femoral venous access – may use left and right femoral veins if four or more venous sheaths required.
- CS cannulation may be performed from femoral, internal jugular, or subclavian approach with fixed or steerable catheters (📖 p. 52).
- Specific long sheaths may be required for TSP access (📖 p. 88) and to improve catheter stability during ablation, particularly of right free wall APs (📖 p. 366).

Basic catheter setup (📖 p. 50)

- Josephson quadripolar (quad) electrode to high RA and RV apex.
- Josephson quad to His, or Cordis 'His-hugger'.
- A composite catheter with appropriately positioned electrodes for pace/sense function from both His and RV apical regions is also available.
- Deflectable or fixed curve multi-polar electrode to CS. Ten poles (decapolar) for left-sided pathways/unknown SVT mechanism are recommended. Closely spaced electrodes may be used to 'bracket' the left-sided AP with a higher degree of accuracy.
- A more minimal approach with a 'roving' catheter between RV and RA may be undertaken for simplicity. However, more catheters may be required if the arrhythmia mechanism is complex.

Paediatric patients

- Arterial access to monitor BP (4 F femoral or radial arterial line).
- Limit the maximum number of sheaths per femoral vein to two. Smaller French paediatric catheters can be obtained. Our suggested practice is to use standard 'adult' EP catheters if age > ~9 years or weight >30 kg.

Diagnostic EPS

Baseline intervals (Fig. 12.7)
- If there is manifest pre-excitation:
  - Short HV interval (<35 ms) is present. The His deflection may even be after the onset of the QRS complex, leading to a negative HV interval.
  - If the manifest AP is left-sided there will be short AV times in the CS electrode catheter with the electrode pair closest to AP having the earliest V signal.
- If the AP is latent or concealed the baseline intervals will be normal.

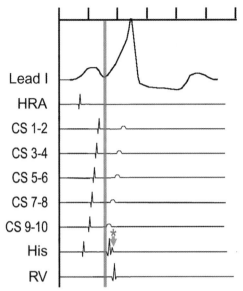

Fig. 12.7 Sinus rhythm and ventricular pre-excitation. The earliest ventricular electrograms are in the His and CS 9-10 electrodes and they time out with the onset of the delta wave (grey line), indicating a septal AP position. The His bundle egram (*) occurs shortly after the delta wave onset and V component, producing a negative HV interval.

Antegrade curve (📖 p. 68)

- Pacing site: HRA or CS; 600/500 ms S1 drive train according to the resting heart rate.
- S2 decreasing in 20 ms increments until 300 ms, then in 10 ms increments to AV node and AP refractoriness.
- Typical findings in manifest pre-excitation:
  - With shortening S2, AVN decrements but AP conduction non-decremental.
  - AH prolongs, but AV interval remains the same – thus, the degree of pre-excitation increases and the HV shortens or becomes more negative.
  - When the AP ERP is reached, pre-excitation disappears. If the AVN is non-refractory, there is a long AH, normal HV interval, and narrow QRS (Fig. 12.8).
  - If the AVN ERP is longer than the AP ERP, AV block occurs once the AP ERP is reached.
- AV nodal duality may be present (📖 p. 140) – this may represent another tachycardia mechanism or be coincidental. Likewise, the AP may or may not be part of the clinical tachycardia mechanism.
- During incremental atrial pacing, when the antegrade AP ERP is reached the QRS becomes narrow only if AP block occurs before AVN block. If the AP ERP is shorter than the AVN ERP, AV block occurs.
- Atriofascicular APs (📖 p. 378):
  - Demonstrate decremental antegrade conduction properties.
  - Typically, increasing degrees of pre-excitation produces a LBBB QRS configuration (<150 ms duration) with earliest V signal at RV apex (the insertion site of the atriofascicular connection).

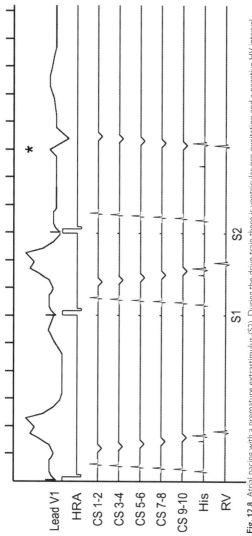

Fig. 12.8 Atrial pacing with a premature extrastimulus (S2). During the drive train there is ventricular pre-excitation and a negative HV interval. Following the S2, antegrade conduction down the AP is blocked. The AVN still conducts, with a longer AH interval and a narrow QRS (*). The AP ERP is the longest S2 that results in AP block.

Lead V1

HRA

CS 1-2

CS 3-4

CS 5-6

CS 7-8

CS 9-10

His

RV

S1

S2

Retrograde curve
- Pacing site: RV apex; 600/500 ms S1 drive, according to resting heart rate.
- S2 decreasing in 20 ms increments until 300 ms, then in 10 ms increments to AV node and/or AP refractoriness.
- Typical finding is non-decremental conduction (Fig. 12.9):
  - Retrograde AP conduction may dominate from the onset, especially if there is no retrograde AVN conduction.
  - Alternatively there may be an interplay between AVN and AP retrograde conduction resulting in progressive emergence of non-decremental AP conduction, e.g. with left lateral APs, retrograde conduction may initially appear midline when the AVN dominates. However, as the S2 shortens, two retrograde wavefronts appear until eventually the AP (eccentric pattern) dominates.
- Earliest atrial activation indicates AP atrial insertion site:
  - CS distal with left lateral AP.
  - CS proximal with postero-septal AP (right or left).
  - His electrode with mid/anteroseptal AP; may be difficult to identify parahisian pathway as activation sequence similar to AVN (parahisian pacing useful, 📖 p. 150).
  - HRA with right lateral AP.
- Beware possibility of two APs.
- Atriofascicular (and some other antegradely conducting) APs do not conduct retrogradely (📖 p. 378).

AP effective refractory period
- Definition:
  - Antegrade AP ERP is the maximum local A-A interval resulting in antegrade AP block (i.e. signified either by the appearance of non-pre-excited QRS with long AH interval indicating slow pathway conduction, or AVN block if slow pathway already refractory).
  - Retrograde AP ERP is the maximum local V-V interval resulting in retrograde AP block (i.e. signified either by block in retrograde, eccentric conduction, or change from non-decremental to decremental, midline conduction if retrograde AVN conduction still present).
- Minimum pre-excited RR interval is an important prognostic marker (<250 ms, increased risk of VF, 📖 p. 257).
- Strictly, this should be determined with the patient in AF. Atrial pacing during isoprenaline infusion is a reasonable alternative, but not validated by prospective trial data.

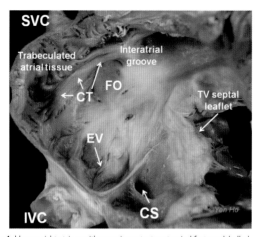

Plate 1 Human right atrium with some important anatomical features labelled. The tricuspid valve (TV) orifice is seen on the right. The coronary sinus (CS) os, the eustachian valve (EV), and the fossa ovale (FO) are marked. The crista terminalis (CT) is a curved ridge that runs from the interatrial groove between the smooth posterior wall and the anterior trabeculated atrial tissue. Orientation of the specimen is almost equivalent to a straight antero-posterior projection with the superior vena cava (SVC) at the top and the inferior vena cava (IVC) at the bottom. (Image kindly provided by Professor S. Yen Ho, Imperial College, London, UK.) (📖 Fig. 2.1, p. 9.)

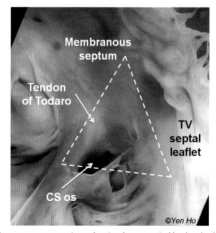

Plate 2 Human necropsy specimen showing the anatomical landmarks that make up the triangle of Koch (dashed lines). The compact AV node lies at the apex of the triangle with the slow pathway fibres running along the right side of the triangle (📖 Chapter 11 on AVNRT). Note the Thebesian valve at the CS os, which is a fenestrated structure and can sometimes obstruct access to the CS. TV – tricuspid valve; CS – coronary sinus. (Image kindly provided by Professor S. Yen Ho, Imperial College, London, UK.) (📖 Fig. 2.2, p. 11.)

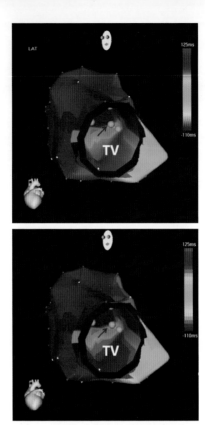

Plate 3 CARTO local activation timing (LAT) map (top) and isochronal map (bottom) of the right atrium in LAO view. The activation sequence demonstrates a typical (counter-clockwise) right atrial flutter. TV – tricuspid valve annulus (black ring). The blue balls on the posterolateral wall (seen through the TV, red arrow) show the location of the crista terminalis. (📖 Fig. 6.1, p. 101.)

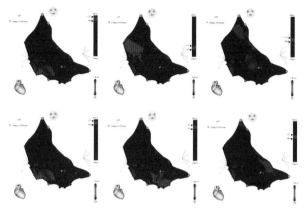

Plate 4 CARTO propagation map of the right atrial flutter from Fig. 6.1. (📖 Fig. 6.2, p. 103.)

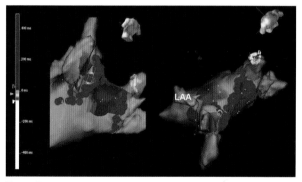

Plate 5 Diagnostic landmarking of the left atrium during left atrial appendage (LAA) pacing to demonstrate a line of block on the atrial roof. The left infero-posterior view is shown on the left image; the superior view is shown on the right image. The colour scale refers to timing relative to a CS reference. Caudal to cranial activation of the posterior left atrium is demonstrated on the left image. (📖 Fig. 6.3, p. 105.)

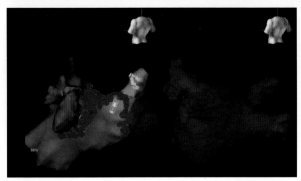

Plate 6 NavX geometry of the left atrium and its DIFF image segmented from a cardiac MRI. It is possible to simultaneously display the circular mapping catheter in the right upper pulmonary vein (yellow). The tip of the ablation catheter is shown in green. Ablation lesions around the pulmonary veins and a roof line are shown as red dots. (☐ Fig. 6.5, p. 113.)

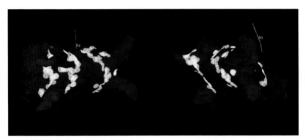

Plate 7 An Ensite Fusion case of atrial fibrillation ablation. An MRI of the left atrium has been fused with the NavX geometry. The fused image provides accurate anatomical guidance for targeting ablation therapy (white dots). Note that a reference catheter has been positioned in the ascending aorta. (☐ Fig. 6.6, p. 113.)

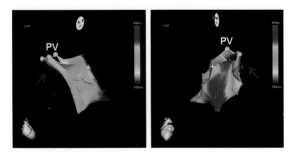

Plate 8 CARTO map of RVOT VT. An area of early activation (red area indicated by red arrow) is seen just below the pulmonary valve (PV). RAO projection on the left and LAO on the right. (☐ Fig. 22.13, p. 515.)

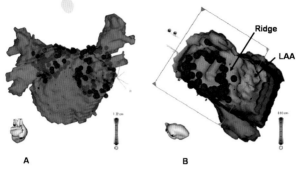

A   **B**

Plate 9 A CARTO merge case of atrial fibrillation ablation. An MRI of the left atrium has been merged with the CARTO shell. Panel A shows a PA view of the left atrium. Circumferential ablation lesions (red dots) have been delivered around the left and right pulmonary veins in pairs. In panel B, the image has been clipped to allow direct endocardial visualization of the left pulmonary venous ostia (LPV) and left atrial appendage (LAA). The LAA ridge can be demonstrated between the LAA and the left pulmonary veins. (📖 Fig. 6.7, p. 115.)

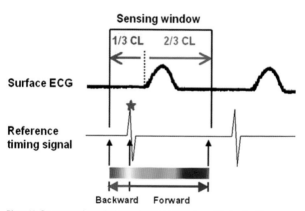

Plate 10 Sensing window calculation: forward and backward timing durations are measured relative to a reference timing signal. The onset of the window is taken before tachycardia onset from the surface ECG (approximately 1/3 of the tachycardia cycle length) to include potential diastolic activity in a re-entry circuit. In this example, the sensing window covers 100% of the tachycardia cycle length. (📖 Fig. 6.8, p. 121.)

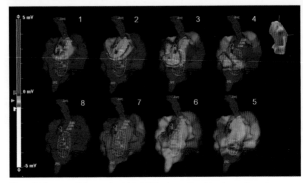

Plate 11 Isopotential map of a right atrial tachycardia arising from a focus in the superior crista terminalis adjacent to the sinus mode. The sequence of depolarization is marked in order of from image 1 to 8. The green SAN labels mark the sinus node. The green numbers 6–10 mark the crista terminalis. Activation begins inferior and posterior to the sinus node (1) and spreads inferiorly and to the septum but is blocked by the crista terminalis (2–4) before passing through a gap (green number 10, 5) and spreading anteriority (6–8). (📖 Fig. 6.9, p. 123.)

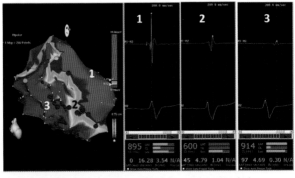

Plate 12 CARTO bipolar voltage map of the left ventricle in sinus rhythm (modified RAO view). This patient has a prior inferior infarction with a large scar in the infero-posterior left ventricle. Representative sites from different regions are selected for display. 1 – normal myocardium (3.54 mV); 2 – probable border zone (1.04 mV); 3 – likely scar (0.30 mV). (📖 Fig. 6.10, p. 125.)

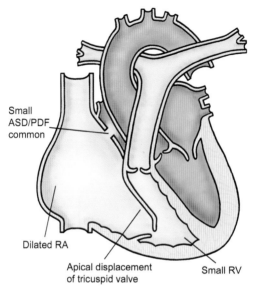

Plate 13 Diagrammatic representation of Ebstein's anomaly. This is often associated with other cardiac defects (PFO, ASD, VSD, and RVOT obstruction). (📖 Fig. 18.10, p. 385.)

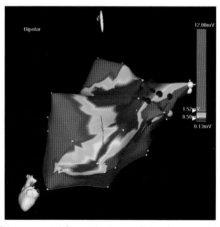

Plate 14 Substrate map in left ventricle. An area of low voltage is seen on the basal lateral wall (red colour). The white balls mark the mitral valve annulus (MVA) and the blue ball an area of double potentials (DPs). The best pace maps for the clinical VT (which was fast and haemodynamically unstable) were in the region of the very basal scar and therefore a set of ablation lesions (red balls) were performed around the margin of the low voltage area, extending through the area of DPs and to the MVA. This rendered the VT non-inducible. (📖 Fig. 22.8, p. 503.)

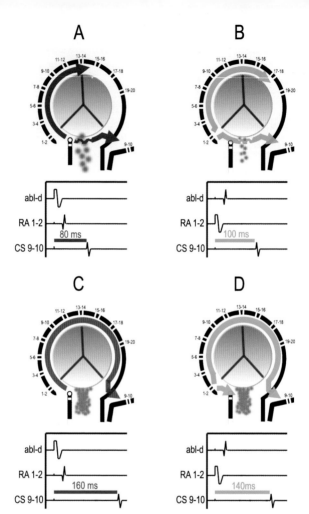

Plate 15 Differential pacing on the lateral side of the ablation line and recording in CS proximal (9-10). Incomplete isthmus block: Pacing from adjacent to the ablation line (A) produces a shorter stimulus to CS 9-10 time than pacing from a more lateral position (RA 1-2). Complete isthmus block: Pacing from adjacent to the ablation line (A) produces a longer stimulus to CS 9-10 time than pacing from a more lateral position (RA 1-2). (📖 Fig. 19.6, p. 409.)

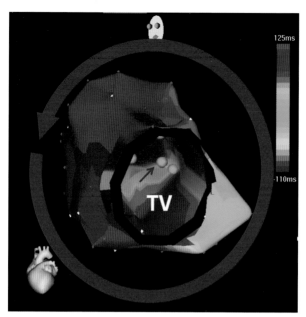

Plate 16 An isochronal activation map of the right atrium during typical atrial flutter displayed in an LAO view. The colours represent activation timings. The entire cycle length of the tachycardia is spread around the tricuspid valve in a counter-clockwise direction (red to yellow to green to blue to purple) with the head meeting the tail. (📖 Fig. 19.8, p. 413.)

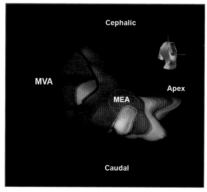

Plate 17 Left ventricular geometry created using a multi-electrode array (MEA). The colours represent electrical activation (📖 Chapter 6). The torso in the top right corner depicts the orientation of the chamber. MVA – mitral valve annulus. (📖 Fig. 22.9, p. 505.)

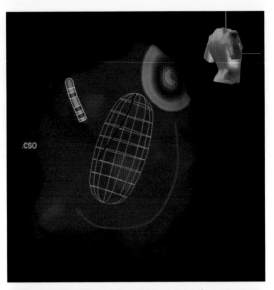

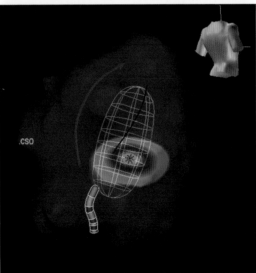

Plate 18 Non-contact mapping during sinus node modification. Top panel: Sinus node activation initially shows earliest activation from high lateral RA, above crista terminalis, down around atrium. Bottom panel: After ablation the activation originates lower in the RA, around the lower end of the crista terminalis. (📖 Fig. 21.9, p. 477.)

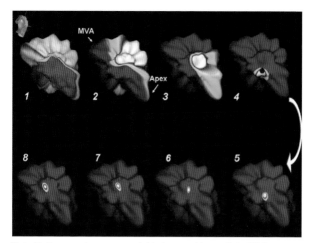

Plate 19 A reverse-time sequence of eight isopotential maps during VT. In (1) the left ventricular virtual endocardium is translucent and the multi-electrode array position can be seen. The translucency has been removed in the rest of the maps. Systolic activation is shown during VT in (1) and (2). The VT is then mapped backwards in time. (3) and (4) show the probable exit site of the VT. (4) to (8) show slow conduction (inferred from the small distance covered by the activation on the isopotential maps during a time period of 150 ms). This presumably represents part of the diastolic pathway for the VT circuit. Ablation at the exit site (marked by a red circle on map 4) terminated VT and rendered it non-inducible. MVA – mitral valve annulus. (📖 Fig. 22.10, p. 507.)

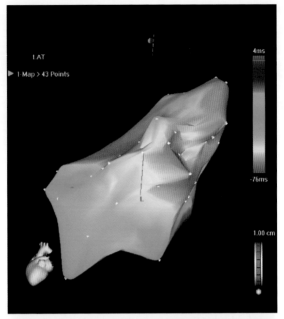

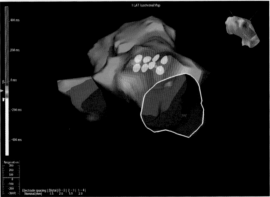

Plate 20 Top panel shows CARTO map of focal VT in the left ventricle. Bottom panel shows a NavX map of a focal VT near the mitral valve annulus (MVA). Circles represent the ablation lesions that terminated VT. Earliest activation during tachycardia in red on the CARTO map and white on the NavX map. (📖 Fig. 22.7, p. 501.)

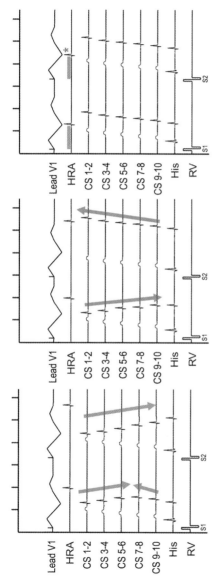

Fig. 12.9 Left: Pacing from the RV apex. During the slower drive train there are two wavefronts, one going up the midline, the other through a left lateral AP, producing a chevron shape. With the S2 the AVN decrements or may indeed block and all retrograde activation is eccentric via the AP (earliest A is distal CS). Middle: In this example there is activation through a left lateral AP during the S1 drive train (eccentric activation, earliest distal CS) and then AP block with retrograde conduction through the AVN with the S2. Right: In this example the presence of retrograde conduction through a right free wall AP is hard to detect during the S1 drive train but becomes clear when looking at earliest, non-decremental activation in the HRA catheter with the S2 (*).

Electrophysiological characteristics during sinus rhythm

Parahisian pacing (📖 p. 150)

Septal APs with retrograde conduction have similar atrial activation sequences to retrograde conduction through the AV node. Parahisian pacing can be used to identify the presence of a retrogradely conducting septal AP, although this does not confirm that it is involved in the clinical tachycardia mechanism.

Other manoeuvres

- Ventricular pacing at TCL:
  - For retrogradely conducting APs the VA time is similar to that during tachycardia.
- Atrial pacing at TCL:
  - The AH time is similar to that during tachycardia. This is a useful differentiation from atypical AVNRT, where the AH time during pacing at TCL is usually longer than the tachycardia AH.
- For retrogradely-conducting right-sided APs, the VA time during pacing at the RV apex > VA time during pacing at the RV base.
- Multiple retrogradely-conducting accessory pathways are suggested by >1 pattern of retrograde atrial activation separate from an AVN pattern.

Induction of AVRT

Arrhythmia induction may occur during atrial or ventricular stimulation.

Orthodromic AVRT (Fig. 12.10)

- During the antegrade curve or atrial incremental pacing, AP block before AVN ERP allows antegrade conduction solely down through the AV node, usually at the point at which the decremental properties of the node result in a long AH time.
- If conduction through the AVN followed by ventricular activation is long enough for the AP to have now recovered, retrograde conduction up the AP to the atrium is now possible, completing one loop of the re-entrant circuit.
- If the AVN has recovered, conduction again occurs antegradely just through the AVN to the ventricles and re-entry continues, perpetuating tachycardia.
- During ventricular pacing the same principles apply, but with AVN block and retrograde AP conduction at initiation, allowing antegrade AVN activation from the wavefront of atrial activation originating from atrial site of AP insertion.

Antidromic AVRT (Fig. 12.11)

- During antegrade curve, the AVN block occurs before AP, and ventricular activation is solely through the AP (maximal pre-excitation).
- AVN recovery permits retrograde atrial activation through the normal conduction system completing one loop of the tachycardia circuit.

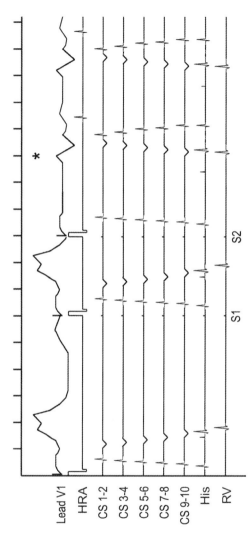

Fig. 12.10 Onset of orthodromic AVRT. The S2 blocks antegradely in the left lateral AP so there is no pre-excitation (*). There is decremental conduction through the AV node with a long enough AH, HV, and ventricular conduction time that by the time ventricular depolarization reaches the ventricular insertion of the AP and travels up through it to the atrium, the atrial myocardium has recovered and there is retrograde activation (earliest A in CS 1-2). The AV node recovers in time to conduct the retrograde P wave through to the ventricle and tachycardia continues.

Orthodromic AVRT: EP characteristics

- Obligatory 1:1 A:V association during tachycardia.
- Shortest VA time >60 ms:
  - During tachycardia, the atria and ventricles are activated in series. Thus, the activation wavefront must travel through the AVN, His-Purkinje network, and ventricular myocardium before reaching the AP insertion site to reciprocate to the atria; a VA time >60 ms is the minimum required for such a circuit.
  - This contrasts with typical slow-fast AVNRT where simultaneous atrial and ventricular activation result in a VA time of <60 ms (📖 p. 160).
- Constant V-to-A conduction times despite TCL variations:
  - In the absence of new onset BBB, 'wobbles' in the TCL may occur due to changes in antegrade AVN conduction properties. However, retrograde AP conduction is constant, so the VA time remains unchanged.
- A His-synchronous VPB advances tachycardia (proves pathway presence but not participation in the tachycardia, 📖 p. 166).
  - Note: May need to pace in the LV if there is a left lateral AP, due to long conduction times from RV apex pacing site to the AP ventricular insertion site.
- Ipsilateral BBB prolongs the His (or V)-to-A time by ≥25 ms (Fig. 12.11). The TCL is usually also prolonged; however, there may be compensatory shortening of the A-H time due to AVN decremental properties that makes this less obvious.
- Reproducible tachycardia termination by PVCs during His refractoriness without conduction to atrium:
  - When His is refractory, VPBs cannot reach the AVN.
  - Reliable tachycardia termination points to the ventricular myocardium (and AP) as a critical limb of the tachycardia.
  - The absence of atrial activation at tachycardia termination excludes the possibility of atrial tachycardia with bystander AP.
- Response to ventricular entrainment (📖 p. 172):
  - V-A-V at offset, with ongoing tachycardia.
  - PPI-TCL not >115 ms when pacing at RV apex. The shortest PPI occurs with right-sided APs.
  - VA interval during V entrainment within 85 ms of tachycardia VA interval.

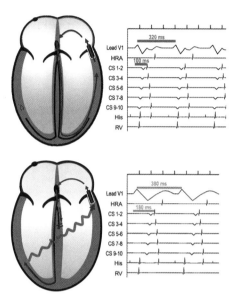

Fig. 12.11 Top: Orthodromic AVRT via a left lateral AP with a TCL of 320 ms and VA time of 100 ms. Bottom: With ipsilateral (in this case left) BBB the route through the ventricle to the AP insertion is longer and slower, thus the TCL and the VA time are prolonged to 380 and 180 ms. The TCL may not prolong as much as the VA time due to a slight shortening of the AH time as it has longer to recover due to the longer TCL. The local VA time at the AP insertion site does not change. Contralateral BBB does not produce this phenomenon as it does not alter the quickest route from the AVN to the AP insertion.

Antidromic AVRT: EP characteristics

- Obligatory 1:1 AV relationship.
- The QRS morphology in tachycardia is consistent with maximal pre-excitation as ventricular activation is solely via the AP.
- The retrograde His deflection may be absent due to being buried within the His catheter's V electrogram.
- Changes in the VH interval (when seen) precede changes in TCL. This is due to the tachycardia circuit consisting of antegrade ventricular activation via an AP and septal activation via the His and AVN. An increase in the VH interval due to ipsilateral retrograde BBB prolongs the TCL by ≥25 ms.
- HA times during antidromic AVRT must be >70 ms if retrograde activation is through the AVN.
- Ventricular activation is advanced by atrial extrastimuli near the AP insertion with advancement of subsequent His and atrial activation and proves the presence of an AP. This is an extension of the principle relating to changes in VH interval, above. A long excitable gap in the atrium allows tachycardia advancement via appropriately timed APBs.
- The differential diagnoses include: VT with 1:1 AV association; atrial tachycardia with bystander AP; AVNRT with bystander AP; pathway-to-pathway AVRT.

Other key features supporting a diagnosis of antidromic AVRT

- The AVN must have excellent retrograde conduction to support tachycardia. If the AP does not conduct retrogradely it may be possible to confirm this by demonstrating 1:1 VA conduction during RVA pacing at the TCL. If the AP does conduct retrogradely and the AP retrograde ERP is shorter than the antidromic TCL this can only be confirmed after successful AP ablation.
- Antidromic AVRT is more likely to occur with lateral, free wall APs owing to the extra conduction time (approximately 50 ms) to and from the AVN/distal His-Purkinje fibres and the AP atrial and ventricular insertion sites. The time from the atrial insertion point of the AP to the retrograde His is usually in the order of 150 ms.
- The V-H time during tachycardia should be identical to the V-H time when pacing at the AP ventricular insertion site at the TCL.

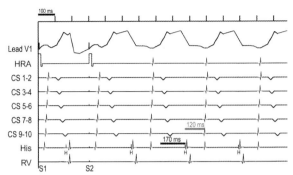

Fig. 12.12 Onset of antidromic AVRT. The S2 blocks antegradely in the AV node but still conducts to the ventricle through the left lateral AP producing maximal pre-excitation. There is retrograde conduction up through the AV node producing a midline atrial activation pattern. The VH time is 170 ms and the HA time 120 ms. The retrograde P wave is in turn conducted antegradely through the AP and tachycardia continues.

Antidromic AVRT may also be induced with ventricular pacing that results in retrograde block in the AP but slow enough retrograde conduction up through the AVN so that by the time the retrograde P wave reaches the AP it has recovered and conducts antegradely to the ventricle.

Common atrial flutter

Introduction

Common atrial flutter was the first macroreentrant atrial tachyarrhythmia to be successfully treated by catheter ablation based on a clear understanding of the three-dimensional activation sequence and the anatomical boundaries that are critical to maintenance of the re-entrant circuit. The treatment strategy involves linear ablation of a normal structure, the cavotricuspid isthmus, with the aim of transecting the re-entrant circuit at its most vulnerable point (⬚ Chapter 19). Demonstrating isthmus conduction block by electrophysiological techniques is now accepted as the key endpoint of treatment, predictive of a low incidence of recurrence unlike the alternative endpoint of flutter termination/non-inducibility. However, achieving and/or confirming isthmus block may be challenging in a minority of cases. Although isthmus ablation is highly effective for treating atrial flutter, it is now clear that this patient population is susceptible to developing other atrial arrhythmias, particularly atrial fibrillation, which occurs in >30% during medium to long-term follow-up, a point that always needs to emphasized to patients beforehand.

Anatomical considerations

The re-entrant circuit of typical atrial flutter involves the entire right atrium (Fig. 13.1). The key anatomical features are:

- Posterior boundary formed by the IVC, SVC, and crista terminalis (a functional barrier to transverse conduction by virtue of its anisotropic properties). The crista terminalis eventually becomes the eustachian ridge, a fibrous structure extending past the IVC orifice towards the CS ostium.
- Anterior boundary formed by the tricuspid annulus.
- The cavotricuspid isthmus (IVC-TA isthmus) is essential for macroreentry, enabling closure of the circuit in the low RA. It is *not* a diseased/slow conduction zone but is the preferred target for ablation because compared to other parts of the circuit it is:
  - Relatively narrow.
  - Accessible/straightforward to stabilize ablation catheter for continuous linear lesions.
  - A relatively safe area for ablation.
- IVC-TA isthmus runs from the low anterior to the low septal RA, i.e. anterolateral to posteromedial direction. The posterior rim is composed of the IVC orifice and eustachian ridge. Interrupting isthmus conduction may be straightforward or difficult depending on a number of factors:
  - Width may vary from a few millimetres to >3 cm.
  - Variable myocardial thickness may be >1 cm.
  - Highly variable muscle composition/orientation with circular fibres, longitudinal muscle bundles from the crista terminalis, and membranous tissue.
  - Prominent eustachian ridge hampering access to the myocardial tissue in the sub-eustachian recess or pouch (📖 p. 8).

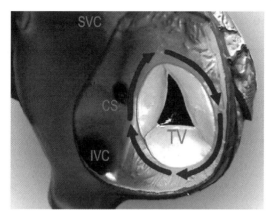

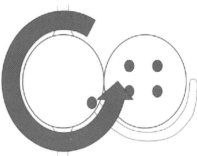

Fig. 13.1 Typical atrial flutter circuit and anatomical relationships. The image shows a view into the right atrium with the free wall removed. The flutter circuit rotates around the tricuspid valve. TV = tricuspid valve, IVC = inferior vena cava, SVC = superior vena cava, CS = coronary sinus.

Role of the electrophysiology study

Electrophysiological testing serves three potential functions during atrial flutter ablation procedures: (i) induction of clinical arrhythmia (in patients with paroxysmal atrial flutter); (ii) confirmation of the diagnosis of common flutter with isthmus-dependency; and (iii) assessment of IVC-TA isthmus conduction and identification of the key endpoint of bidirectional conduction block. However, clinical practice differs markedly between individual operators with respect to the electrode configuration used, how much evaluation is carried out prior to ablation, and the method of assessing isthmus block.

- The commonest configuration is a steerable multi-polar catheter such as the 20 or 24-pole Halo (2-4-2 mm spacing) positioned close to the anterior/superior tricuspid annulus to record RA activation, plus another in the CS. In addition, the ablation catheter is available for pacing and recording in/adjacent to the isthmus region. It is important to check the orientation of the RA mapping catheter in both LAO and RAO projection to avoid recording erroneous activation patterns during flutter or pacing.
- Simpler 2-catheter configurations can be used, for example a multi-polar RA catheter plus ablation catheter (i.e. no CS), or an ablation catheter plus CS catheter.
- For patients in atrial flutter at the start of the procedure it is advisable to check:
  - Activation of the RA (counter-clockwise or clockwise sequence) corresponding to the entire flutter cycle length (Fig. 13.2).
  - Concealed entrainment to check participation of the IVC-TA isthmus in the arrhythmia with a post-pacing interval (PPI) close to the tachycardia cycle length (Fig. 13.3) (□ p. 28).
- For patients in sinus rhythm at the start of the procedure, ideally the clinical arrhythmia should be induced by atrial extrastimuli and/or burst pacing, followed by confirmation of the activation sequence and isthmus-dependency as above. However:
  - Flutter may be non-inducible.
  - Aggressive programmed stimulation may induce non-clinical arrhythmias, particularly AF, with the possible need for DC cardioversion.
  - Some operators prefer to undertake isthmus ablation empirically (i.e. with no attempt at flutter induction plus verification) during pacing if prior ECG recordings have shown the typical flutter morphology, as isthmus-dependency is then very likely.
- Assessment of isthmus conduction is covered in the ablation section (□ p. 402).

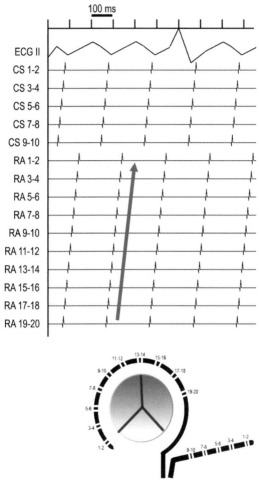

Fig. 13.2 Schematic of CS and multi-polar catheter and corresponding electrograms during atrial flutter.

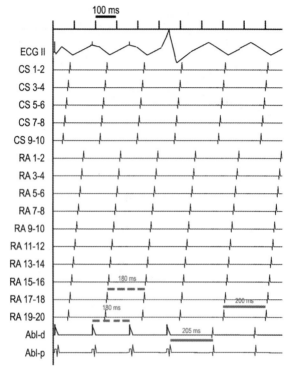

Fig. 13.3 Entrainment from the isthmus using Abl-d during atrial flutter. The first four beats show burst pacing at 180 ms entrains the tachycardia as demonstrated by the atrial cycle length (dotted line). When pacing stops the post-pacing interval (time from last pacing spike on Abl-d to first return electrogram in the same catheter) is 205 ms. The flutter cycle length is 200 ms. As the PPI – TCL is <30 ms it means the pacing site is within the tachycardia circuit.

Atrial tachycardia and AF

Introduction and terminology

The first part of this section concerns *regular* or *organized* atrial tachyar-rhythmias arising *entirely* within the atria, i.e. not dependent on the AV junction for re-entry like AVNRT and AVRT. The term includes **atrial flutter (AFl)** and **atrial tachycardia (AT)** but not atrial fibrillation.

- The distinction between AFl and AT used to be of little clinical importance – it was based exclusively on ECG criteria, with a rate cut-off around 240–250 bpm and the presence of isoelectric baselines between atrial deflections in AT but *not* AFl. These correlate poorly with the underlying mechanisms/anatomical substrates defined by EPS, which provide the targets for specific catheter ablation treatments.
- The Joint ESC/NASPE Arrhythmia Working Group proposed a new classification (Sauodi *et al.*, 2001), which has now been generally adopted. The major distinction is between **focal atrial tachycardia (FAT)** and **macroreentrant atrial tachycardia (MRAT)**.
- **Focal atrial tachycardia** is characterized by rhythmic atrial activation arising from a small area or focus, with centrifugal spread, represented as a 'hot spot' on 3-D mapping systems (📖 p. 120). The mechanism may be automaticity, triggered activity or 'microreentry' (📖 p. 120).
- **Macroreentrant atrial tachycardias** involve re-entrant activation around a 'large' central obstacle or area of block (typically several centimetres in diameter), which may be due to fixed anatomical/pathological structures (veins, valve annuli, scars etc.) and/or areas of functional block. There is no point of origin or site of earliest atrial activation ('hot spot') and the circuit produces a 'head-meets-tail' pattern on 3-D mapping (📖 p. 120). MRATs are most usefully classified in relation to atrial anatomy to define targets for ablation. **Typical** (syn. 'common') **atrial flutter** is a right atrial MRAT involving the cavotricuspid (IVC-TA) isthmus with characteristic ECG features (see below). This term continues to be generally used. **Atypical** (syn. 'uncommon') **atrial flutter** is used more loosely, either to describe any organized atrial tachyarrhythmia without the ECG features of typical flutter or any form of MRAT not dependent on the IVC-TA isthmus. The terms type I and type II flutter are obsolete and should be avoided (the latter defined on the basis of rapid rate >350 bpm and inability to demonstrate entrainment).
- Another arrhythmia considered within this category is **sinus node re-entrant tachycardia**, and sometimes also the **syndrome of inappropriate sinus tachycardia**.

Joint ESC/NASPE Working Group's revised classification of regular atrial tachyarrhythmias (modified): Indications for ablation

Focal atrial tachycardia (FAT)

- Microreentrant or 'small loop' re-entry.
- Abnormal automaticity or triggered activity.

Macroreentrant atrial tachycardia (MRAT)

- Typical atrial flutter.
- Reverse typical atrial flutter.
- Scar or lesion-related macroreentrant tachycardia.
- Other right atrial forms of macroreentry:
  - Lower loop re-entry.
  - Upper loop re-entry-
- Left atrial macroreentry:
  - Peri-mitral flutter.
  - Peri-venous flutter.
  - 'Small loop' re-entry.
  - Coronary sinus macroreentry.

Sinus node tachyarrhythmias

- Sinus node re-entrant tachycardia.
- Syndrome of inappropriate sinus tachycardia.

Saoudi N, Cosio F, Waldo A et al. (2001) Working Group of Arrhythmias of the European of
    Cardiology and the North American Society of Pacing and Electrophysiology. A classification
    of atrial flutter and regular atrial tachycardia according to electrophysiological mechanisms
    and anatomical bases: a statement from a Joint Expert Group from the Working Group of
    Arrythmias of the European Society of Cardiology and the North American Society of Pacing
    and Electrophysiology. *Eur Heart J* **22**(14): 1162–82.

Epidemiology

- Common atrial flutter develops in the same patient populations as atrial fibrillation. These arrhythmias often co-exist in the same patient, possibly reflecting a common atriomyopathy. They may occur in individuals with no evidence of underlying heart disease or in association with ischaemic heart disease, valvular disease, cardiomyopathy, and other causes of atrial pressure or volume overload. Incidence increases with age (male > female).
- Left atrial flutters seldom occur without prior surgical atriotomy, extensive ablation for AF, or congenital heart disease because the LA has no natural lines of conduction block to facilitate macroreentry (cf. crista terminalis in the RA).
- Idiopathic focal atrial tachycardias account for a significant proportion of SVT in childhood/adolescence and may result in incessant tachycardia and rate-related cardiomyopathy.
- Pulmonary vein tachycardia is an important cause of paroxysmal AF in younger adults with no structural heart disease ('focally driven AF').
- Focal atrial tachycardia may develop due to microreentry in patients with structural heart disease and/or prior ablation or surgery.
- Sinus node re-entrant tachycardia (SNRT) is very commonly detected incidentally during EPS/ablation procedures for other forms of SVT but is seldom the principal/sole cause of paroxysmal tachycardia.

Clinical presentation

ECG appearances may be regular or irregular, narrow complex tachycardia, broad complex tachycardia, or (rarely) 'polymorphic' broad complex tachyarrhythmia due to variable bundle branch block. Atrial tachyarrhythmias can manifest in more ways than junctional SVTs.

- Paroxysmal tachycardia.
- Persistent tachyarrhythmia with palpitation and/or symptoms of reduced functional capacity (dyspnoea, decreased effort tolerance, fatigue, and presyncope).
- Syncope is uncommon but may occur with 1:1 conduction of atrial activity to the ventricles, particularly during exercise or treatment with class I drugs (paradoxically due to slowing of the atrial rate).
- 'Silent' atrial tachyarrhythmias may be detected in asymptomatic patients on routine ECGs or Holters or via implanted devices (pacemakers and ICDs).
- 'Silent' atrial tachyarrhythmias may present in ICD patients through causing inappropriate shock therapies.
- Atrial tachyarrhythmias may present with thromboembolic complications (stroke, TIA etc.).
- Persistent tachyarrhythmia may result in heart failure due to rate-related cardiomyopathy (syn. tachycardiomyopathy), including in children or adolescents.
- In association with sinus node disease in so-called 'bradycardia-tachycardia syndrome'. Symptomatic bradyarrhythmias (syncope or presyncope) may be the predominant feature.

Investigations

- ECG confirmation is essential in all cases, if possible full 12-lead ECG tracing for proper evaluation of P wave morphology.
- If presentation is with a regular tachycardia, IV adenosine to differentiate from junctional SVT (and VT if broad complex tachycardia).
- Complete evaluation for underlying heart disease, including echocardiography in all cases plus stress testing, coronary angiography, CMR etc., as clinically indicated.
- Holter ECG monitoring if suspected bradycardia-tachycardia syndrome.

Classification, mechanism, and ECG features

Focal atrial tachycardia

- Commonest sites are crista terminalis and pulmonary veins.
- Idiopathic FAT usually occurs in childhood and adolescence.
- Microreentrant FAT is increasingly seen as a recurrent arrhythmia after left atrial ablation procedures for AF (📖 Table 14.2).
- Classical ECG appearance is discrete P waves separated by isoelectric baseline in *all* leads (Fig. 14.1), but this is often obscured by QRS-T.
  - Tachycardia cycle length is usually ≥250 ms but can be as short as ≤200 ms (i.e. overlaps MRATs).
  - It may exhibit rate increase ('warm-up') at tachycardia onset or decrease ('cool down') prior to termination.
  - If visible, P wave morphology can be used to approximately localize the focus prior to EPS (Fig. 14.2).
- Activation mapping shows centrifugal spread from a site of earliest activation (hot spot on 3-D map).
  - Typically no atrial electrical activity for a significant portion of tachycardia cycle length, corresponding to isoelectric baseline on the surface ECG.
  - With complex intra-atrial conduction disturbances, atrial activation may spread over a much greater proportion of tachycardia cycle length and mimic MRAT.
- FAT due to microreentry may exhibit initiation/termination by programmed stimulation, and manifest/conceal entrainment, whereas FAT due to abnormal automaticity is provoked by catecholamine infusion with post-overdrive suppression by pacing. In practice, distinguishing FAT mechanism at EPS is not often possible and does not alter management.

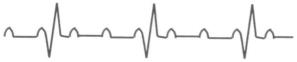

Fig. 14.1 Surface ECG of focal atrial tachycardia typically shows discrete P waves.

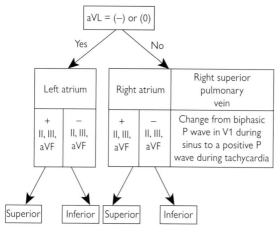

Fig. 14.2 Algorithm for determination of focal atrial tachycardia chamber of origin. Reproduced from Tang et al. (1995) Use of P wave configuration during atrial tachycardia to predict site of origin. J Am Coll Cardiol, **26**: 1315–1324, with permission from Elsevier.

Typical (syn. common) atrial flutter

- Commonest MRAT. Re-entrant activation of a right atrial circuit bounded anteriorly by the tricuspid annulus by a posterior boundary formed by the IVC, SVC, and crista terminalis (a functional barrier to transverse conduction by virtue of its anisotropic properties). The crista terminalis eventually becomes the eustachian ridge, a fibrous structure extending past the IVC orifice towards the CS ostium.
- The cavotricuspid isthmus (IVC-TA isthmus) is essential for macroreentry, enabling closure of the circuit in the low RA, but it is *not* a diseased/slow conduction zone.
- Activation is counter-clockwise in 90% of cases and clockwise in 10% of cases, so-called **reverse typical atrial flutter**.
- Typical flutter produces a 'sawtooth' ECG pattern sequence in the inferior limb leads (down-sloping plateau, sharper negative deflection, then sharp positive deflection with overshoot) and frequently a positive flutter wave in V1. Cycle length is typically around 200 ms (300 bpm) but very variable (Fig. 14.3).
- The ECG pattern in reverse typical flutter is often broad positive deflections in the inferior leads and/or wide negative deflections in V1 (Fig. 14.4).
- Concealed entrainment (Fig. 13.3) can be produced by pacing from the inferior isthmus but also from the low posterior right atrial wall.

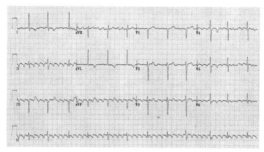

Fig. 14.3 Typical (counter-clockwise) flutter 12-lead ECG. Atrial activation manifests as continuous activity on the surface ECG.

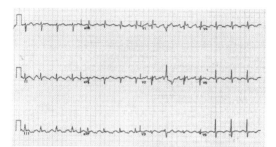

Fig. 14.4 Reverse typical (clockwise) flutter 12-lead ECG.

Lesion or scar-related MRAT

- The central obstacle is usually a right atriotomy scar, suture line, or septal prosthetic patch (Fig. 14.5), with other boundaries being formed by the IVC or SVC.
- Commonest form is macro re-entry around an incision scar of the lateral RA wall with descending activation of the anterior RA and upper/lower pivot points provided by the gaps or isthmuses between the atriotomy and SVC/IVC.
- Often co-exists with typical atrial flutter.
- Complex ECG patterns, varying between typical flutter and focal atrial tachycardia. In fact, the site of surgery (atriotomy) has greater predictive value for the mechanism of MRAT than any specific ECG pattern.
- Demonstration of concealed entrainment from the isthmuses may be difficult due to lack of local capture or termination of the arrhythmia.

Other right atrial MRATs

- All uncommon without prior surgery or ablation.
- 'Lower loop re-entry' MRAT is a variant of typical atrial flutter:
  - Anterior limb is still formed by the IVC-TA isthmus.
  - Upper turnaround is in the posterior RA rather than the roof due to breakthrough of the crista terminalis.
  - This results in colliding wavefronts on the upper lateral RA wall (ascending via the crista and descending via the septum).
  - Also treated by IVC-TA isthmus ablation.
- 'Upper loop re-entry' MRAT involves rotation around the SVC with similar short-circuiting via the crista terminalis. This MRAT does *not* involve the IVC-TA isthmus.

Left atrial MRAT

- These arrhythmias are very rare without prior surgery or ablation but have become increasingly common and important as sequelae of left atrial circumferential ablation (LACA) procedures for AF (📖 p. 466).
- Organized atrial tachyarrhythmias occur in 5–40% of post-LACA patients in different series. Approximately half are due to microreentrant FAT, usually involving gaps and/or areas of slow conduction in the lesions used to encircle the pulmonary veins.
- Peri-mitral flutter is the commonest left atrial MRAT, involving the isthmus between the mitral annulus and left inferior PV (Fig. 14.6).
- Re-entry around the ipsilateral veins using the gap between the superior PVs (left atrial roof) is the other common post-LACA MRAT.

Small loop re-entry (SLRT)

- Depending on the size of the re-entrant circuit, post-LACA FATs may overlap left atrial MRATs – the term 'small loop' re-entry is often used.
- One form of SLRT involves the musculature of the coronary sinus and the atrial septum (also described as CS flutter).

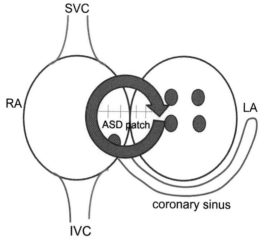

Fig. 14.5 Surgical or other scars create both areas of slow conduction and an area of block facilitating reentry. In this example there is a macroentract circuit around an atrial septal defect (ASD) patch (arrow). RA = right atrium, LA = left atrium.

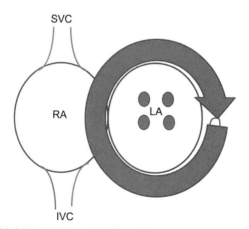

Fig. 14.6 Atrial activation in peri-mitral flutter. The macroreentrant circuit rotates clockwise around the mitral annulus (arrow) in the left atrium.

Sinus node tachyarrhythmias

Although not traditionally regarded as atrial tachyarrhythmias, these conditions most logically fall within that spectrum and are included in the modern classification.

Sinus node re-entrant tachycardia (SNRT)

SNRT is a microreentrant tachycardia involving the sinus node and/or upper crista terminalis, with sudden onset and offset but P wave morphology identical to or similar to sinus rhythm (Fig. 14.7). May be induced and terminated by programmed stimulation and terminated by adenosine. Readily amenable to catheter ablation (📖 p. 462).

Syndrome of inappropriate sinus tachycardia (IST)

IST is often characterized as an automatic focal tachycardia within the sinus node at supraphysiological rates and with an inappropriate response to autonomic changes. In addition, the exit site moves down the crista terminalis with increasing sympathetic tone. In contrast to SNRT, IST does not exhibit abrupt onset/offset and cannot be induced/terminated by programmed stimulation. Not amenable to curative catheter ablation, but sinus node modification is rarely used in severe drug-refractory cases. IST overlaps with postural orthostatic tachycardia syndrome (POTS), a form of dysautonomia.

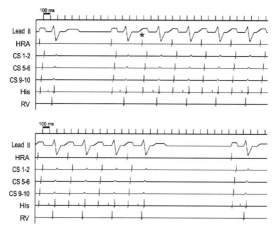

Fig. 14.7 Onset and offset of sinus node re-entry. In this case spontaneously occurring, the first beat of tachycardia (*) is seen to have a very similar activation pattern to the previous sinus beats but the P wave morphology is subtly different. Termination also occurs spontaneously and sinus rhythm is seen to restart after a short pause.

Invasive electrophysiological testing

The primary objective is to identify the mechanism of the arrhythmia as a prelude to catheter ablation. Diagnosis is based on ECG appearance as well as conventional electrophysiologic techniques and/or 3-D mapping (see Tables 14.1 and 14.2).

Assessment is more straightforward in persistent atrial tachyarrhythmias – with paroxysmal arrhythmia by programmed atrial tachyarrhythmias, inducibility of the **clinical** stimulation, ± catecholamine infusion is less reliable than with junctional SVTs. Non-inducibility, inducibility of non-sustained arrhythmias, or inducibility of non-clinical arrhythmias are common problems and may preclude mapping and ablation except in cases of presumed common atrial flutter.

Catheter setups

- Standard four-catheter configuration (HRA, His, CS, and RV) is usually sufficient to make a broad diagnosis of atrial tachycardia/flutter.
- RA Halo, CS, and roving catheters may all be used for activation mapping circuits and entrainment (see below).
- 3-D electroanatomical mapping systems (📖 p. 120) may be used to create isochronal, propagation, and scar maps for diagnosis.

Electrophysiologic techniques

- Activation mapping using conventional electrodes, particularly activation sequence of RA Halo (clockwise, counter-clockwise, chevron) and CS (proximal → distal or distal → proximal).
- Activation/propagation maps using 3-D electroanatomical systems.
- Recording of widely split double potentials (WSDP) at site of functional block (e.g. crista terminalis) or anatomical block (e.g. surgical scar, ablation line) to delineate macroreentrant circuit.
- Transient entrainment (📖 p. 28) to confirm that pacing site is involved in re-entrant circuit. Interpretation may be complex.

Responses to transient entrainment

- Easier to check for 'fusion' vs. 'concealed' entrainment with multi-electrode catheters *in situ* as P wave fusion is difficult to gauge from surface ECG (unlike with ventricular entrainment).
- Use pacing CL only slightly faster than tachycardia CL to avoid significant conduction delay and spurious prolongation of return cycle, i.e. PPI.
- Ideally check transient entrainment several times at each site to confirm consistent finding.
- Too aggressive pacing risks terminating/degenerating tachycardia.
- Concealed entrainment with PPI = tachycardia CL confirms that pacing site is within re-entrant circuit.
- Entrainment with fusion and PPI > tachycardia CL suggests pacing site outside re-entrant circuit.
- Concealed entrainment with PPI > tachycardia CL suggests pacing site is at a bystander location connected to re-entrant circuit.

- In theory microreentrant FATs should exhibit consistent transient entrainment with fusion and long PPI, but often the PPI varies because of variable conduction block/delay if pacing site is remote from arrhythmia focus.

Differentiating atrial tachycardias from other SVTs

- Atrial rate > ventricular rate rules out most junctional forms of SVT other than AVNRT with infra-His block (📖 p. 236).
- If 1:1 AV relationship, cycle length variation with A-A consistently leading H-H and V-V suggests atrial tachycardia (📖 p. 162).
- If 1:1 ventricular entrainment during tachycardia results in either VA dissociation or entrainment ending with a V-A-A-V response, likely diagnosis is atrial tachycardia (Fig. 7.18).
- Adenosine terminates junctional tachycardias but transiently slows atrial tachycardia if given at adequate dose (but note SNRT is an exception).

Identifying tachycardia mechanism

Differentiation of FAT vs. MRAT

- Depends on endocardial activation mapping, either standard or 3-D, to confirm centrifugal spread from site of earliest activation ('hot spot' on 3-D mapping).
- Unipolar recording may show negative QS pattern at focus (📖 p. 56).
- Usually an electrically silent period of atrial cycle length (= isoelectric baseline on surface ECG) but note that with complex intra-atrial conduction disturbance, atrial activation may extend over longer period and mimic MRAT.
- Activation mapping may be hampered by paucity of endocardial electrograms, especially if prior surgery/ablation.
- Microreentrant FAT circuit may extend over more than a single 'point' location.
- Response to entrainment (📖 p. 298) often inconsistent, or may produce consistently long PPIs if pacing site is not close to focus.
- In one study, CS pacing at 10, 20, and 30 ms shorter than tachycardia cycle length differentiated MRAT and FAT on the basis of variability in PPI: <10 ms for MRAT vs. >30 ms for FAT.

Establishing mechanism of MRAT

- Activation mapping delineates macroreentry circuits and site of earliest activation in focal tachycardias.
- Entrainment demonstrates PPI = TCL within a macroreentry circuit and long PPI > TCL outside the circuit. Focal tachycardias exhibit variable PPIs.

Table 14.1 Characteristics of right atrial tachyarrhythmias

Tachycardia	Surface ECG	Electrograms	Mechanism	Entrainment	Electroanatomy
Cavotricuspid isthmus (counter-clockwise)	P waves positive in V1, sawtoothed II, aVF, III	Proximal to distal CS. Proximal to distal RA	Macroreentry	Concealed from TVA points, consistent long PPIs from distal CS	Counter-clockwise round TV annulus (entire CL), dependent on CTI
Cavotricuspid isthmus (clockwise)	P waves negative in V1, sawtoothed II, aVF, III	Proximal to distal CS. Distal to proximal RA	Macroreentry	Concealed from TVA points, consistent long PPIs from distal CS	Clockwise round TV annulus (entire CL), dependent on CTI
Upper loop re-entry	Positive P waves inferiorly	Proximal to distal CS activation	Macroreentry	Long PPIs from CS and CTI	Whole CL round SVC os
Lower loop re-entry	Negative P waves inferiorly	Proximal to distal CS activation	Macroreentry	As for CTI dep. flutter	Whole CL round IVC os
Post incisional	Variable	Usually proximal to distal CS	Macroreentry	Concealed entrainment from around scar	Whole CL around scar
Atrial tachycardia	Variable. Isoelectric interval between P waves	Proximal to distal CS activation	Microreentry or automaticity	Usually variable. May be consistent with long PPIs if microreentrant tachycardia	Centrifugal spread

Table 14.2 Characteristics of left atrial tachyarrhythmias (usually post-LACA)

Tachycardia	Surface ECG	Electrograms	Mechanism	Entrainment	Electroanatomy
PV tachycardia	Positive P waves V1-6	Flat CS activation, RA late	Triggered activity or automaticity	Variable PPIs	From PV or antrum, centrifugal spread from focus
Post-LACA focal tachycardias	Variable	Variable	Microreentry, triggered activity, or automaticity	Usually variable PPIs	From venous antrum, CS, roof, septum, or LAA base, centrifugal spread from focus
Peri-mitral clockwise	P waves negative in V1, Sawtoothed II, aVF, III	Distal to proximal CS	Macroreentry	Concealed from MVA points (including CS). Consistent long PPIs for RA	Counter-clockwise round MV annulus (entire CL)
LA roof flutter	Regular tachy with discrete P waves	Flat CS activation	Macroreentry	Concealed entrainment from LA roof and either distal or proximal CS	LA roof and one pair of veins (right or left). Whole CL in LA
Peri-mitral counter-clockwise	P waves positive in V1. Sawtoothed II, aVF, III	Proximal to distal CS	Macroreentry	Concealed from MVA points (including CS). Consistent long PPIs for RA	Counter-clockwise round MV annulus (entire CL)

Atrial fibrillation

The underlying mechanism of atrial fibrillation has yet to be completely elucidated.

Early hypotheses
- Proposed that AF was caused by multiple random wavelets colliding with each other (Fig. 14.8).
- Subsequently theory suggesting rapidly firing foci may cause AF (Fig. 14.8).

Factors predisposing to AF
- Atrial enlargement (for example, secondary to mitral valve disease or hypertension).
- Fibrosis of atrial tissue (resulting in slowing of intra-atrial conduction).
- Altered autonomic tone, especially increased sympathetic activity.

Heterogeneity of atrial refractoriness and slow conduction times (allowing time for the myocardium to regain excitability between each wavefront) help to perpetuate the process, leading to persistent atrial fibrillation.

Identification of AF and role of EP study
- Can usually be made from the 12-lead ECG and rarely needs an EP study to verify diagnosis.
- Overlap between atrial fibrillation and pulmonary vein foci now recognized and part of ablation strategy.
- Where conduction of atrial fibrillation is rapid, consider accessory pathway, but normally readily apparent on ECG also.
- Induction of AF is performed during assessment of accessory pathway risk stratification.

Recent developments
Various foci have been identified/hypothesized to be involved in initiation and maintenance of AF (Fig. 14.9) more recently. These are mainly on the basis of ablation strategies targeting these mechanisms (see Chapter X). However, none of these is completely successful in eradicating AF and it remains likely that the process is multi-factorial. Genetics presumably plays a role too but as yet this is poorly understood.

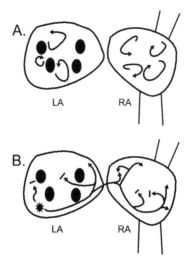

Fig. 14.8 Diagrammatic representations of the early hypotheses for AF initiation. (A) The multiple wavelet and (B) the rapidly firing foci models.

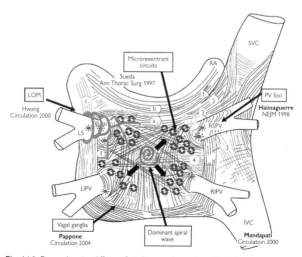

Fig. 14.9 Figure showing different foci that may be implicated in AF initiation and maintenance.

Ventricular tachycardia

Mechanisms

The commonest of the broad complex tachycardias (📖 p. 190), VT usually occurs as a result of re-entry related to a ventricular cardiomyopathic process, e.g. infarction, or arises from an area of ventricular automaticity/triggered activity (📖 Chapter 3).

Re-entry

These arrhythmias rely on a scar (or area of functional block, 📖 p. 18) around which a circuit revolves, and islands of viable myocytes within the scar provide a slowly conducting substrate. A critically timed premature beat (in this case a ventricular beat) initiates the tachycardia and an excitation wave that spreads around the circuit. This is maintained by the different properties of the various components of the circuit (📖 p. 19).

Automaticity

Automaticity refers to the spontaneous nature of cardiac muscle cell depolarization. All cardiac tissue has the ability to initiate an action potential; however, only some of the cells are designed to do so routinely, including the SA node, AV node, His bundle, and Purkinje fibres. Any other part of the heart that initiates an impulse is an ectopic focus. This may cause a single premature beat or produce a sustained arrhythmia. Conditions that increase such ectopic automaticity include sympathetic nervous system stimulation.

Triggered

The difference between automatic and triggered activity is mainly in the way that the latter may be initiated by programmed stimulation and terminated by pacing manoeuvres more commonly associated with a re-entrant tachycardia. However, triggered activity occurs by a non-re-entrant mechanism that appears to be primarily due to delayed after-depolarizations that arise from altered cellular calcium handling and ionic currents.

Fibrillation

Ventricular fibrillation (VF) is rapid, disorganized, asynchronous ventricular contraction. Although originally described as simultaneous independent multiple wavelets that follow random, continuously changing pathways through the myocardium, it is now clear from experimental evidence that the instability of 'rotors' of cardiac excitation are the organized centres that underlie the mechanism that sustains VF.

Monomorphic vs. polymorphic VT

The principal mechanistic difference between these two forms of VT is that whereas monomorphic VT is mostly caused by re-entry as described above, polymorphic VT (or Torsades de Pointes) is often based on ionic mechanisms inducing prolonged repolarization and early after-depolarizations.

Infarct-related VT

Infarct-related VT is typically re-entrant in nature. Components of the re-entrant circuit that are common to all infarct-related VT are outlined opposite (Fig. 15.1).

Entry and exit sites

A VT circuit will have both entry and exit sites – it is often very difficult to locate the entry site of a VT circuit. In a proportion of VT circuits it is possible to map at least part of the diastolic pathway and in the majority the exit site can be located. However, the exit site may be quite a large area and/or there may be multiple exit sites.

Diastolic pathway

The diastolic pathway of a VT circuit represents a critical area of slow conduction that is needed to maintain re-entry. During tachycardia these pathways are protected from extraneous systolic wavefronts by lines of block and the integrity of these is essential for sustaining VT. There is evidence that even small changes in the conduction characteristics of these pathways or their morphology can terminate VT. These critical 'diastolic' components that maintain re-entrant circuits are often complex, difficult to map, and highly variable between individuals. Patients need to be maintained in tachycardia to map/localize these diastolic pathways, which can be difficult when VT is not tolerated haemodynamically.

Types of infarct-related VT re-entry

A common example of a VT circuit is characterized as a figure of eight pattern, with clockwise and counter-clockwise rotating wavefronts that share a small common central isthmus of tissue where the diastolic pathway is located (Fig. 15.1).

Practical note

Although the area of slow conduction and block may be a fixed obstacle such as scar, it is also possible for areas of 'functional' block to occur because of the conductive properties of that tissue. In its simplest form, tissue may allow conduction at long cycle lengths but as this shortens it does not propagate the impulse, resulting in block of conduction.

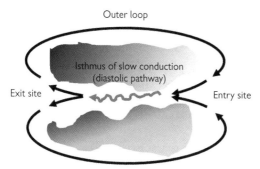

Fig. 15.1 An example of a very common VT circuit showing an area of scar tissue (grey) with a channel or 'isthmus' of slowly conducting tissue. Activation arrives at the entry site to this slowly conducting isthmus and travels along it (the diastolic pathway). It exits as shown and then activates the rest of the ventricle travelling around the outer loops. If there is another anatomical barrier or area of scar with normal conducting tissue, this loop is referred to as an inner loop (📖 p. 493).

Non-ischaemic scar-related VT

VT may also be associated with other forms of structural heart disease that are non-ischaemic, e.g. arrhythmogenic right ventricular cardiomyopathy (ARVC), hypertrophic cardiomyopathy, and idiopathic dilated cardiomyopathy. These are thought to have similar mechanisms to the infarct-related VT, with the substrate provided by less discrete scarring or myocardial disarray. This means that: (a) control by either pharmacology or ablation is difficult with progressive disease; and (b) multiple morphologies of VT are more likely to exist in the same patient.

ARVC

Patients with ARVC may present with palpitations, syncope, right heart failure, ventricular tachycardia, or sudden cardiac death (SCD).
- Commonly presents between the ages of 12–45 years.
- Accounts for 3–4% of sporting SCD.
- Most commonly characterized histopathologically by fatty replacement of mid-myo/epicardium of the RV free wall (fibrosis and thinning) but can affect any part of RV, and also involve LV (Fig. 15.2).
- ECG abnormalities include anterior T wave inversion, epsilon waves (late depolarizations) (Fig. 15.3), and parietal block.
- Diagnosis based on fulfilling a certain number of criteria including those described above.[1]
- 2–3% incidence of SCD/year (despite medication).

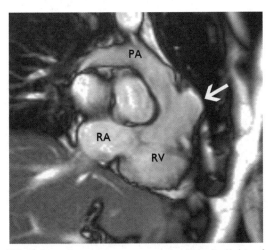

Fig. 15.2 Cardiovascular magnetic resonance scan showing localized bulging of the right ventricular outflow tract (arrow). RV – right ventricle; RA – right atrium; PA – pulmonary artery.

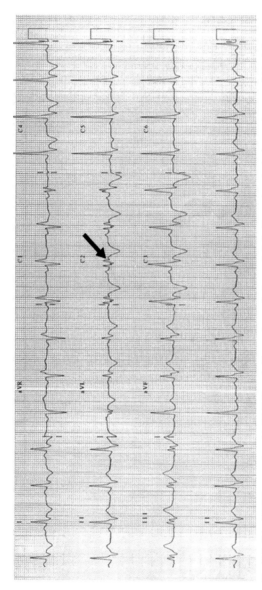

Fig. 15.3 12-lead ECG from a patient with ARVC. Extensive T wave abnormality is seen, including T wave inversion in the anterior precordial leads. Late depolarizations are also seen, particularly on the end of the QRS complex in lead V2 (arrow).

Hypertrophic cardiomyopathy

A hereditary cardiac muscle disorder with an estimated incidence of 1:500. The clinical course is heterogeneous with affected individuals often being asymptomatic and presenting with aborted sudden cardiac death (mortality 1% p.a.). Ventricular tachycardia may occur and represents an adverse prognostic indicator in this population (Fig 15.4).

Idiopathic dilated cardiomyopathy

Ventricular tachycardia in these patients is common (prevalence of up to 60% of patients). Patients with VT in this group have more impaired ventricular systolic function than those that do not. However, mortality is more closely related to the degree of impairment of ventricular function than to the presence of ventricular arrhythmia itself.

Reference

1. McKenna WJ, Thiene G, Nava A, et al. (1994) Diagnosis of arrhythmogenic right ventricular dysplasia/cardiomyopathy. Br Heart J, **71**: 215–218.

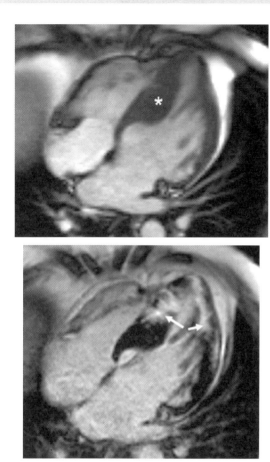

Fig. 15.4 Cardiovascular magnetic resonance scan in a patient with hypertrophic cardiomyopathy. Top: Diastolic image in the horizontal long axis (four-chamber) view showing asymmetrical hypertrophy (septum thicker than lateral wall) characteristic of the condition (*). Bottom: Late enhancement image in the same position, ten minutes post-gadolinium injection. Significant areas of mid-wall fibrosis can be seen (white/high signal, arrowed), compared to the normal black myocardium. (Image kindly provided by Dr Saul Myerson, John Radcliffe Hospital, Oxford, UK.)

Bundle branch re-entrant VT

In patients with conduction delay in the His-Purkinje system, macro-reentry involving the right and left bundles can result in sustained VT (Fig. 15.5). This bundle branch re-entry is important to recognize as it responds poorly to pharmacological therapy, has high recurrence rates, can cause syncope, and may be eliminated by catheter ablation.

- In order to sustain bundle branch re-entry there must be delay in the normal conduction of the left bundle of the Purkinje system. This will usually be manifest by interventricular conduction delay on the ECG during sinus rhythm (LBBB) with or without AV delay (prolongation of the PR interval) (Fig. 15.6).
- During tachycardia (Fig. 15.6) often LBBB (similar to SR ECG).
- Rarely a RBBB morphology may be seen when activation is in the opposite direction.
- The left ventricle is dilated (non-ischaemic dilatation is more common than ischaemic).
- Ablation is potentially curative.
- **But** patient profile may still warrant pacemaker/ICD/CRT.

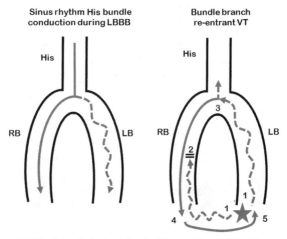

Fig. 15.5 The His bundle (His), right bundle (RB), and left bundle (LB) of the Purkinje fibres are shown on the left during sinus rhythm with left bundle branch block (LBBB) and on the right during bundle branch re-entrant VT. Conduction during sinus rhythm propagates from the His to the RB normally. Contrary to the nomenclature, LB conduction is not blocked but only slowed in LBBB, as shown by the dashed arrow. On the right, a ventricular ectopic (shown as a grey star) initiates slow conduction retrogradely in the LB, and across and retrogradely in the RB (1). The retrograde conduction in the RB blocks (2). The slow conducting retrograde LB wavefront reaches the RB and this conducts antegradely (3). This antegrade conduction reaches the distal portion of the RB (4) and spreads to the distal LB (5). By this time the LB is able to conduct retrogradely again and the re-entrant circuit is completed.

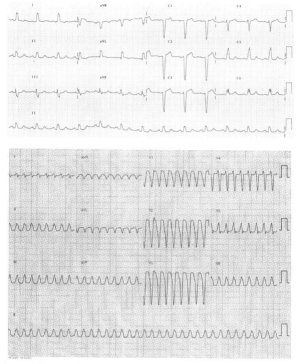

Fig. 15.6 The top ECG shows sinus rhythm with a slightly prolonged PR interval and left bundle branch block with a QRS duration of approximately 120 ms. These conduction abnormalities are common in patients with bundle branch re-entrant VT (shown in the lower ECG). The bottom ECG shows bundle branch re-entrant VT with a very similar QRS morphology to sinus rhythm.

Right ventricular outflow tract tachycardia

This is a common arrhythmia in patients without heart disease and is characterized by isolated or repetitive burst of non-sustained VT. In the early phase this may simply be ectopics.

- Most common form of idiopathic VT (75–90%).
- LBBB pattern.
- Strongly positive inferior complexes (inferior axis) (Fig. 15.7).
- May see similar morphology ectopy on non-tachycardia ECG (Fig. 15.8).
- Equal incidence in men and women.
- Presentation commonly between the ages of 30 and 50.
- Normal ventricular function.
- Adrenergically driven.
- Responsive to β-blockers or verapamil in 25–50% of cases (abolition of all symptoms).
- Recurrent symptoms in 30–40% of patients during long-term drug therapy.
- Catheter ablation is successful in 80–90% of cases.
- This may represent a spectrum of cardiac disease. Some cases may be the first sign of the major differential diagnosis of ARVC, and this needs to be considered in many cases (Table 15.1).

Table 15.1 Factors differentiating RVOT VT from ARVC

	RVOT VT	ARVC
Family history of arrhythmia or sudden cardiac death (SCD)	No	Frequently yes
Arrhythmias	VEs, non-sustained VT, or sustained VT at rest or with exercise	Same
SCD occurrence	Rare	1% per year
QRS axis	Positive in ECG leads III and AVF, negative in lead AVL	Inferior or superior
T-wave morphology	T wave upright V_2–V_5	T wave inverted beyond V_1
QRS duration	<110 ms in V_1, V_2, or V_3	>110 ms
(T-wave morphology and QRS duration 84% sensitivity and 100% specificity)		
Epsilon wave V_1–V_3	Absent	Present in 30%
Signal averaged ECG	Normal	Usually abnormal
Echocardiogram	Normal	Increased RV size and/or wall motion abnormalities
RV ventriculogram	Usually normal	Usually abnormal
MRI	Usually normal (but data in literature are conflicting)	Increased signal intensity of RV free wall; wall motion abnormalities with CINE MRI
Response to therapy	Acute: vagal manoeuvres, adenosine, β-blockers, verapamil Chronic: β-blockers or verapamil and class I anti-arrhythmic drugs	Sotalol Amiodrone and β-blockers
>1 VT morphology seen	Rare	Commonly seen
RF Ablation	Usually curative	Seldom curative; may modify substrate to permit anti-arrhythmic drugs to be effective Arrhythmias of different morphology tend to occur

VE – ventricular ectopic; RF – radiofrequency.

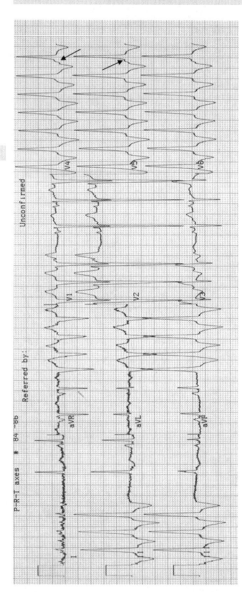

Fig. 15.7 12-lead ECG from a patient with idiopathic RVOT VT. Runs of a broad complex tachycardia are seen with a left bundle branch block morphology and an inferior axis (positive QRS in leads II, III, and aVF). The presence of dissociated P wave activity (arrows) confirms VT.

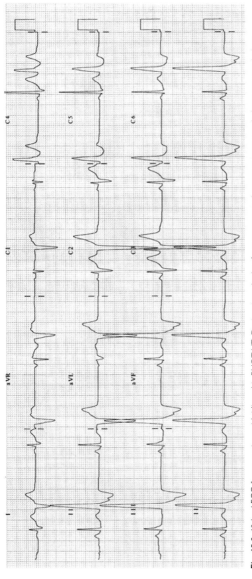

Fig. 15.8 12-lead ECG from a patient with idiopathic RVOT VT. During sinus rhythm frequent ventricular ectopy is seen with the same morphology as the VT.

Fascicular tachycardia

This form of VT (also commonly referred to as idiopathic left ventricular tachycardia) is seen in patients without heart disease and characterized by the following:

- RBBB pattern (Fig. 15.10).
- Mostly leftward axis (often the vector is 'straight up', i.e. QRS isoelectric in lead I and negative in aVF; positive in aVR and aVL).
- Relatively narrow QRS (aVL).
- Classified into three types: RBBB/LAD (common/'posterior' 90–95%) (ECG); RBBB/RAD (uncommon/'anterior'); and narrow QRS/normal axis (rare/'upper septal').
- Origin of tachycardia mostly close to left posterior fascicle (with a small region of re-entry) in the common type (Fig. 15.9).
- 60–80% of cases are in men.
- Presentation commonly between the ages of 15 and 40.
- Normal ventricular function.
- Tachycardia is verapamil sensitive.
- Purkinje potentials may be seen (activation via region of slow conduction of abnormal Purkinje tissue linked to the posterior fascicle).
- Catheter ablation successful in at least 90% of cases.
- Incessant cases may lead to tachycardia-related cardiomyopathy.
- Relatively uncommon and therefore should not be over-diagnosed.

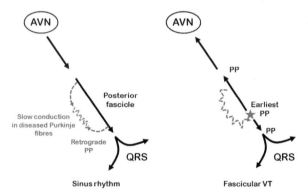

Fig. 15.9 Conduction through the posterior fascicle and Purkinje fibres showing the mechanism by which (common) left posterior fascicular VT occurs. During sinus rhythm conduction is seen through the posterior fascicle but also slowly through diseased Purkinje fibres both antegradely and retrogradely. It is this slow retrograde conduction that gives rise to a retrograde Purkinje potential (PP) (📖 p. 522). A premature ventricular ectopic (shown as a grey star) triggers a re-entrant circuit that involves antegrade conduction via the diseased, slowly conducting Purkinje fibres and retrograde conduction through the posterior fascicle. The earliest PP is now seen as the posterior fascicle is activated.

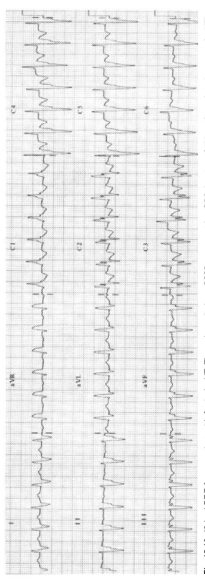

Fig. 15.10 12-lead ECG from a patient with fascicular VT. The tachycardia has a RBBB pattern with a QRS duration of 130 ms (i.e. relatively narrow for VT) and classical 'straight up' axis (isoelectric in lead I and negative in lead aVF).

Idiopathic ventricular fibrillation

Idiopathic ventricular fibrillation is defined as ventricular fibrillation that occurs in a structurally normal heart. It has a reputed incidence of approximately 1% of all cases of out-of-hospital arrest, as well as 3–9% of the cases of ventricular fibrillation unrelated to myocardial infarction, and 14% of all ventricular fibrillation resuscitations in patients under the age of 40. This suggests a primary electrical disease. An example of this is the long QT syndrome (LQTS) in which the altered membrane ionic channel function underlies QT prolongation (Fig. 15.11). The altered channel activity is due to mutations in genes encoding ion channels and predisposes the affected individual to ventricular arrhythmias, particularly polymorphic VT and VF (Fig. 15.11). Likewise, Brugada syndrome is another 'normal heart' disorder characterized by a sodium channel abnormality, and is again associated with malignant ventricular arrhythmia. The importance of identifying these patients not only lies in the appropriate risk stratification and treatment of the primary case, but also in the screening of family members who may be affected. Ablation of these patients has been described when polymorphic VT or VF are recurrent despite anti-arrhythmic medication.

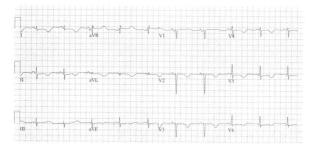

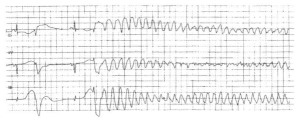

Fig. 15.11 12-lead ECG from a patient with long QT syndrome (top). The QT is measured as 540 ms, which even when corrected for the sinus bradycardia gives a QTc of 535 ms. The upper limit of normal is 450 ms (although some overlap exists between normal and affected individuals above this value). R-on-T in the same patient causes polymorphic VT/VF (bottom).

Part 4

Catheter ablation techniques

Ablation of the atrio-ventricular (AV) junction

Indications for ablation

In patients with atrial fibrillation where rate control is required, AV nodal blocking agents such as β-blockers, calcium channel blockers, and digoxin are used. Where medical therapy proves ineffective or causes severe adverse effects, catheter ablation of the AV junction (commonly referred to as AV node ablation) is an important and effective means of achieving ventricular rate control. However, a permanent pacemaker must be implanted because the junctional escape rhythm after ablation is typically slow and unreliable (📖 p. 332).

Originally the first procedures performed were in patients with tachycardia-bradycardia syndrome (paroxysmal or persistent atrial fibrillation where ventricular rates are sometimes slow enough to warrant pacemaker implantation anyway, but where fast ventricular response rates are also seen and not adequately controlled with medical therapy). The first AV junction ablations were performed with a direct current shock but this has been replaced by radiofrequency (RF) energy ablation. Cryoablation of the AV junction has been described but is not widely used.

Currently the indications for AV junction ablation include:
• Patients with AF and poorly controlled ventricular rates despite maximal medical therapy (although consideration may be given to primary ablation of the AF itself in some).
• Control of ventricular rate in patients with AF and a cardiac resynchronization therapy device (to maximize biventricular pacing).

Pacing issues with AV junction ablation

Before AV junction ablation, appropriate measures for ventricular pacing need to be in place. There are different approaches to this, as described below.

Temporary pacing and AV junction ablation, followed by permanent pacemaker insertion

A temporary pacing electrode is placed in the right ventricular apex before ablation of the AV junction, and then a permanent pacemaker system is implanted.

Advantages: No risk of displacing a permanent pacemaker lead during catheter manipulation for AV junction ablation (which may be of particular concern in a patient with a cardiac resynchronization therapy device); no risk of pacing failure through inhibition of permanent pacemaker by RF energy during ablation (see below).

Disadvantages: Possibility of acute permanent pacemaker lead displacement in a patient who has been rendered pacing-dependent by AV junction ablation; may be unexpected problems with implanting permanent pacemaker system, e.g. unusual anatomy in a patient who is now pacing-dependent.

Permanent pacemaker implantation and subsequent AV junction ablation

A permanent pacemaker system is implanted some weeks prior to AV junction ablation.

Advantages: Acute permanent pacemaker malfunction is avoided; no unexpected problems with permanent pacemaker implantation.

Disadvantages: Possibility of permanent pacemaker lead displacement with catheter manipulation during AV junction ablation; interaction between RF energy and pacemaker may occur and cause pacemaker inhibition at same time as AV junction is ablated causing asystole.

Practical note

If a permanent pacemaker has already been implanted then some operators will still choose to insert a temporary pacing electrode and inactivate any pacing by the permanent system to avoid the risk of pacemaker inhibition during RF energy delivery. If a temporary pacing wire is not used, the pacemaker pacing parameters should be checked before the procedure to make sure it is functioning satisfactorily (sensing and pacing threshold) and then programmed to either VVI or VOO mode at 40 to 50 beats per minute before ablation. The indifferent electrode (skin patch for the ablater) should be placed as far as possible from the pacemaker, avoiding the pacemaker in the circuit, i.e. place the patch on the outer thigh rather than the shoulder that is commonly used. The pacing parameters should be checked again after ablation.

Post-AV junction ablation pacemaker programming

A risk of ventricular tachyarrhythmia and sudden cardiac death has been noted in the first few weeks after AV junction ablation even with effective ventricular pacing at rates of 60 beats per minute. To prevent this the pacemaker is programmed to a lower rate of 80 to 90 beats per minute and then reduced by 10 beats per minute every month to a standard lower rate of 60 beats per minute.

Standard right-sided femoral approach

This is normally the first approach for AV junction ablation and is acutely successful in 95% of cases. The target for ablation is the compact node region (📖 p. 235). It is *not* common practice to place a diagnostic catheter in the His position for the right-sided approach to AV junction ablation. Instead, a combination of fluoroscopic markers and electrogram characteristics are used to identify this region.

Fluoroscopic positioning

The ablation catheter (either a D or F curve catheter, depending upon the size of the right atrium and right ventricle) is deflected slightly and advanced into the right ventricle (easiest in the RAO projection). The deflection on the catheter is then relaxed and the catheter rotated in a clockwise direction to maintain contact with the septum and to allow it to rise anteriorly/superiorly. The catheter is then gradually drawn back towards the atrium to an anatomical position that is just proximal and inferior to where a His catheter would normally be (Fig. 16.1). The catheter tip may again need to be deflected slightly to follow the course of the AV conduction system and stop it prolapsing out into the high right atrium.

Electrogram appearance

When the ablation catheter is in the right ventricle a typical ventricular electrogram is recorded (Fig. 16.2). As the catheter is withdrawn (described above), a large His electrogram is initially seen (Fig. 16.2). This may in fact be a right bundle potential and is not the ideal site for ablation (📖 p. 346). The catheter is then withdrawn further into the right atrium to record a clear atrial electrogram with an A:V ratio of 1:1 or 1:2 and a small His (less than 0.15 mV amplitude), which represents the optimal ablation site (Fig. 16.2).

Practical note

The above description assumes mapping during sinus rhythm. A large proportion of these patients will be in persistent AF and mapping is more difficult with variable atrial electrogram amplitudes and obscuration of the His electrogram. An example is shown in Fig. 16.3.

Ablation

Once a stable, optimal position has been found, RF is commenced. A standard 4 mm-tip catheter is often used initially with power settings of 50 to 60 W and temperature limited at 55 to 65°C. During RF energy application, accelerated junctional rhythm occurs (similar to that seen during slow pathway ablation for AVNRT but faster), followed by slowing of the ventricular response and subsequently AV block and pacing from whichever means of pacing is present. Ideally AV block occurs within 5–10 seconds of reaching target powers and temperatures (Fig. 16.4). RF energy is then delivered for a total of 60 seconds normally.

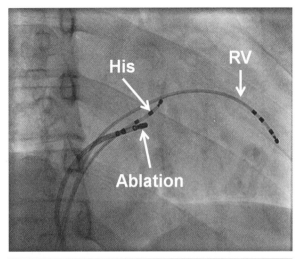

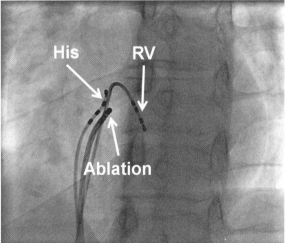

Fig.16.1 Fluoroscopic images showing catheter positions during AV node ablation using a standard right femoral approach. Top: Right anterior oblique projection (RAO). Bottom: Left anterior oblique projection (LAO). The catheters shown are the ablation catheter (Ablation), His catheter marking the position of the His bundle (His), and the right ventricular catheter (RV). Note that the ablation catheter is positioned at the proximal end of the His catheter electrodes in the RAO view and septally in the LAO view.

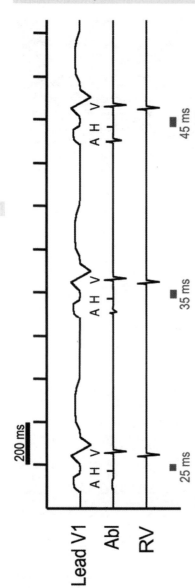

Fig. 16.2 From left to right: The first ablation catheter signal has a very small atrial signal and a short HV interval, indicating that it is actually the RBB potential being recorded. Ablation here will cause RBBB, not CHB. The middle electrograms are more annular and represent the distal His bundle. The right-hand signal is the optimal site, with a large atrial signal and typical HV interval. At this site the AVN should be successfully ablated and may even result in a narrow complex escape rhythm.

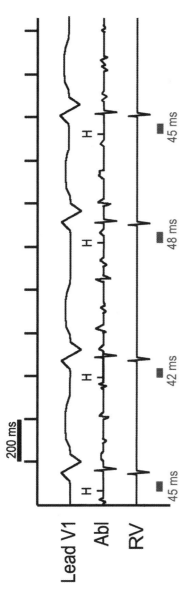

Fig. 16.3 Identification of the optimal site for AVN ablation during atrial fibrillation. The His bundle electrogram can be differentiated from the rapid fibrillatory atrial electrograms by its almost constant HV interval. It may sometimes (but not always) be a shorter, sharper electrogram.

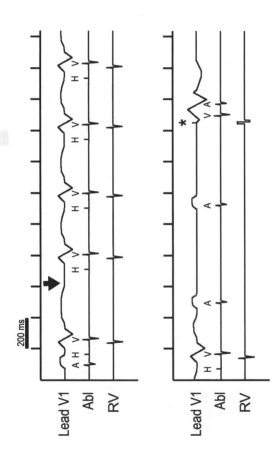

Fig. 16.4 Delivery of RF energy at the optimal site. Immediately after RF energy is turned on (arrow) there is a rapid junctional rhythm as the heat 'excites' the AV node (top line). Complete heart block then develops (bottom line), with non-conducted P waves and ventricular pacing (*). If the ventricular escape rhythm is faster than the temporary pacing rate this may be seen instead.

Left-sided or transaortic approach

This approach is generally used where the right-sided approach has been unsuccessful. It is also used by some operators as the first choice in patients where a cardiac resynchronization device has been recently implanted before AV junction ablation and concern exists regarding pacemaker lead displacement (particularly the left ventricular/coronary sinus lead).

Technique description

A diagnostic catheter may be placed on the right side in the His position to help guide ablation. The curve of the ablation catheter used depends on the size of the left ventricle but in a normal heart a B curve is used whilst a very dilated ventricle may need a D curve catheter. The ablation catheter enters the left ventricle retrogradely and retroverted and may then be positioned in this configuration by rotation of the catheter towards the septum and withdrawal of the catheter towards the aortic valve – use of the LAO and RAO projections helps ensure a septal and basal position (Fig. 16.5). Alternatively, once in the left ventricle the catheter may be straightened towards the inferior apical septum and then withdrawn towards the area on the septum just below the non-coronary cusp of the aortic valve (Fig. 16.5). The His electrogram needs to be differentiated from the left bundle branch electrogram. The left-sided His should occur at the same time as the right-sided His, whilst the left bundle branch electrogram is typically 1–1.5 cm inferior to the His, has an A:V ratio of less than 1:10 (i.e. very small A), and a short interval to the ventricular electrogram (20 ms).

Practical note

As with all left-sided ablation, the patient needs to be anticoagulated with heparin during catheter manipulation and ablation, and then post-procedure with either aspirin (as for left-sided accessory pathway ablation, 📖 p. 392) or warfarin if indicated anyway.

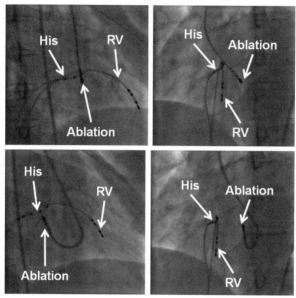

Fig. 16.5 Fluoroscopic images showing catheter positions during AV node ablation using a left-sided, transaortic approach. Top and bottom left: Right anterior oblique projection (RAO). Top and bottom right: Left anterior oblique projection (LAO). The catheters shown are the ablation catheter (Ablation), His catheter marking the position of the His bundle (His), and the right ventricular catheter (RV). The top two panels show a direct approach to positioning the ablation catheter across the aortic valve, whilst the lower two panels show the ablation catheter inverted in the left ventricle to reach the same position. The orientation of the catheter chosen for ablation depends upon which gives the best signal and which is most stable. Note that the ablation catheter is in line with the His catheter electrodes in the RAO views but separated by the thickness of the septum in the LAO views.

The subclavian approach

This approach is infrequently used, but with the increase in AV junction ablation and cardiac resynchronization therapy device implantation, an approach that allows both to be performed at the same time using the subclavian vein route alone has been described.

Technique description

Having gained access to the subclavian vein and placed the right ventricular pacing lead in the usual fashion, a sheath is used with an ablation catheter (Fig. 16.6) and it is positioned in the same region as for the standard right-sided approach (□ p. 334). This may be technically challenging as the catheter is less stable than with a femoral approach but it removes the need for a femoral venous puncture.

Table 16.1 Comparison of different approaches to AV junction ablation

Standard right-sided approach	Left-sided approach	Subclavian approach
Most common and familiar	Usually when right-sided approach has failed. May be used if concern re: right-sided approach, e.g. in CRT patients and risk of lead displacement	Limited to a small number of cases where this is needed
Small His electrogram at target site (<0.15 mV)	HV interval >30–40 ms	Same His electrogram as standard right-sided approach
A:V ratio of 1:1 or 1:2	A:V ratio ~ 1:10	Same A:V ratio as standard right-sided approach
Antero/mid-septal position on tricuspid annulus	Site <1–1.5 cm below aortic valve, i.e. above left BB	Position same as standard right-sided approach but different angulation so need to ensure good contact
Right bundle branch		**Left bundle branch**
Absent or minimal atrial electrogram		A:V ratio ≤1:10
BB-V interval <30–35 ms		BB-V interval ≤20 ms
		Site 1–1.5 cm below aortic valve

HV – His-to-ventricular; A:V ratio – atrial-to-ventricular electrogram ratio; BB – bundle branch; BB-V – bundle branch-to-ventricular.

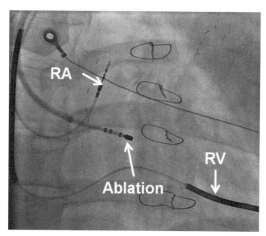

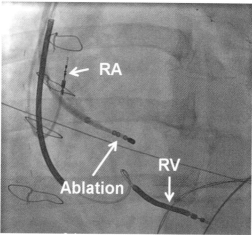

Fig. 16.6 Fluoroscopic images showing catheter positions during AV node ablation using a subclavian approach. Top: Right anterior oblique projection (RAO). Bottom: Left anterior oblique projection (LAO). The ablation catheter (ablation) is in a steerable sheath that has been introduced from the left subclavian vein (and the sheath was subsequently used to place a lead in the coronary sinus for cardiac resynchronization therapy). A right atrial pacing lead (RA) and right ventricular pacing/defibrillator lead (RV) are also seen, and were implanted during the same procedure before the AV node was ablated.

Outcomes and post-procedure management

Outcomes

Overall 100% acute success of AV junction ablation is possible. A recurrence of AV conduction is seen in up to 5%. Many studies have demonstrated improvement of quality of life in AF patients with palpitations, dyspnoea, and reduced exercise tolerance secondary to fast ventricular response rates. Reversal of tachycardia-induced cardiomyopathy has also been described.

Practical note

Although patients are rendered pacing-dependent after AV junction ablation, the more proximal the ablation site within the AV conduction system, the more likely that there will be some form of residual escape rhythm, rather than asystole.

Post-procedure management

Complications due to AV junction ablation are rare. Post-ablation polymorphic ventricular arrhythmias were initially documented but have been effectively eradicated by appropriate pacemaker programming (📖 p. 333). It is possible to damage pacemaker leads either directly or indirectly through interference during RF energy application so if a permanent pacemaker was *in situ* before ablation, it should be checked thoroughly at the end of the procedure. Anticoagulation with coumarins after the procedure should be continued. Increasingly these procedures are routinely performed whilst the patient continues to take their normal coumarin dose and with an international normalized ratio (INR) between two and three, as the risks of perforation/bleeding complications are very low.

Common pitfalls and troubleshooting

Inability to record a clear His signal

- The most common and frustrating problem encountered.
- May be due to anatomical reasons, e.g. an intramyocardial course of the His or scar/fibrosis. A systematic search of the septum superiorly and inferiorly and/or use of a separate multi-polar catheter may help identify a small His electrogram.
- Pacing from the distal electrodes of the ablation catheter at high outputs can be used to look for QRS narrowing, indicating that the catheter is in the region of the proximal His bundle.
- If a His electrogram cannot be identified then anatomical ablation may be performed on the right and then left side. Use of irrigated tip/large tip catheters may be necessary. Practically, a line of ablation lesions is made on the septum, perpendicular to the presumed location of the His, which may cause enough damage to the nodal tissue to generate complete AV block.
- Continuous atrial activity of AF also obscures the His electrogram. Cardioversion may restore sinus rhythm for long enough to allow identification/confirmation of the presence of a His electrogram and therefore guide AV junction ablation.
- Multiple ineffective lesions create local oedema and make recording His electrograms/delivering RF energy to target tissue difficult. Careful mapping for the optimal ablation site (with good stability) should therefore be performed before any ablation energy is delivered.

Failure to achieve complete AV block despite clear His electrogram recordings

- This may be because of instability/poor contact of the ablation catheter. With a right-sided approach, use of a preformed, long sheath may help.
- Ablation at the maximal His deflection on the right side may create right bundle branch block only. In this case mapping and ablating more proximally with a larger atrial signal may help achieve complete block. Alternatively the left bundle branch may be targeted once right bundle branch block is achieved but this is a more diffuse structure and complete ablation may require a series of lesions on the left side.
- Where there is pre-existing bundle branch block, ablation of the contralateral bundle branch may create complete AV block.
- Rarely, where right- and left-sided ablation are unsuccessful, mapping and ablation in the non-coronary cusp where a His potential is recorded can create complete AV block.

Loss of ventricular pacing during ablation

- This may be due to electromagnetic interference and pacemaker inhibition where a permanent pacemaker is being used. Programming to VOO mode will normally correct this. A temporary pacing wire may also be inserted if asynchronous pacing is not wanted.

- Loss of temporary pacing usually indicates temporary pacing wire displacement. It is prudent to have the ablation catheter ready to pace at a cycle length of 600 ms at full output so that if this occurs, the catheter can be quickly advanced into the ventricle and used to pace until the temporary wire is repositioned. If displacement of the temporary wire occurs repeatedly, an active fixation temporary wire can be used.

In patients with congenital heart disease or prosthetic valves the anatomical variation may make ablation of the AV junction awkward and all the previously mentioned problems *are more common in these patients*. The solutions to these problems are still the same.

Ablation of atrio-ventricular nodal re-entrant tachycardia (AVNRT)

Ablation of AVNRT

Indication
The following should ideally be present in all patients before proceeding with ablation:
- A clinical history of palpitations consistent with AVNRT.
- ECG documentation of a narrow complex tachycardia consistent with AVNRT during clinical episodes.
- Electrophysiological evidence of dual AV nodal physiology.
- Reproducibly inducible tachycardia with the characteristics of AVNRT during electrophysiological testing.

Many electrophysiologists would also perform a slow pathway modification in patients with clear ECG documentation of a supraventricular tachycardia consistent with AVNRT and electrophysiological evidence of dual AV nodal physiology, even if they were unable to induce tachycardia during an EPS. However, in this setting the endpoint of ablation is more difficult to define.

The presence of dual AV nodal physiology in the absence of either ECG documentation of tachycardia during an attack or inducible AVNRT during EPS is usually not sufficient to proceed to ablation.

Complications
Patients should be consented for the following specific complications of AVNRT ablation:
- 0.5% risk of complete heart block.
- 5% risk of recurrence.

In addition all patients undergoing an electrophysiological study for a narrow complex tachycardia should be warned of the risk of:
- Access site complications:
  - Inadvertent arterial puncture.
  - Femoral vein: groin haematoma.
  - Subclavian vein: pneumothorax.
- Heart attack.
- Stroke.
- Death (1/1000).

Techniques – typical AVNRT

Fast pathway ablation

This was the initial approach to treatment of AVNRT, but is no longer used because of a high risk for development of both complete heart block and incessant atypical AVNRT.

Slow pathway modification

This is the standard approach for ablative treatment of AVNRT. Typically a medium curve radiofrequency ablation catheter will be used in addition to a catheter marking the His position and a coronary sinus catheter. Often further catheters will be placed in the right ventricle and the high right atrium (Fig. 17.1). Ablation of typical slow/fast AVNRT is usually performed during sinus rhythm.

Two complementary approaches may be used to identify suitable ablation sites:

Ablation of slow pathway potential

Careful mapping of the posterior portion of the triangle of Koch can lead to detection of a slow pathway potential discrete from the His potential and local atrial electrograms. Ablation at this site is associated with a high chance of success, as long as it is a reasonable distance from the His catheter and no His signal can be identified on the ablation catheter. This approach can, however, be very time-consuming and equal success can usually be achieved by the use of an electroanatomical approach.

Electroanatomical approach

This uses a combination of anatomical landmarks and typical electrograms to identify a suitable ablation site. The ablation catheter is positioned at the level of the coronary sinus os between the coronary sinus and the tricuspid valve annulus. At a good ablation site a typical electrogram morphology is seen with a small atrial bump followed by a larger sharp ventricular spike (A:V ratio of between 1:2 and 1:10). The atrial signal in the ablation catheter should be later than that seen in the His catheter (at least 20–30 ms) (Fig. 17.1).

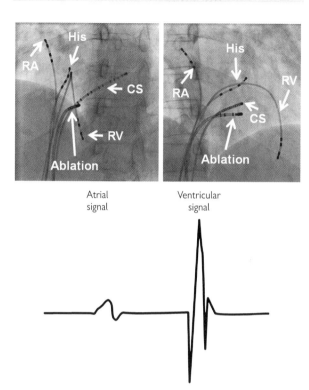

Fig. 17.1 Upper panel – typical catheter setup seen prior to ablation of AVNRT by the electroanatomical approach. Left fluoroscopic image shows left anterior oblique projection; right image shows right anterior oblique projection. The catheters shown are in the right atrium (RA), His position (His), the right ventricle (RV), and coronary sinus (CS). The ablation catheter is in a typical low position for slow pathway ablation, near the CS os. If this site is unsuccessful then the ablation catheter is moved superiorly and anteriorly, but the closer the catheter is moved to the His, the greater the risk of AV block. Lower panel – typical electrogram at this point showing 'bump' (atrial electrogram) and 'spike' (ventricular electrogram).

Ablation

Once a suitable site has been identified radiofrequency ablation is performed. Ablation parameters vary between operators, but a typical approach would be to use temperature-limited ablation with a maximum power of 40 W and temperature of 60°C, increasing the power for subsequent burns if necessary. During the burn the atrial and ventricular electrograms must be watched closely.

- Successful ablation is associated with the development of junctional rhythm during the burn (Fig. 17.2) that gradually slows and then returns to sinus rhythm. The burn should be continued for a minute to ensure complete ablation and further consolidation lesions may be necessary (📖 p. 356).
- A fast junctional rhythm (Fig. 17.3) or the presence of either ventricular electrograms that are not conducted to the atrium or atrial electrograms without corresponding ventricular signals suggest damage to either the fast pathway or the compact AV node, and **the burn must be stopped immediately to prevent the damage becoming permanent**.

Practical tip

Whilst ablating it is often easiest to focus on only one or two electrograms. To ensure 1:1 VA/AV conduction it is common to concentrate on an atrial electrogram (HRA) and a single surface electrogram positioned one above the other – as long as a one-to-one relationship is maintained without excessive acceleration it is usually safe to continue. Intermittently the His catheter electrograms should be checked to ensure no gross AH prolongation.

If no junctional rhythm is obtained initially the ablation catheter may be moved more anteriorly and superiorly. However, the closer the ablation catheter is to the compact AV node the greater the risk of inducing complete heart block.

Practical tip

It is sometimes possible to abolish slow pathway conduction without any junctional rhythm during ablation itself, therefore if RF applications have been delivered in a good anatomical position with good signals as described above then test antegrade conduction again before further RF.

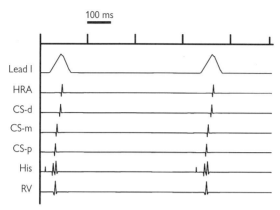

Fig. 17.2 Slow junctional rhythm induced during slow pathway modification. The presence of a slow junctional rhythm during ablation predicts a successful outcome.

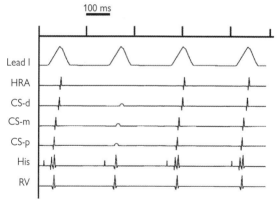

Fig. 17.3 Fast junctional rhythm with loss of atrial capture seen during slow pathway modification. The first, third, and fourth beats show both ventricular and atrial electrograms. The second beat shows only ventricular activity. This suggests injury to the fast pathway with retrograde block. The burn must be stopped immediately to prevent development of complete heart block.

Endpoints

Slow pathway ablation

In some patients complete loss of slow pathway conduction is seen with the loss of the characteristic features of AV node dual physiology and no echo beats. Following ablation of the slow pathway the electrophysiological characteristics of the fast pathway with shortening of its refractory period become apparent.

Slow pathway modification

Whilst complete loss of slow pathway conduction is an ideal endpoint, frequently slow pathway modification will result in nearly as good clinical outcomes with a lower risk of complications. Thus if tachycardia is no longer inducible it is often appropriate to stop even in the presence of single echo beats and some preserved slow pathway conduction. However, the presence of multiple echo beats or persistently inducible tachycardia suggest a low chance of clinical success and further consolidation ablation lesions are necessary.

Practical tips for slow pathway modification

- AVNRT is often associated with a large CS orifice, which can make catheter stability difficult. Consider using a long sheath to aid stability.
- Atrial and ventricular ectopics can give the appearance of VA or AV block during ablation. However, a cautious approach is safest.
- Occasionally slow pathways can only be successfully targeted within the CS or even the LA.

How to avoid complete heart block in **AVNRT** ablation

- Always check the ablation site in two different projections (LAO and RAO). The ablation catheter must be on the septum, but a safe distance from the AV node. A prominent eustachian ridge can result in a failure of a burn to induce a junctional rhythm until the ablation catheter is at the level of the AV node.
- Start low (infero-posteriorly) and work up towards the AV node if unsuccessful.
- Continuously watch the electrograms during ablation to ensure 1:1 VA/AV conduction.
- Stop burning immediately if non-conducted beats or a fast junctional rhythm are seen.
- If in doubt about speed of junctional rhythm or AV/VA conduction, always stop and reassess.
- Be cautious in patients with poor fast pathway conduction on the antegrade curve. They may be dependent on their slow pathway for normal conduction.
- Remember, a repeat procedure is usually preferable to a pacemaker.
- Always consent the patient for complete heart block. Even in the best hands it can never be completely avoided.

Alternative approaches

A number of alternative approaches to ablation for typical AVNRT have been described. They may be particularly useful in cases where ablation at more inferior sites has been unsuccessful and ablation is being planned near the AV node.

Cryotherapy

The use of cryotherapy in slow pathway modification is thought to be associated with a lower risk of complete AV block but has a higher recurrence rate. Once a suitable site is identified with the mapping catheter, it is cooled to −30°C. This temperature is maintained for a few seconds to ensure no AH prolongation suggestive of fast pathway damage. Once stability of the AH interval is confirmed, the cryocatheter is then frozen to −70°C to apply a therapeutic freeze. If AV nodal or fast pathway block is demonstrated during the initial freeze the catheter is re-warmed and an alternative site chosen. Generally at least three freezes are required.

Practical tip: There is no junctional rhythm seen during any freeze application, unlike RF. Also, the ratio of A:V on the mapping catheter for successful cryotherapy normally requires a slightly larger atrial component (often nearer 1:1 and inside the CS os, on the roof).

Multiple short burns

Rather than applying a single prolonged radiofrequency burn, multiple short burns may be applied at a single site, with each burn being terminated as soon as a junctional rhythm is induced. Once a junctional rhythm can no longer be induced and the conventional endpoints have been achieved, no further burns are applied.

Ablation within the CS os and left atrium

Occasionally AVNRT remains inducible even after radiofrequency ablation at the usual site. In this instance further burns may be required either within the roof of the coronary sinus or very rarely within the floor of the left atrium.

Techniques – atypical AVNRT

This is best performed during tachycardia at the site of earliest atrial activation in both fast-slow and slow-slow AVNRT. This is usually within the triangle of Koch or in the proximal coronary sinus.

Successful ablation is associated with early termination of tachycardia during the burn. However, the burn should be continued for a full minute at this site to ensure complete treatment, as long as the catheter has not been displaced by the termination of tachycardia.

Practical tip: Programming the stimulator to pace the atrium at a cycle length slightly longer than the tachycardia cycle length during the burn may minimize displacement as tachycardia terminates. As for slow pathway modification, careful attention should be placed on the electrograms during ablation to look for evidence of VA or AV dissociation or a fast junctional rhythm. If these occur ablation should be discontinued immediately.

Ablation of accessory pathways and atrio-ventricular re-entrant tachycardia (AVRT)

Ablation of accessory pathways

AP localization: principles

- Mapping may be undertaken using any combination of the following three methods:
  - During manifest pre-excitation, mapping of the earliest V signal relative to the onset of the delta wave/QRS, either during sinus rhythm or atrial pacing. Left-sided APs often need faster pacing rates due to latency (ideally pacing close to the insertion site of the AP, i.e. using CS electrodes).
  - For concealed APs, map the earliest A signal during ventricular pacing (shortest stim-A time). Left lateral APs may require left ventricular pacing or a faster cycle length to avoid mapping retrograde AVN conduction.
  - During orthodromic AVRT, map the earliest A signal (shortest VA time when measuring from the onset of the surface QRS).
- Both unipolar and bipolar recordings may be useful:
  - Unipolar recordings may provide more precise AP localization, since bipolar electrode spacing inevitably increases recording area and therefore reduces accuracy.
  - Unipolar recordings may also differentiate between endocardial and epicardial insertion of AP (QS complex noted at endocardial insertion sites vs. RS complex for epicardial APs, 🔲 p. 56).
  - Bipolar recordings reflect timing and may more clearly demonstrate local electrogram components and AP potentials.
- Mapping during sinus/atrial pacing in manifest pre-excitation targets the ventricular AP insertion point. Mapping during ventricular pacing localizes the atrial AP insertion point. APs with an oblique course may have their atrial and ventricular insertions a few cm apart and local VA times may be misleading.
- Ideal pre-ablation signal characteristics (Fig. 18.1):
  - 1:1 A:V ratio, unless in a mid/anteroseptal location, where a dominant V signal reduces the risk of CHB (🔲 p. 370).
  - A stable electrogram morphology (minimal beat-to-beat variation).
  - A lack of isoelectric interval between the atrial and ventricular components, with local A-V or V-A interval <40 ms.
  - During manifest pre-excitation: for left-sided APs, the earliest V signal ≤0 ms pre-delta; for right-sided APs, earliest V ≤–10 ms pre-delta.
  - Presence of a 'pathway potential' (a small spike between the atrial and ventricular components).
- Loss of AP conduction should occur within 1–6 seconds of RF delivery. If the AP disappears after this the ablation catheter may not be quite on the AP or the AP may be epicardial. If there is no effect noted after 10 seconds, it may be best to stop ablation and map for a better signal.

Table 18.1 Pros and cons of different approaches to AP ablation

Mapping technique	Pros	Cons
Earliest V during sinus rhythm or atrial pacing	Good catheter stability	Only useful for manifest pre-excitation
Earliest A during ventricular pacing	Good catheter stability	Only useful for retrogradely conducting APs
Earliest A during AVRT	Useful if incessant tachycardia Best method for parahisian APs as ablation of AP or AVN will terminate tachy and allow immediate assessment	Ablation catheter may be displaced immediately after AP block, due to abrupt rate slowing following conversion to sinus rhythm

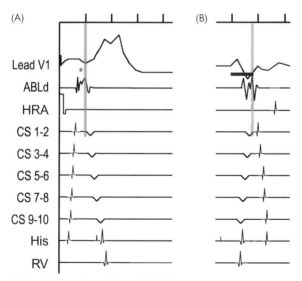

Fig. 18.1 Ablation site for a left lateral AP. (A) During atrial pacing the ablation catheter electrogram shows a sharp atrial signal followed immediately by a slurred ventricular signal. The two are fused with a small potential between them (*), which is a pathway potential. The V signal times out with the onset of ventricular activation (the beginning of the delta wave on the surface ECG, grey line). (B) During tachycardia the ablation catheter shows two components, a ventricular signal fused with an atrial signal that is also the site of earliest atrial activation and the shortest VA time (red line). A small pathway potential can be seen between the V and A.

Accessing left-sided accessory pathways

Trans-septal approach to ablation of left-sided APs

- For details of how to perform TSP, 📖 p. 90.
- Preformed sheaths allow catheter direction towards particular parts of the annulus (Fig. 18.8). Use the CS catheter to 'bracket' the AP and determine the correct sheath shape (Fig. 18.3).
- Clockwise sheath rotation moves the catheter towards the posterior atrium, while anticlockwise rotation directs the catheter towards the mitral annulus and ventricle.
- The RAO view is useful to position the catheter tip on the mitral annulus. The LAO view is then used to view the mitral annulus as a 'clock face' to guide mapping and ablation.
- Once a correct A:V ratio has been obtained, detailed mapping is undertaken by small movements of the catheter and sheath.
- A 'B curve' (small sweep) catheter is often chosen for small precision movements of the tip during mapping.

Transaortic approach to ablation of left-sided APs

- Directed at sites beneath the MV annulus.
- A tightly curved ablation catheter is prolapsed across the aortic valve.
- On entering the LV cavity, maintaining the 'J' curvature the catheter is rotated anticlockwise, turning the tip posteriorly towards the MV annulus.
- Opening the catheter then engages the sub-annular area.
- Mapping is undertaken via incremental movements in this position, or repetitively sliding along the annulus before dropping down beneath it (Fig. 18.2).
- Anterolateral and lateral positions are often unstable for the transaortic approach.
- A 'B curve' (small sweep) catheter is often the first choice to permit easier prolapse across the aortic valve, although a 'D curve' (medium sweep) may be required if there is insufficient catheter reach.

Table 18.2 Pros and cons of trans-septal and transaortic approaches

Approach	Pros	Cons
Trans-septal	Often greater operator familiarity with catheter manipulation via this route	Often difficult to access left postero-septal space, even with pre-shaped sheaths
	Pre-shaped sheaths permit stable mapping and ablation	
Transaortic	Avoids risks of TSP (📖 p. 88)	Risk of damage to coronary arteries and aortic valve
	Good access to left postero-septal space	Contraindicated by presence of peripheral vascular or aortic valve disease, or AVR

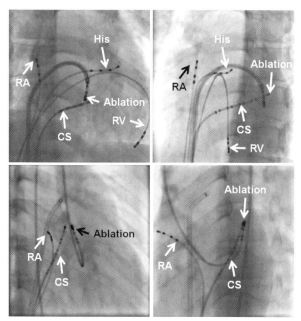

Fig. 18.2 Fluoroscopic images showing catheter positions during left lateral AP ablation using a trans-septal approach (top) and retrograde transaortic approach (bottom). Top and bottom left: Right anterior oblique projection (RAO). Top and bottom right: Left anterior oblique projection (LAO). The catheters shown are in the right atrium (RA), the His position, the right ventricle (RV), and the coronary sinus (CS). The ablation catheter is positioned to find an appropriate annular signal (📖 Fig. 18.7). Note that the ablation catheter is in line with the distal CS poles where the earliest atrial signal was recorded during maximal pre-excitation. A pre-formed sheath has been used to reach the desired area on the mitral valve annulus.

Ablation of specific anatomical accessory pathways

Left free wall APs

- Access the MV annulus either via a TSP (📖 Chapter 5), or transaortic route (📖 p. 364).
- TSP necessitates the choice of long pre-shaped sheaths to better direct ablation catheter to the AP insertion point.
- Advance the CS catheter proximally or distally to 'bracket' the site of earliest atrial activation to better localize the AP and guide the choice of sheath (Fig. 18.3).
- 2–500 U IV heparin boluses should be administered to achieve a target ACT ~250 seconds during mapping and ablation.
- RF power generally 50 W, target temperature 60–65°C, with standard ablation catheters. Occasionally irrigated-tip ablation catheters (📖 p. 42) are required for deep-seated/epicardial APs.

Right free wall APs

- Access is via the right femoral route as first choice.
- A right subclavian/internal jugular vein approach may allow better AP localization if unsuccessful from the femoral route.
- The flat TV annulus and lack of radiographic markers can present a challenge during ablation.
- Often a long sheath may be required to improve catheter stability (SR0 – 4).
- A multi-polar Halo catheter positioned around the TV annulus may be useful to 'bracket' the AP and to act as a radiographic marker.
- 2 F Cardima duodecapolar catheters may be advanced into the right coronary artery to map the RV free wall if coronary anatomy permits (RCA dominance).
- Longer curve ablation catheters sometimes provide extra reach to map the TV annulus.
- Cryoablation may help catheter stability by fixing the ablation catheter tip to the annulus (📖 p. 44).
- RF energy is chosen as the first choice energy source. 50 W power, target temperature 60–65°C.
- NavX or CARTO 3-D mapping systems may be useful in redo cases, especially where mechanical block complicated the first attempt.

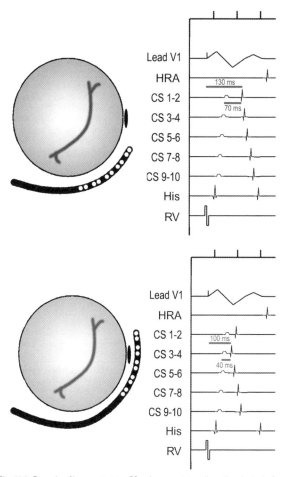

Fig. 18.3 Example of how optimizing CS catheter position allows 'bracketing' of AP and may better guide ablation. In the upper figure, a proximally positioned CS catheter displays the earliest retrograde atrial signal during ventricular pacing at CS 1-2. This is misleading, however, which becomes apparent in the lower figure where the CS catheter has been advanced more distally and the earliest atrial signal is now at CS 3-4 (the AP is 'bracketed') with a shorter VA time both from the surface ECG and locally in the CS catheter. This allows a better guide to AP location and positioning of the ablation catheter.

Paraseptal APs

- Most paraseptal APs are ablated in the right atrium/TV annulus. Some, however, have their successful ablation sites in the coronary sinus or in the left atrium (Fig. 18.4).
- Conventional RF energy is generally the first choice. A 'D curve' (medium sweep) catheter is usually used.
- Some APs may be 'epicardial' (middle cardiac vein territory) or deep within the postero-septal space. A switch to irrigated-tip RF ablation is required in up to 25% of cases.
- Mapping the CS before undertaking TSP may permit ablation of APs with apparent left-sided insertion, but entirely from venous access.
- A CS venogram may demonstrate a diverticulum. In such cases the AP is commonly found at the neck of the diverticulum. For venography use a MP1 or AL1 or 2 catheter from the femoral approach with a contrast-filled luer-lock syringe. Rarely a balloon occlusion catheter is required for a good quality CS venogram.
- RF power generally 30–50 W depending upon the proximity to the AVN.
- Beware risk of damage to RCA/AV nodal artery during ablation.

Table 18.3 Indicators of successful ablation site

Right side favoured	Left side favoured
Negative delta in V1 R > S transition in V2 or V3	R > S in V1
Long RP tachycardia	Earliest atrial activation during orthodromic AVRT at mid-CS
Difference between VA at His and shortest CS VA interval <25 ms*	Difference between VA at His and shortest CS VA interval >25 ms*

*This finding is due to the closer proximity of right-sided APs to the His catheter, thus the difference in VA intervals between the His and earliest CS A will be small. Conversely, left-sided AP insertion results in a greater distance and therefore timing difference between the earliest atrial signals.

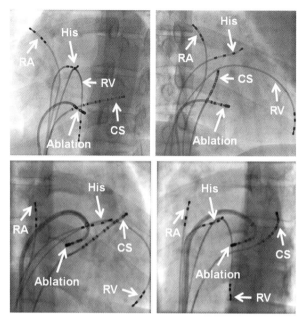

Fig. 18.4 Fluoroscopic images showing catheter positions during para(postero) septal AP ablation using a right-sided and left-sided approach. Top and bottom left: Right anterior oblique projection (RAO). Top and bottom right: Left anterior oblique projection (LAO). The catheters shown are the ablation catheter (ablation), His catheter marking the position of the His bundle (His), and the right ventricular catheter (RV). The top two panels show a right-side approach to positioning the ablation catheter, with the tip lying just inside the CS os, whilst the lower two panels show the ablation catheter inserted into the left atrium via a trans-septal puncture to reach a similar position. The orientation of the catheter chosen for ablation depends upon which gives the best signal and which is most stable. The transaortic retrograde approach could also be used.

Mid/anteroseptal APs (Fig. 18.5)

- The ideal ablation site signal has a relatively large V component to reduce the risk of compact AVN ablation.
- A small His deflection may be seen at sites of successful ablation (<0.1 mV).
- Cryoablation may be first choice in view of the ability to undertake a 'test freeze', plus improved catheter stability once the ice ball is formed (📖 p. 44).
- If RF energy is chosen, power titration commencing at 10–15 W (📖 box 'Power titration for the ablation of mid/anteroseptal APs') with a gradual increase depending on effect is advised.
- If ablation is undertaken during sinus rhythm it is important to look for increasing degrees of pre-excitation, which suggests the AVN, not the AP, is being affected. Sinus rhythm ablation has the advantage of minimizing the risk of catheter displacement.
- If energy is delivered during tachycardia then ablation of the AP and/or the AVN will terminate tachycardia. It is important to see whether pre-excitation persists (suggesting AVN block) or a narrow QRS complex with normal AH interval is present (suggesting AP block).
- If fast junctional beats occur, this indicates heating of the compact AVN and RF energy should be terminated before AV block occurs.
- These pathways may be very superficial – mechanical block resulting from catheter manipulation may cause difficulty during ablation (occurs in ~40% of cases). Slow movements of the ablation catheter are recommended during mapping. If mechanical AP block occurs, the catheter is kept in the same position to allow RF application at this site when conduction recovers.

Power titration for the ablation of mid/anteroseptal APs

- Once an appropriate, stable catheter position has been identified as above, commence ablation at 10 W (target temperature 60–65°C).
- If no response after 10 seconds, increase power to 20 W.
- If AP block occurs, continue RF application for ~45 seconds minimum.
- If junctional beats occur, stop RF and reposition catheter to a more ventricular position.
- If no response at 20 W after 10 seconds, reposition catheter to find an earlier ventricular signal.
- Once AP block achieved with RF, move ablation catheter away from septum since mechanical pressure may cause AP block.

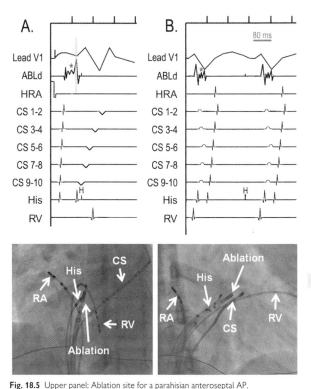

Fig. 18.5 Upper panel: Ablation site for a parahisian anteroseptal AP.
(A) During atrial pacing the ablation catheter electrogram shows a sharp atrial signal followed immediately by a pathway potential and slurred ventricular signal. The V signal times out with the onset of ventricular activation (the beginning of the delta wave on the surface ECG, grey line). A small His egram is seen following the V. The earliest V signal in the diagnostic catheter is in the His catheter, which is fractionally later. (B) During tachycardia the ablation catheter shows two components, a ventricular signal fused with an atrial signal, which is also the site of earliest atrial activation and the shortest VA time (grey line). A small pathway potential can be seen between the V and A, as well as a His egram.

Lower panel: Typical catheter setup seen prior to ablation of parahisian AP. Left fluoroscopic image shows left anterior oblique projection; right image shows right anterior oblique projection. The catheters shown are in the right atrium (RA), His position (His), the right ventricle (RV), and coronary sinus (CS). The cryoablation catheter is being used with a long sheath for extra support.

Signs of successful ablation

Elimination of pre-excitation in cases of manifest, antegradely-conducting APs, or a return to midline, decremental conduction or VA block in concealed APs, are the two sought-after signs of acute procedural success. The time to AP block is an important determinant of success, with a lower rate of recurrence noted for APs blocked immediately after RF application (<5 seconds).

- Following successful ablation, programmed stimulation should be repeated (also with isoprenaline) to identify alternative tachycardia substrates (e.g. AVNRT, SNRT).
- A 20–30 minute waiting period is recommended, since recurrent AP conduction may occur within this time period. A longer period is recommended in redo cases, or when the time to AP block was >10 seconds (30–60 minutes' wait).
- Adenosine is useful in confirming AP block, particularly in cases of concealed, septal APs where VA conduction through the AVN is present following ablation. Adenosine may also uncover a previously unidentified second AP.
  - IV administration of 12–18 mg (depending on the patient's weight) should be sufficient to cause AV block and result in VA and AV block during ventricular and atrial pacing if AP conduction is abolished.

Troubleshooting the difficult case

Left free wall

Problem	Cause	Solution
No early signals	Inability to access target site	Change approach: trans-septal versus transaortic
		Use alternative pre-shaped sheath
	Epicardial AP	Map within CS or LAA
		Pericardial access
	Ligament of Marshall connection	Map LA anterior to LSPV
Recurrent AF	AVRT degeneration, or recurrent APBs	IV flecainide (up to 50 mg in 10 mg increments)
		Internal cardioversion
Unsuccessful energy delivery	Poor catheter stability	Change approach: trans-septal versus transaortic
		Use alternative pre-shaped sheath
	Low power delivery	Use irrigated RF or cryoablation

Right free wall

Problem	Cause	Solution
No early signals	Inability to access target site	Change approach: inferior versus superior
		Use pre-shaped sheath
		Change catheter reach
	Difficulty identifying annulus	Use multi-electrode Halo catheter or duodecapolar Cardima catheter within RCA
	Epicardial AP	Map RAA
		Pericardial access
Unsuccessful energy delivery	Poor catheter stability	Change approach: inferior versus superior
		Try cryoablation
		Use alternative pre-shaped sheath
	Low power delivery	Use irrigated RF or cryoablation
Mechanical block	Superficial AP	Move away from site of block, then carefully re-map
		Use 3-D electroanatomical mapping systems

Paraseptal APs

Problem	Cause	Solution
No early signals	Incomplete mapping	Map proximal CS and tributaries
		Map left heart
	Epicardial AP	Perform CS venography and map within CS (📖 p. 368)
	Slow and/or decremental antegrade conduction	Map AP potentials
		Map pathway potential
		Map shortest AV interval during atrial pacing
		Map site of electrogram polarity reversal
Low power delivery	Low blood flow or ablating within CS	Use irrigated RF; cryoablation is an alternative
Epicardial connection near RCA	AP in proximal CS system	Use cryoablation

Anteroseptal/mid-septal APs

Problem	Cause	Solution
Large His potential at site of earliest signal	Parahisian pathway	Power-titrated RF (📖 p. 370)
		Try cryoablation, to allow 'test-freezes'
Accelerated junctional rhythm during RF	Heating of AV nodal tissue	Stop RF and reposition catheter
RBBB during RF	Lesion too distal	Stop RF and reposition catheter
Mechanical AP block	Superficial AP	Wait for recurrent AP conduction without moving catheter, if possible

Uncommon and unusual variants

These were formerly called 'Mahaim-type' accessory pathways, following the initial description by Mahaim et al. (1938) of anatomical connections between the AV node and upper septum. However, subsequently **atriofascicular** pathways were determined to be the commonest of these so-called atypical accessory pathways, which also include **nodofascicular**, **nodoventricular**, and **fasciculoventricular** pathways (Fig. 18.6). Overall, atypical APs comprise <3% of accessory AV connections.

Epicardial APs may be difficult to map endocardially as the earliest atrial or ventricular signal may not accurately reflect the true epicardial insertion site and pathway potentials may not be present. If they pass through the coronary sinus musculature the earliest atrial signal during V pacing or orthodromic AVRT may be in the CS and precede any left atrial signal. Their depth may also make it challenging for RF energy to reach them with enough power for complete tissue destruction. **Appendage-to-ventricular APs** present similar challenges.

Congenital heart disease such as **Ebstein's anomaly** and a **persistent left-sided superior vena cava** are associated with APs (which may be **multiple**) and can make mapping and catheter stability a challenge.

Reference

Mahaim I, Benatt. Nouvelle recherches sur les connexions superiors de la branche gauche du faisceau de His-tawara. *Cardiologia* 1938; **1**:61–120.

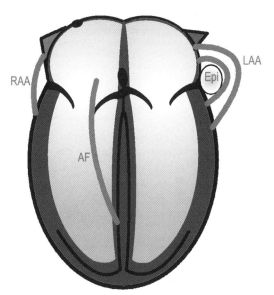

Fig. 18.6 Uncommon AP positions include epicardial pathways through the coronary sinus musculature (Epi), epicardial pathways from the appendage to a ventricular insertion site a little way from the annulus (LAA and RAA), and atriofascicular APs that have their atrial insertion typically near the coronary sinus os and their ventricular insertion into the right bundle branch (AF).

Atriofascicular APs

Atriofascicular and related atypical APs demonstrate decremental, antegrade-only conduction properties. The atrial insertion is commonly in the anterior or lateral RA (rarely posterior or septal RA), with a distal ventricular insertion into the right-sided fascicles, although other RV sites such as the free wall are possible.

ECG clues

- Baseline pre-excitation may not be evident on surface ECG due to slow, decremental, antegrade conduction comparable with the AVN. Alternatively, a subtle LBBB-type appearance may exist (lack of septal Q in I, aVL, V5, and V6, 🕮 Fig. 18.7).
- Antidromic AVRT is the tachycardia mechanism and produces a LBBB-type QRS complex as a result of the RV ventricular insertion.
- The tachycardia QRS duration is typically <150 ms; QRS axis 0–75 degrees; late R > S transition at V4/5.

Specific electrophysiological findings at baseline

- Atrial pacing produces pre-excitation with a relatively long AV interval. Right atrial pacing produces more pre-excitation than left atrial pacing. An AP potential may be found around the TV annulus.
- There is decremental antegrade conduction proximal to AP potential, with fixed AP-to-V interval.
- No retrograde AP conduction.
- Ventricular activation is earlier at RV apex than RV base (His catheter) when maximally pre-excited due to earlier activation of the RV apex from the relatively apical AP insertion into the fascicles.

Specific electrophysiological findings during tachycardia

- QRS should be <145 ms with rapid QRS onset in I and/or V1 due to utilization of the RBB.
- Ventricular activation is earlier at RV apex than RV base.
- His-synchronous APBs delivered when the septum is refractory advance the V and subsequent A.
- The tachycardia VH interval is <50 ms, frequently <20 ms. The V onset is at the fascicular AP insertion and subsequent retrograde His activation occurs rapidly via the normal conduction system.
- There is retrograde RBB activation before the His.
- There is an increase in VA and VH with RBBB, without a change in pre-excitation. This reflects the participation of the RBB in the retrograde limb of the tachycardia.
- The HA in tachycardia = HA with RV pacing. If the tachycardia is AVNRT with a bystander AP, SVT HA < HA with RV pacing.
- VH in tachycardia < VH with RV pacing. This is due to insertion of the AP directly into the fascicle and resulting rapid retrograde His activation, compared to the situation during RV pacing of retrograde His activation from a site distant to the fascicle, resulting in a longer interval.

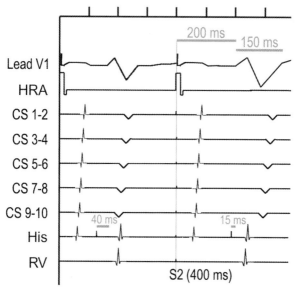

Fig. 18.7 Pre-excitation through an atriofascicular AP. During a relatively slow drive train there is preferential conduction through the AVN due to the atriofascicular pathway's long conduction time, producing a relatively normal QRS complex and HV interval of 40 ms. The premature S2, however, decrements more in the AVN than the AP and pre-excitation with a LBBB morphology emerges with a long PR interval of 200 ms and shorter HV time of 15 ms.

Catheter ablation of atriofascicular pathways

- Map when maximally pre-excited either during atrial pacing or AVRT (greater catheter stability during atrial pacing).
- Identify discrete AP, or 'Mahaim' potential at tricuspid annulus (Fig. 18.8).
- Shortest stimulus to delta interval may also be used, if no AP potentials are identified.
- Historically mapped using atrial extrastimuli to identify the site resulting in the greatest advancement of the next QRS complex with a fixed coupling interval. This is time-consuming and no longer recommended.
- RF application recommended as for conventional APs (📖 p. 366).
- RF at target site may result in a non-sustained pre-excited rhythm due to increased automaticity as AP heating occurs.
- Ablation success rate 90–95% when mapping 'M' potentials, with 5% recurrence rate.

Nodoventricular and nodofascicular connections

These are very rare forms of accessory AV connections, arising from the AV node and inserting into the right ventricular myocardium and distal RBB, respectively.

- They may result in narrow or broad complex SVT.
- AV dissociation may occur, since the upper turnaround for re-entry is contained within the AV node, so the atrial myocardium is not an obligate participant in the tachycardia circuit.
- A key distinction from atriofascicular APs is that APBs delivered during septal refractoriness will not advance the tachycardia. Since the AV node itself is participating in the tachycardia, APBs will only advance the tachycardia when septal activation itself is advanced.
- During antidromic tachycardia, the VH interval is short (<50 ms) for nodofascicular, or intermediate (50–80 ms) for nodoventricular APs in the absence of RBBB. This again relates to the proximity of the insertion point into the normal conduction system being the determinant of retrograde His activation and therefore the VH interval.

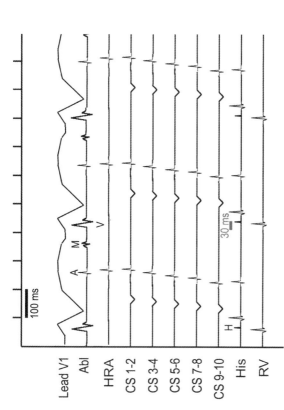

Fig. 18.8 AVRT due to an atriofascicular AP. The QRS morphology is LBBB. Retrograde activation is midline through the AV node. There is a negative HV interval (VH of 30 ms). An ablation catheter at the TV annulus near the CS os displays a pathway 'M' potential just before the onset of the QRS complex.

Coronary sinus 'epicardial' APs

A myocardial coat around the CS is present in all individuals, comprising bands of muscle arising from both atria. In most cases, this extends to the great cardiac vein, providing electrical continuity and possibly a substrate for AP conduction via insertion into the epicardial ventricular myocardium. Muscular sleeves may also cover the terminal portions of the middle and posterior cardiac vein, in 3% and 2% of hearts, respectively.
- Associated CS diverticulum in 21% (Fig. 18.9). The AP is often found at the neck.
  - Near-field high-frequency potentials, generated by the extensions of the CS muscular 'coat', are often present, occurring before the earliest recorded far-field ventricular potential.
- RF is both safe and effective within CS.
- Powers may be limited to 30 W maximum to minimize risk of damage to adjacent structures, particularly the RCA and its AV nodal branch:
  - Coronary angiography may be required to define anatomy.
  - Cryothermal energy delivery may be undertaken as an alternative, if too close to arterial branches.
- If unable to achieve adequate power due to poor blood flow around the catheter tip, irrigated-tip ablation may be needed.
- Damage to the CS is rare; however, thrombosis, stenosis, and perforation have been reported.

Atrial appendage-to-ventricular APs

This is a recognized variant of epicardial AV connection, representing <0.5% of all cases presenting for ablation of WPW syndrome. Anatomically they constitute a band-like muscular structure most commonly extending from the underside/apex of the RAA and inserting into the RV myocardium 5–10 mm apical to TV annulus.
- Pre-excitation patterns are consistent with anterior or anterolateral APs, with previously failed endocardial approach.
- Earliest retrograde atrial activation earlier at the appendage than the annulus.
- Relatively long tachycardia VA (consistent with longer, epicardial course).
- Earliest ventricular activation 5–10 mm towards the apex.
- Need for high energy delivery within the appendage to achieve success.
- Irrigated RF may be required.
- 3-D electroanatomical mapping systems may be beneficial:
  - Earliest retrograde atrial activation may then be more readily mapped and visualized for ablation.
  - Sub-xiphoid, epicardial access may also be required in rare cases.

Table 18.4 ECG clues to coronary sinus APs

Finding	Sensitivity (%)	Specificity (%)	PPV (%)
Steep negative delta lead II	87	79	50
Steep positive delta aVR	61	98	88
Deep S wave in V6 (R ≤ S)	70	87	57

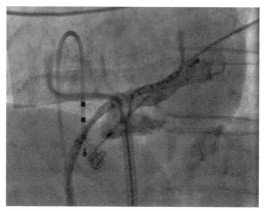

Fig. 18.9 Figure showing coronary sinus venography and diverticulum.

Ebstein's anomaly

This is the most common congenital defect associated with WPW syndrome. Ebstein's is characterized anatomically by apical displacement of the TV, with 'atrialization' of the right ventricular myocardium between the 'true annulus' and anomalous attachments of TV leaflets (Fig. 18.10).

• AVRT seen in 20–30%.
• Increased risk of sudden death in the presence of pre-excitation and symptomatic atrial arrhythmias (fibrillation or flutter).
• Multiple APs in up to 50%.
• APs right-sided in 96% – usually right posterior or posterolateral location.
• Baseline, non-pre-excited ECG usually RBBB – absence should raise suspicion of AP connection.
• Standard approach as for right-sided APs (📖 p. 366).
• Sources of difficulty include:
  • Presence of abnormal, fractionated electrograms along atrialized ventricular myocardium in ~50%.
  • Catheter instability – may be exacerbated by tricuspid regurgitation.
  • Multiple APs.
• Overall acute success in 76–90%.

Persistent left-sided SVC

This is the most common systemic venous anomaly, resulting from failure of involution of the left cardinal vein during embryological development.

• Incidence: 0.5% (4% of those with congenital heart disease).
• Associated with ASD, tetralogy of Fallot, AV canal defect, and partial anomalous pulmonary venous connections.
• Left SVC to LA connection, between LAA and left-sided PVs.
• Anastomosis with CS results in a left SVC to CS fistula.
• Rarely accompanied by absence of right SVC.
• Dilated CS on echocardiography.
• Usually discovered during CS cannulation (Fig. 18.11):
  • Inferior/jugular approach – CS catheter freely passes to left subclavian vein.
  • Left subclavian approach – abnormal course of catheter posteriorly to the left side of the heart.
• May complicate ablation of left-sided APs.
• Sources of difficulty:
  • Poor CS electrode contact making AP localization difficult.
  • Dilated CS may be at a site distant from MV annulus.

A single catheter approach may be required instead, with careful mapping of the MV annulus, if CS not a useful guide to ablation.

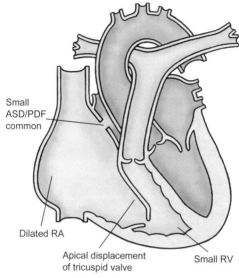

Small
ASD/PDF
common

Dilated RA

Apical displacement
of tricuspid valve

Small RV

Fig. 18.10 Diagrammatic representation of Ebstein's anomaly. This is often associated with other cardiac defects (PFO, ASD, VSD, and RVOT obstruction). (📖 Plate 13 for colour version.)

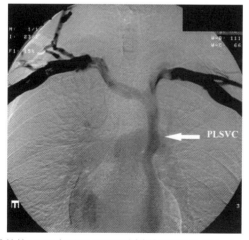

PLSVC

Fig. 18.11 Venogram showing a persistent left SVC draining down into a large CS and absent right SVC.

Multiple APs

These are defined as having a separation of at least 1–3 cm at the AV junction, based on an approximate distance during mapping. However, there may be difficulty in differentiating multiple from oblique or broadly inserting APs.

• Incidence 3–15%.
• Usually unilateral.
• Most frequently two APs present.
• Higher incidence suggested in patients with right free wall or posterior AP.
• Greater risk of sudden death in symptomatic patients.

Clues to diagnosis

• Associated with Ebstein's anomaly and a history of antidromic AVRT.

Invasive electrophysiological findings

• >1 pattern of ventricular pre-excitation during atrial pacing or AF.
• >1 pattern of atrial activation during RV pacing or AVRT.
• Pathway-to-pathway tachycardia (Fig. 18.12).
• Mismatch (>1 cm) between antegrade and retrograde limbs of the tachycardia circuit.
• Switch from orthodromic to antidromic AVRT, and vice versa.
• During pathway-to-pathway tachycardia, bundle branch block does not affect the TCL.

Approach to ablation

• Recognition of the presence of >1 AP is essential to avoiding primary ablation failure.
• A completed RF application at target sites should be undertaken before remapping.
• Close observation of the surface ECG for changes in pre-excitation pattern during RF application is essential in order to avoid multiple, incomplete RF applications.
• Multi-polar mapping catheters (CS or Halo catheters for left and right-sided APs, respectively) are also useful to identify subtle changes in intracardiac activation sequence.
• Procedure duration, number of RF applications, and radiation dose are higher than for single APs.
• Acute success rate 86–98%; recurrence rate 8–12%.

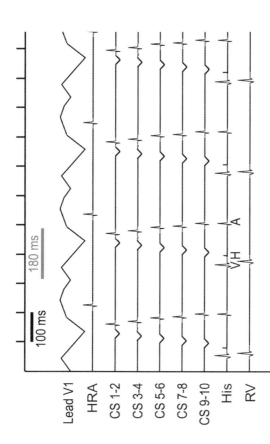

Fig. 18.12 Pathway-to-pathway tachycardia. There is a wide QRS consistent with ventricular pre-excitation with earliest ventricular activation in the His catheter, suggesting a right-sided AP. The negative HV interval (actually a VH interval) confirms antegrade activation is not through the AVN. The retrograde atrial activation pattern is eccentric with the earliest A in the distal CS, suggesting a left lateral AP as the retrograde limb.

Oblique APs (Fig. 18.13)

APs frequently follow an oblique course. Using a definition of a change in the local VA or AV interval of ≥15 ms during pacing from either side of the AP, Jackmann et al. demonstrated oblique APs to be present in 87% of patients with a single left- or right-sided AP.

Using such pacing manoeuvres, Jackmann et al. were also able to demonstrate an AP potential in 89% of cases and undertake successful ablation with a median of one RF application in 99 patients with an AP potential, versus 4.5 applications in 12 patients without an AP potential. Therefore, in cases where RF application at the shortest VA interval has been ineffective, attempts should be made to change the local VA by pacing either side of the AP and repeat mapping and ablation with a longer VA interval.

Reference

Otoma K, Gonzalez MD, Beckman KJ et al. (2001) Reversing the direction of paced ventricular and atrial wave fronts reveals an oblique course in accessory pathways and improves localization for catheter ablation. *Circulation*, **104**: 550–6.

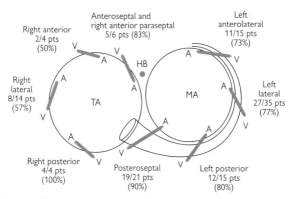

Fig. 18.13 Frequency of obliquely-orientated APs. Reproduced with permission from Otomo K, Gonzalez MD, Beckman KJ, *et al.* (2001) Reversing the direction of paced ventricular and atrial wavefronts reveals an oblique course in accessory pathways and improves localization for catheter ablation. *Circulation*, **104**: 550–556.

Permanent junctional reciprocating tachycardia (PJRT)

This is a rare form of tachycardia most commonly seen in newborns and infants, although it has been reported in rare adult cases. It is usually incessant due to the long tachycardia cycle length. It results from a concealed AP with slow conduction from the ventricle to atrium. The AP, which only conducts retrogradely, has decremental properties. The antegrade limb of the re-entrant circuit is the AV node and His-Purkinje system. The AP is usually in the right paraseptal region with the atrial insertion close to the coronary sinus ostium; however, other sites have been reported. Incessant tachycardia in the very young may result in tachycardia cardiomyopathy. The limited success of drug therapy means catheter ablation is frequently the treatment option of choice.

Key features
- No pre-excitation at baseline.
- An incessant long RP tachycardia (📖 p. 182).
- Initiation is with a VPB during sinus rhythm when the His is refractory – distinguishes PJRT from atypical AVNRT (📖 p. 242).
- During entrainment the VA interval prolongs due to the decremental properties of the AP.
- During tachycardia the A may be advanced with a His-synchronous VPB; however, the decremental properties of the AP may mean that the A is actually *delayed*.
- During tachycardia the VA interval increases with ipsilateral BBB.
- Ablate at the site of earliest atrial activation (with reference to P wave onset or a fixed CS electrode position) (Fig 18.14).

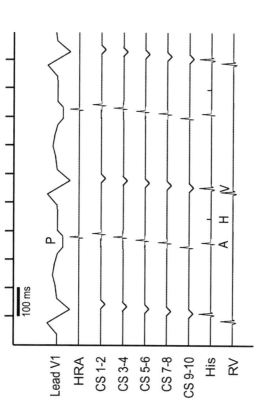

Fig. 18.14 PJRT. There is a regular, narrow complex long RP tachycardia. Earliest atrial activation is in the proximal CS (9-10).

Post-procedural management and advice

With modern technology and appropriate pre-operative work-up, advice, and hospital facilities, most cases may now be undertaken as day-case procedures.

Immediate post-operative management

- 12-lead ECG on return to ward to exclude AP recurrence and compare with pre-procedural ECG for evidence of damage to normal conduction system.
- CXR if subclavian access used to exclude pneumothorax.
- The value of post-procedural echocardiography in all cases has not been established, although many operators perform bedside scans in the EP lab before returning the patient to the recovery ward, particularly if TSP has been performed.
- Close haemodynamic monitoring for four hours, with bed rest. Tachycardia and hypotension may indicate pericardial effusion or femoral bleeding, although this rarely develops at this stage in otherwise uncomplicated cases.
- Four hours' bed rest followed by gentle mobilization if groin puncture sites appear satisfactory.
- A further ECG at six hours post-ablation, followed by an explanation of the procedure, advice, and hospital discharge.

Counselling and advice

- Driving – DVLA guidelines now state a two-day ban from driving. However, one week to allow healing of groin puncture sites seems prudent. The DVLA need not be notified.
- Exercise – normal activity may resume after one week, allowing healing of groin puncture sites. Keen sportsmen and women, particularly if exercise is high-impact, should desist for up to two weeks.
- Medications – anti-arrhythmic medications are stopped before the ablation procedure and should no longer be required. Aspirin 75 mg/day is recommended for all left-sided procedures for six weeks; some operators also recommend aspirin for right-sided ablation procedures.

Follow-up
- Outpatient follow-up generally arranged at 3–4 months following successful ablation. This allows sufficient time for an AP or arrhythmia recurrence to be documented, either as manifest AP conduction or recurrent symptoms.
- It is essential to obtain ECG documentation at the time of any recurrent symptoms to exclude benign palpitations (increased heart beat awareness during sinus rhythm), benign atrial or ventricular ectopy, and alternative arrhythmia mechanisms.
- Unsuccessful procedures may be scheduled for redo ablation following explanation of the reasons for failure.
  - Careful planning is required to identify the optimal redo approach, choice of energy (irrigated versus conventional RF or cryothermal energy), use of different access approaches (TSP vs. retrograde transaortic, jugular vs. femoral, epicardial vs. endocardial), the role of electroanatomical mapping systems, and assistance of additional colleagues.

Ablation of common atrial flutter

General information

Certain issues that frequently arise in respect of patients undergoing ablation for common atrial flutter are summarized below.

Patient information – risks/benefits

- Isthmus ablation abolishes common atrial flutter in >95% of cases but 5–10% will need redo procedures for recurrence of the arrhythmia.
- Long-term efficacy is limited by a significant incidence of atrial fibrillation (or atypical flutter), probably >30% within five years.
- Overall risk of fatality is 1/2000, although this may be higher in patients with advanced significant co-morbidity.
- Low risk of AV block, certainly <0.5%, but cases do occur, particularly with ablation towards the septal side of isthmus.
- Generally a more painful procedure than most SVT ablations because of the requirement to generate an extensive linear lesion. Deeper sedation/analgesia is needed unless cryoablation is used.

Peri-operative anticoagulation

- Can usually be withdrawn 3–5 days beforehand in patients with paroxysmal atrial flutter, unless there are other high-risk features (prior history of cerebral emboli, prosthetic heart valve etc.).
- Patients in persistent atrial flutter should be therapeutically anticoagulated for four weeks beforehand and continue warfarin peri-operatively. Provided the INR is below 3.0, ideally 2.0–2.5, the risk of haemorrhagic complications such as tamponade appears to be small. Anticoagulation should usually continue for three months post-operatively, although it can be withdrawn sooner in patients at low risk of thromboembolism.
- Patients with persistent atrial flutter but no prior anticoagulation requiring urgent ablation can undergo TOE to exclude left atrial thrombus. Following ablation, therapeutic anticoagulation for at least one month (usually three months) is required.

Anti-arrhythmic drug treatment

- There is no strict requirement to withdraw anti-arrhythmic medication beforehand, except in patients with paroxysmal atrial flutter in whom induction of the arrhythmia is deemed essential to check the mechanism, isthmus-dependence.
- Rate-controlling medications (β-blockers, digoxin etc.) should not be withdrawn in case that precipitates haemodynamic deterioration before or during the ablation.
- Following successful isthmus ablation, anti-arrhythmic drugs are normally withdrawn immediately unless required for a separate arrhythmia such as AF or VT.

Ablation technique

Ablation of the IVC-TA isthmus involves an electroanatomical approach, irrespective of the type of ablation catheter and mapping technique used. The standard method is to stabilize the ablation catheter over the isthmus region and then create a linear lesion by dragging the tip back from the ventricular margin of the tricuspid annulus to the rim of the IVC (Fig. 19.1). Patients who are in atrial flutter at the start of the procedure should convert back to sinus rhythm during creation of the linear lesion (confirming isthmus-dependency) but **ablation should always be continued until the primary endpoint of bidirectional isthmus conduction block is achieved** (⌸ p. 402).

Key points:
- Most commonly the lesion crosses the midpoint of the isthmus (i.e. the 6 o'clock point of the annulus in the LAO 45° projection; ⌸ Fig. 19.1) – more anterolaterally (beyond 7 o'clock) the isthmus is broader and thicker; at the septal end (beyond 5 o'clock) RF applications may be more painful and there is some risk of injury to the AV node. However, the precise orientation varies between individuals depending on local anatomy and the need to achieve a stable catheter position.
- To achieve stability requires a large curve ablation catheter (e.g. F curve or ≥3 cm) and/or long support sheath (e.g. SR0).
- The ablation catheter is advanced to the right ventricle, deflected onto the RA floor, and withdrawn until the bipolar signal exhibits a dominant V with a small A electrogram.
- RF application for 30–60 seconds, expecting to see diminishing atrial electrogram amplitude. The catheter is withdrawn towards the IVC until a fresh area of sharp atrial electrograms is reached and then RF application continues. As the tip is retracted, the bipolar electrogram becomes A dominant and the V signal disappears. RF application continues until the rim of the IVC is reached, at which point no local electrogram can be recorded.
- The linear lesion may be created by a succession of point-by-point applications with interruption of current delivery in between, or by continuous RF application during a slow drag-back of the catheter. The point-by-point technique allows more accurate analysis of the local atrial electrogram.
- Even once flutter terminates during RF application (Fig. 19.2), ablation must continue until isthmus conduction block is demonstrable, the primary endpoint.
- If the initial linear lesion fails to achieve isthmus block, the options are to deliver a new linear lesion in a more lateral or septal orientation, or 'spot welding' – searching for gaps or breakthrough sites in the original line, typically fractionated, polyphasic electrograms (Fig. 19.5). This technique requires high recording gain (e.g. 0.2 or 0.1 mV) and is the preferred approach for ablation when atrial flutter has recurred after an acutely successful isthmus ablation.

(A)   (B)

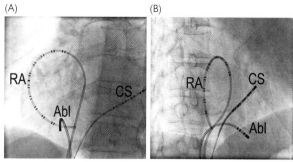

Fig. 19.1 Fluoroscopic views of typical catheter positions for cavotricuspid isthmus ablation. (A) Left anterior oblique view: The 20-pole multi-polar catheter (RA) encircles the tricuspid annulus with the distal poles (1–2) adjacent to the lateral aspect of the proposed ablation line and the proximal poles in the high atrium anterior to the superior vena cava. The ablation catheter (Abl) is at the 6 o'clock position. There is a ten-pole catheter in the coronary sinus (CS). (B) Right anterior oblique view: This demonstrates that the multi-polar catheter is in the anterior right atrium, between the crista terminalis and tricuspid annulus, and that the ablation catheter is at the annulus – this would be confirmed by seeing a large ventricular and small atrial electrogram in the distal ablation catheter poles.

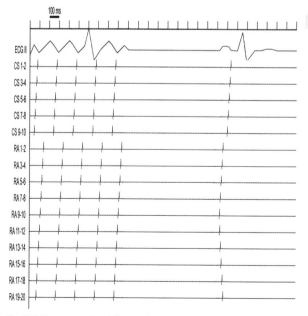

Fig. 19.2 Termination of atrial flutter and restoration of sinus rhythm.

Choice of ablation catheter and power source

The standard 4 mm-tip RF ablation catheters used so successfully for procedures requiring a single-point lesion (accessory pathways, slow pathway modification etc.) are less effective for creating the confluent linear lesions with conduction block needed for interrupting macroreen-trant circuits such as common atrial flutter. Therefore the most commonly used technologies (with pros and cons) are:

- Large 8 mm-tip RF ablation catheters:
  - Allow higher power delivery (typically 70–150 W) for more extensive, deeper lesions.
  - Fewer catheter movements to complete linear lesion.
  - May be difficult to achieve proper coaptation to isthmus in some cases.
  - 8 mm electrode is less good for identifying residual 'gaps' in the line of block (characterized by complex multi-phasic electrograms) for 'spot welding' (📖 p. 398).
- Irrigated or cooled 4 mm-tip RF ablation catheters:
  - Deliver more extensive, deeper lesions.
  - Better coaptation with awkward isthmus anatomy.
  - 4 mm tip is ideal for 'spot welding' of residual gaps (📖 p. 407).
  - Clearly shown to facilitate isthmus ablation compared to standard catheters by RCTs.
- Cryoablation catheters (large tip, e.g. 10 mm):
  - Painless lesion generation (therefore ideal for patients with relative contraindications to sedation/opiate analgesia, e.g. severe respiratory disease).
  - Stable catheter position due to icing effect (📖 p. 44).
  - Poor electrogram resolution for 'spot welding'.

Ablation endpoints – assessment of cavotricuspid isthmus conduction

Bidirectional isthmus conduction block is now the accepted endpoint for ablation of common atrial flutter, predicting a low incidence of recurrent flutter (<10%) compared to the traditional endpoint of flutter termination/non-inducibility (>30%). In addition, adopting isthmus block as the endpoint enables ablation to be performed in sinus rhythm during continuous pacing and is not dependent on induction of the arrhythmia in patients with paroxysmal atrial flutter. Some general points about evaluation of isthmus conduction are summarized below:

- All assessment techniques depend on pacing from both sides of the ablation line, either adjacent to the isthmus itself (usually performed via the ablation catheter) or at the low lateral RA and low septum (usually performed via the distal poles of the Halo catheter and the proximal poles of the CS catheter, respectively).
- Assessment of isthmus conduction and block may be challenging in a significant minority of cases regardless of the method used, particularly differentiation of incomplete isthmus ablation with conduction delay (i.e. still potentially able to support flutter) from complete isthmus block. Correct catheter positioning is vital to avoid the appearance of 'pseudo-block' (Fig. 19.3).
- Pacing close to the ablation line minimizes the chance of failure to detect residual slow isthmus conduction.
- The term 'bidirectional' conduction block refers to abolition of trans-isthmus conduction in both clockwise (septal → lateral) and counter-clockwise (lateral → septal) directions. In practice, unidirectional conduction block is seen in <5% of ablation procedures and so some operators only test conduction in one direction (most commonly clockwise) and accept that as a surrogate for bidirectional block. This applies particularly to cases performed using 3-D-mapping systems, as mapping of the reverse activation map may be time-consuming (📖 p. 412).
- Although this chapter describes assessment of isthmus conduction using a multipolar halo catheter to record RA activation on a beat-to-beat basis during ablation, CTI ablation procedures are commonly performed with a two-catheter set-up (CS plus ablation catheter, without 3D mapping. Isthmus conduction is assessed after ablation using the ablation catheter to record or pace at sites lateral to the ablation line. Beat-to-beat changes in isthmus conduction may still be detected during ablation from 'splitting' of the local electrogram recorded via the ablation catheter (📖 p. 404).

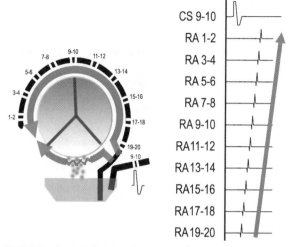

Fig. 19.3 Pseudo-block. The isthmus has been partially ablated. During pacing from the proximal coronary sinus (CS 9-10) a wavefront still travels slowly through the isthmus in a clockwise direction, but as the 20-pole right atrial catheter has been positioned incorrectly with the distal poles (RA 1-2) high up the lateral wall, it does not record it and only shows the counter-clockwise wavefront activating the RA catheter sequentially from 19-20 to 1-2 and giving the appearance of block. Repositioning the catheter with the distal poles adjacent to the ablation line would show a chevron pattern and reveal isthmus conduction (📖 Fig. 19.4).

Right atrial activation sequence

- Pre-ablation, pacing from low lateral RA or low septum, results in two colliding wavefronts (clockwise and counter-clockwise directions) and a 'chevron' pattern of RA activation (Fig. 19.4).
- This is easier to appreciate with septal or PCS pacing, i.e. clockwise activation across isthmus, because the wavefronts collide along the lateral RA wall and are readily apparent on the multi-polar Halo recording. Pacing from the low lateral RA, the collision occurs in the septal region where it is more difficult to achieve activation mapping with standard Halo-type catheters.
- Successful isthmus ablation eliminates one of the wavefronts, resulting in 'straightening' of the activation sequence – with low septal pacing, abolition of the clockwise trans-isthmus wavefront produces an exclusively counter-clockwise RA activation sequence in the Halo catheter (Fig. 19.4), with cranio-caudal activation of the lateral RA wall.
- This technique is ideally suited for beat-to-beat assessment of isthmus conduction during ablation delivery. In most cases isthmus block is heralded by an abrupt change in activation sequence, although occasionally the sequence may change more gradually over the course of 10–15 seconds of RF power application.
- Differentiating incomplete isthmus ablation with slow residual conduction can still be a problem but is rare if an abrupt beat-to-beat change in RA activation is observed during RF application.

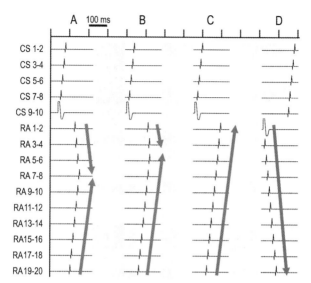

Fig. 19.4 Right atrial activation sequence during pacing before, during, and after ablation. (A) Pre-ablation pacing from proximal coronary sinus (9-10) produces two wavefronts. Conduction travels through the isthmus in a clockwise direction (RA1-2 to 7-8) and around the superior tricuspid valve annulus in a counter-clockwise direction (RA19-20 to 9-10). The two wavefronts collide in the lateral RA wall. (B) After some ablation there is slowing of isthmus conduction but block is not complete as activation still travels through the isthmus in a clockwise direction (RA 1-2 to 3-4). (C) There is now clockwise isthmus block as there is only one wavefront that travels counter-clockwise around the entire length of the multi-polar catheter (RA 19-20 to 1-2). (D) Bidirectional block is confirmed by switched pacing to the low lateral RA wall (RA 1-2) and RA activation is through a single clockwise wavefront that travels from RA 19-20 to 1-2, followed by proximal CS activation.

Widely-split double potentials (DP)

- Isthmus block is characterized by recording split or double electrograms separated by an isoelectric baseline along the entire course of the ablation line. Each component represents arrival of the two activation wavefronts to either side of the line of block, the earlier due to local activation from the adjacent pacing site, the later from activation around the RA septum/lateral wall or vice versa (Fig. 19.5). These can be recorded via the ablation catheter at high-gain settings but may be difficult to detect in up to 30% of cases because of extensive local electrogram destruction.

- Although there are no universally agreed criteria, complete isthmus block is associated with DP isoelectric interval >90 ms along the entire line, whereas any DP interval <90 ms implies some residual conduction. Complete block can probably be assumed if any DP interval >110 ms can be recorded along the ablation line.

- If detectable via the ablation catheter, DP splitting can be used to assess beat-to-beat changes in isthmus conduction during RF application. DP mapping is also useful for assessment of isthmus conduction with minimalist two-catheter technique, including ablation of flutter performed with 3-D mapping (p. 412).

- Spurious DP electrograms may be recorded due to local conduction disturbances unrelated to block of isthmus conduction. Differentiation may require additional techniques such as differential pacing (p. 408).

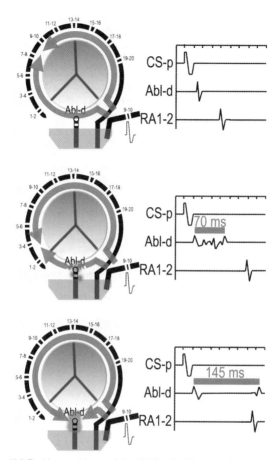

Fig. 19.5 Double potentials recorded on Abl-d on the ablation line during CS proximal (9-10) pacing. Top figure: Before ablation, pacing results in rapid conduction through the isthmus, and a single electrogram in Abl-d, which comes before RA 1-2. Middle figure: Following ablation but incomplete block there is delayed conduction through the isthmus. The slow conduction through the injured myocardium results in a complex fractionated electrogram in Abl-d. The time from beginning to end of the electrogram is 70 ms and it is then followed by RA 1-2. Bottom figure: With complete isthmus block there is an early electrogram in Abl-d from the blocked clockwise wavefront. This is followed by an isoelectric line while the counter-clockwise wavefront travels around the tricuspid annulus before arriving at the lateral side of the line, producing a second electrogram and widely split double potentials measuring 145 ms. The second component comes after RA 1-2.

Differential pacing
- Usually used in conjunction with DP mapping.
- Moving the pacing site further away from the isthmus line should increase the interval to the first (local activation) component but shorten the interval to the second (remote activation) component (Fig. 19.6).
- If the interval to the second potential also increases, that may indicate residual but delayed isthmus conduction.

Trans-isthmus conduction interval
- Pacing adjacent to the ablation line via distal Halo or proximal CS and measure earliest local atrial activation on the opposite side.
- Residual conduction very likely if conduction interval <120 ms.
- Isthmus block likely if conduction interval >140 ms but some overlap with cases of incomplete block/conduction delay.
- Simplest but probably least reliable technique for assessing isthmus conduction, used on its own. Valuable 'screening' technique during ablation with 3-D mapping systems (may reduce the need for time-consuming remaps).

Common errors/pitfalls in assessment of isthmus are:
- Incorrect placement of Halo catheter resulting in misdiagnosis of isthmus block.
- Pacing too far away from ablation line with failure to detect residual conduction.
- Spurious double potentials due to local conduction disturbance unrelated to ablation line.

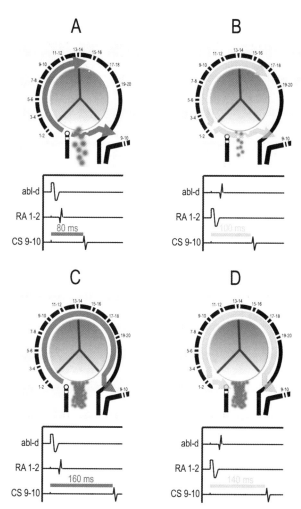

Fig. 19.6 Differential pacing on the lateral side of the ablation line and recording in CS proximal (9-10). Top two panels show incomplete isthmus block (A). Pacing from adjacent to the isthmus line produces a shorter stimulus to CS 9–10 time than pacing from a more lateral position (B). The bottom two panels show complete isthmus block (C). Pacing from adjacent to the line produces a longer stimulus to CS 9–10 time than pacing from a more lateral position (D). (□ Plate 15 for colour version.)

Difficult cases – what to do

In a minority of difficult cases, it may prove impossible to interrupt flutter and/or achieve isthmus block, despite very extensive ablation around the isthmus region. The following possibilities should be considered:

- If in sinus rhythm, reassess isthmus conduction to double-check residual breakthrough.
- If in atrial flutter, reassess activation sequence and response to entrainment etc. in case it is not an isthmus-dependent form (e.g. cristal breakout).
- Consider use of long support sheath (e.g. SR0) to facilitate stabilization of ablation catheter on the isthmus and optimal tip contact.
- If using 8 mm tip or cryoablation, switch to irrigated 4 mm tip.
- Retroflexion technique, i.e. introducing ablation catheter deep into the RV and deflecting the tip maximally back towards the tricuspid annulus to access myocardial tissue within the sub-eustachian recess that may have been 'shielded' by a prominent eustachian ridge (Fig. 19.7).
- Occasionally, extensive ablation may result in acute oedematous changes over the isthmus region that act as a barrier to elimination of viable myocardium. Anecdotal experience suggests that ablation may be straightforward if the patient is brought back after a gap of 4–6 weeks to allow these changes to resolve. In a few of these cases, lesion progression and fibrotic healing may even have produced complete isthmus conduction block by the time of restudy, obviating the need for further intervention.

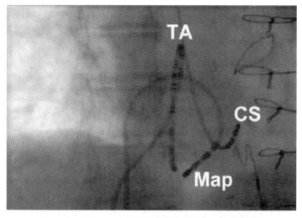

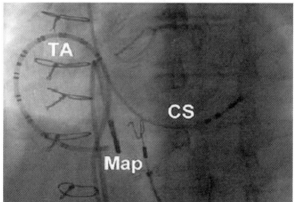

Fig. 19.7 Retroflexion (inversion) of the ablation catheter (Map) to get the tip deep into folds between the pectinate muscles. The top image is in a RAO projection, the bottom image is in an LAO projection.

Ablation of common atrial flutter with 3-D mapping systems

Although ablation of common atrial flutter using conventional electrophysiological techniques (as described) is straightforward, ablation guided by 3-D mapping (📖 Chapter 6) is also widely practised. Potential advantages include reduced radiation exposure, fewer catheters needed, and acquiring greater expertise/experience with 3-D mapping systems generally, which may improve performance when treating more complex arrhythmias (📖 Chapter 6) that cannot be managed by conventional electrophysiological techniques. In addition, cavotricuspid isthmus may be performed adjunctively as part of an AF ablation procedure, in which the 3-D mapping system will already be in use. Key points are:

- Typically requires only the ablation catheter and one other quadripolar/multi-polar catheter for pacing/referencing (e.g. a CS electrode).
- Geometric and activation mapping of the RA may be performed simultaneously or sequentially. Important landmarks to define are the IVC, SVC, CS, His bundle, and tricuspid annulus. Some operators also mark the line of the crista terminalis.
- If the patient is in atrial flutter at the start of the procedure, activation mapping should use a window equal to 90% of the flutter cycle length, with the timing set to the reference catheter such that the 'head-meets-tail' will fall into the area of interest, i.e. the isthmus (Fig. 19.8).
- Even if the RA activation map suggests common atrial flutter, it is advisable to confirm isthmus-dependence by entrainment (📖 p. 284).
- If the patient is in sinus rhythm, it is preferable to obtain a baseline map of RA activation during pacing (from the low lateral RA or proximal CS) for comparison with post-ablation, taking care to exclude the stimulus artefact from the mapping window.
- Ablation may be performed without fluoroscopy by using two projections: (i) LAO with caudal tilt to display the tricuspid annulus and check septal/lateral orientation of the catheter; and (ii) RAO to assess dragback of the catheter tip from TA to IVC.
- Isthmus conduction may be assessed beat-to-beat during RF application by DP splitting if a high-gain setting is used, or between applications by measurement of trans-isthmus conduction time.
- The ablation lesion markers facilitate identification of gaps in the ablation line for 'spot welding' if isthmus conduction is still demonstrable after creation of the initial linear lesion.
- Once the local electrograms are suggestive of conduction block it is appropriate to repeat the activation map to confirm isthmus conduction block, with detailed acquisition immediately adjacent to the isthmus line. As activation mapping can be time-consuming, confirmation of complete conduction block in one direction (most commonly clockwise using proximal CS pacing) is acceptable.

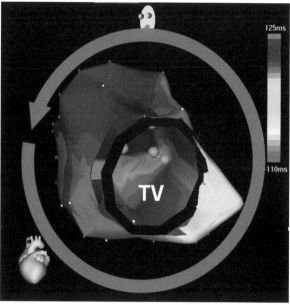

Fig. 19.8 An isochronal activation map of the right atrium during typical atrial flutter displayed in an LAO view. The colours represent activation timings. The entire cycle length of the tachycardia is spread around the tricuspid valve in a coun-ter-clockwise direction (red to yellow to green to blue to purple) with the head meeting the tail. (📖 Plate 16 for colour version.)

Atrial fibrillation ablation

Introduction

Catheter ablation may be performed to achieve rhythm-control of either permanent/persistent AF or paroxysmal AF. It is the most rapidly growing intervention in modern cardiology, reflecting that:

• AF is a common arrhythmia. Incidence increases with age and the prevalence reaches 15% in the over 80s.
• Conventional pharmacological therapy for rhythm-control is relatively ineffective.
• Rhythm-control improves quality of life in those patients with intrusive symptoms despite rate-control (although it has not been shown to increase survival or prevent stroke/embolic complications compared to a rate-control strategy in RCTs).

Current strategies for left atrial ablation to prevent AF have evolved from the catheter-based approached to pulmonary vein-triggered focal AF pioneered by Dr Haissaguerre and the surgical Maze procedures developed by Dr Cox. Particular emphasis has been given to the critical role of the pulmonary veins in the initiation and perpetuation of AF (📖 p. 304). A range of anatomical and electrogram-guided techniques are deployed in various permutations and combinations by individual operators, using different mapping systems and/or ablation technology. As there is currently no consensus about the optimal approach, this chapter will describe the general principles and most commonly used ablation strategies.

These modern AF ablation techniques should only be undertaken by operators with substantial experience in cardiac electrophysiology and ablation. Specific requirements include:

• Proficiency in trans-septal puncture and catheter manipulation (📖 Chapter 5).
• Experience with 3-D electroanatomical mapping (📖 Chapter 6).
• Familiarity with key anatomical relations of the left atrium (Fig. 20.1):
  • Location/orientation of pulmonary veins and common variants.
  • Relationship of LA appendage to left-sided pulmonary veins.
  • Location of mitral annulus, mitral isthmus, and distal CS.
  • Awareness of adjacent structures at risk of iatrogenic injury (especially the oesophagus, phrenic nerves, and coronary arteries).

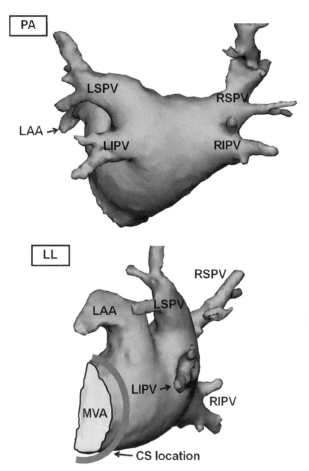

Fig. 20.1 Diagram showing key anatomical relations for left atrial catheter ablation procedures. RSPV – right upper pulmonary vein; RIPV – right lower pulmonary vein; LSPV – left upper pulmonary vein; LIPV – left lower pulmonary vein; LAA – left atrial appendage; MVA – mitral valve annulus; CS – coronary sinus. Upper panel PA (postero-anterior) projection. Lower panel LL (left lateral) projection.

Selection of patients for ablation

Indications

Catheter ablation should be considered in cases with documented paroxysmal or persistent AF and intrusive symptoms, normally after failure to achieve rhythm-control with ≥2 anti-arrhythmic drugs (whether due to inefficacy or intolerance). Patients should be made familiar with risks, overall efficacy, and need for repeat procedures. Only suitable for motivated individuals.

'Non-indications'

- Minimal or no symptoms.
- Rhythm-control achieved by anti-arrhythmic drugs without side-effects (there may be some exceptions).
- Desire to avoid long-term anticoagulation (currently no evidence).
- Desire for long-term 'cure' (limited data on efficacy beyond five years).

Cautions

- Long-standing permanent AF (say >5 years). Decreased efficacy.
- Major structural heart disease – increased procedural risks and lower overall efficacy.
- Age >75 years – increased procedural risks (especially stroke) but efficacy is probably not affected.

Patient preparation

Informed consent
- Success rates:
  - Paroxysmal AF 75–85%.
  - Persistent AF 60–75%.

(Usually defined as rhythm-control off anti-arrhythmic drugs but may include substantially improved rhythm-control ± drugs.)

- Redo rates:
  - Paroxysmal AF 20–40%.
  - Persistent AF 50–75%.
- Complications to be mentioned include:
  - Fatality (1:1000).
  - Stroke (0.5–10%).
  - Tamponade (1–5%).
  - Pulmonary vein stenosis.
  - Vascular injury.
  - Worsening atrial arrhythmias (may be self-limiting).

Pre-operative imaging
Left atrial/pulmonary vein geometry is often assessed by cross-sectional imaging (MR angiography or contrast CT) prior to the procedure. Essential if image-integration mapping is to be used (p. 112).

Management of peri-operative anti-thrombotic treatment
- Transoesophageal echocardiography (TOE) performed (ideally) immediately prior to ablation to exclude intracardiac thrombus.
- Pre-operative anticoagulation with warfarin:
  - For at least four weeks at therapeutic INR if persistent AF.
  - For long enough to achieve stable INR if paroxysmal AF.
- Peri-operatively – two approaches commonly used:
  - Continue warfarin, maintaining INR 2.0–2.5. Any intra-operative bleeding complications treated by reversal with FFP or Beriplex® (human prothrombin complex).
  - Discontinue warfarin three days pre-op and restart immediately afterwards, covering early post-op period with LMW-heparin injections (usually self-administered at home) until INR >2.0.
- Post-operative anticoagulation:
  - Required for at least two months while left atrium re-endothelializes.
  - Greatest risk is early on, hence need to continue warfarin or 'bridge' early post-op period with LMW heparin.

Procedural issues and equipment choices

Sedation vs. GA

The ablation procedure may be performed under sedation or general anaesthesia according to local practice and physician/patient preference. GA may be preferred for redo procedures if the initial left atrial ablation under sedation was poorly tolerated.

Peri-operative anticoagulation

📖 Management of peri-operative anti-thrombotic treatment.

Intra-operative anticoagulation

IV heparin to maintain ACT >300 as soon as left atrial access is obtained (some operators prefer to start heparinization prior to trans-septal puncture).

Irrigation

Continuous irrigation of trans-septal sheath(s) with saline or heparinized saline (>60 ml/hour) is also recommended to minimize thrombus formation and hence procedural stroke risk (also to reduce risk of air embolism). However, this adds to total fluid burden.

Mapping system

- Fluoroscopy-guidance with conventional multi-polar mapping catheters, usually circumferential PV catheter plus CS decapolar catheter.
- 3-D electroanatomical system with geometric mapping.
- 3-D mapping with image integration.
- Integrated circumferential PV mapping/ablation catheters ('**PVAC**', Ablation Frontiers™), usually guided by fluoroscopy.

Ablation technology

- Irrigated-tip RF ablation catheters (most commonly used modality).
- Conventional RF with large (8 mm)-tip catheters.
- Ablation Frontiers™.
- Cryoablation including cryo balloon.

Trans-septal sheaths

- Pre-shaped – cheaper but less manoeuvrable.
- Steerable – more expensive but facilitate catheter stability and placement.

Remote navigation systems

Rationale is to reduce procedure time, improve catheter stabilization (especially around right-sided PVs), and decrease operator radiation exposure.

- Magnetic remote navigation ('**Stereotaxis**') – more expensive and requires larger, customized EP lab.
- Robotic arms ('**Hansen**').

Biophysical parameters for AF ablation

- Assuming use of irrigated-tip (cooled) ablation catheters, standard settings are:
  - Maximum 30 W (power) and 48°C (temp.).
  - Irrigation up to 20 ml/min (ablation), 2 ml/min (background).
- Particular care needed ablating along posterior wall (risk of oesophageal injury), therefore catheter tip should be moved frequently.
- Higher powers may be required for specific situations:
  - Mitral isthmus ablation (□ p. 438) up to 40–50 W near annulus.
  - Cavotricuspid isthmus ablation up to 40–50 W.
  - Rarely up to 35–40 W for difficult PV isolation at antral level and away from posterior wall (usually ablating between the LA appendage and left-sided PVs).
- Lower powers should be used for epicardial ablation via the coronary sinus, usually 20–30 W.
- Continuous impedance monitoring should be used routinely, especially if the catheter tip is being repositioned without interrupting current delivery. Depending on the mapping system used and equipment setup, impedance measurements may vary over a wide range but any sudden increase by >20–30 Ω usually indicates that the catheter has slipped beyond the PV ostium and further current application may risk injury and development of PV stenosis.

Ablation strategies, techniques, and endpoints

Modern left atrial ablation procedures for AF may incorporate: (i) empirical ablation based on anatomical landmarks; (ii) targeted ablation guided by local electrograms; (iii) 'stepwise' approaches combining (i) and (ii). The principal techniques are:

- Anatomical techniques to electrically isolate the pulmonary veins (PVs) from the left atrium (LA), given their critical role in arrhythmogenesis (Fig. 20.2(A)):
  - Segmental ostial PV isolation.
  - Antral PV isolation.
  - PV isolation as part of wide-area circumferential ablation (WACA), also referred to as left atrial circumferential ablation (LACA).
- Isolation of non-PV sites responsible for triggering and maintaining AF (e.g. SVC, crista terminalis, CS, ligament of Marshall).
- Modification of atrial substrate to make AF less sustainable. Ablation is guided by '**rotor mapping**', i.e. lesions delivered at sites exhibiting '**complex fractionated atrial electrograms**' (📖 p. 434) (Fig. 20.2(B)).
- Compartmentalization of the LA to prevent macroreentry and reduce the risk of post-ablation macroreentrant atrial tachyarrhythmias (📖 p. 436). This is achieved as a result of LACA combined with linear ablation, most commonly of the **LA roof** (between the two upper PVs, the '**roof line**') and the **mitral isthmus** (left lower PV to mitral annulus) (Fig. 20.2(C)).

These techniques may overlap to some extent. For example, LACA may not only isolate arrhythmogenic sites within the PV and their antra but also contribute to rhythm-control via incidental LA debulking (by 20–30%) and elimination of rotors and/or ganglionated plexi.

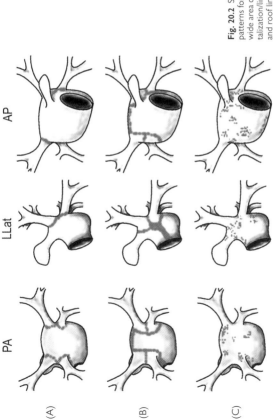

Fig. 20.2 Schematic diagram showing typical lesion patterns for (A) ostial/segmental PV isolation; (B) wide area circumferential ablation with compartmentalization/linear ablation (WACA plus mitral isthmus and roof lines); and (C) electrogram-guided ablation.

AP

LLat

PA

(A)

(B)

(C)

PV isolation techniques

With recognition of the important role of PV/LA interactions in the pathogenesis of AF, empiric isolation of the pulmonary veins has emerged as a key component of AF catheter ablation strategies, either as a stand-alone treatment or in conjunction with other techniques (see below).

The pulmonary veins contain myocardial sleeves extending out from the left atrium that are in electrical continuity with the atrial myocardium (normally bidirectional). This PV musculature may be segmentally distributed and generates sharp, high-frequency endocardial deflections or '**PV potentials**' that can be recorded by multi-polar catheters positioned within the vein (Figs. 20.3 and 20.4). The procedure endpoint or aim is to achieve complete electrical disconnection of all four veins from the left atrium.

Originally ablation was performed at ostial level using a segmental approach until isolation of each vein had been achieved, but increasingly therapy is delivered at antral or atrial level to reduce the risk of PV stenosis. The technical options are described below.

Simple fluoroscopic guidance ('Bordeaux technique')

- Double trans-septal puncture.
- Selective angiography to define PV anatomy/identify location of ostia.
- Deployment of a circumferential PV mapping catheter (Lasso™, Orbiter™, Optima™ etc.) to record the PV potentials and assess electrical isolation on a beat-to-beat basis.
- In segmental ostial isolation, lesions are targeted at site of earliest PV activation.
- Proximity of the ablation catheter to the correct area is suggested by contact artefact in the corresponding poles of the PV circumferential catheter and subsequently by electrical interference in the same poles when RF current is switched on.
- The site of earliest activation typically shifts progressively during ablation until isolation is achieved (Fig. 20.6).

This was the original technique for PV isolation but is seldom used nowadays because of the complexity of LA anatomy and difficulty in judging ostial location, requiring substantial operator experience to undertake without the assistance of 3-D mapping or other modern technologies.

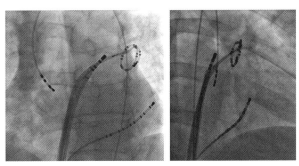

Fig. 20.3 Fluoroscopic images of 'traditional' setup for PV isolation, with PV circumferential mapping catheter in LSPV, ablation catheter, and CS mapping catheter. The quadripolar catheter in the aorta is the reference catheter for the NavX mapping system. LAO on the left, RAO on the right.

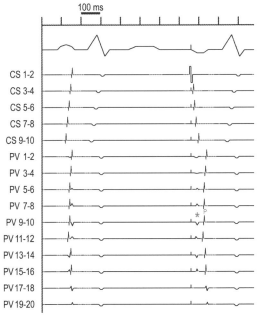

Fig. 20.4 Normal PV electrogram patterns during sinus rhythm (left) and CS pacing (right) to show separation of local PV activity (*P) from far-field atrial activity.

3-D mapping ± image integration

- Essentially the same technique but the 3-D electroanatomical system enables more accurate delineation of the PV ostium/antrum and facilitates navigation/catheter positioning.
- Following trans-septal puncture, either geometric mapping or image integration (📖 Chapter 6) is undertaken to establish left atrium/PV geometry.
- Lesions are targeted at antral and/or atrial rather than ostial sites but ostial segmental ablation may be required in a few cases to achieve PV isolation.
- As lesions are delivered progressively further away from the veins, this method merges into wide area circumferential ablation/LACA (📖 p. 432).
- Single ablation catheter may be used for both ablation and to assess PV isolation but this has some disadvantages:
  - PV isolation cannot be monitored on a beat-to-beat basis.
  - More likely to miss residual PV connections.
  - In cases where PV isolation proves challenging, a circumferential mapping catheter aids identification of breakthrough sites.
  - Cannot use LA appendage pacing to assess far-field signals (Fig. 20.8).

ICE guidance

- Enables very accurate delineation of ostial/antral anatomy. Ideal for PV isolation at antral level.
- Detects 'cavitation' due to excessive thermal injury at catheter tip (increased risk of complications).
- More expensive without convincing data showing superior efficacy to other techniques, so not much used outside USA.

Ablation Frontiers

- Integrated mapping and ablation circumferential PV catheter (PVAC™) positioned with fluoroscopic guidance based on selective angiography (Fig. 20.5).
- RF lesions applied at sites of earliest PV activation.
- If the vein remains connected, the PVAC is rotated and further lesions delivered until isolation is achieved.
- Advantages of this technique include:
  - Speed/simplicity (= shorter procedure times).
  - Avoids the need for 3-D mapping.
  - Single trans-septal puncture.
- Although the PVAC may result in more ostial than antral ablation, results to date suggest a low risk of PV stenosis.

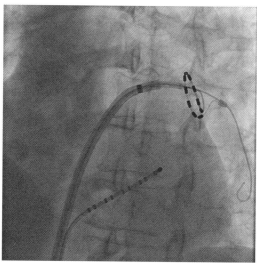

Fig. 20.5 Fluoroscopic image (LAO) of Ablation Frontiers PVAC™ plus CS mapping catheter. The PVAC is in the left superior pulmonary vein and the introducer wire is seen extending into the pulmonary vein.

Determining PV isolation

This is the most commonly used and important electrophysiological end-point in modern AF ablation procedures. All operators must be familiar with the electrogram patterns recorded from within the pulmonary veins and their interpretation, including differentiating PV potentials from far-field signals. PV isolation is indicated by:

- Elimination of all PV potentials recorded via the circumferential mapping (Fig. 20.6) and ablation catheters (or PVAC if using Ablation Frontiers).

  OR

- Entrance block into the PVs with dissociated PV potentials (Fig. 20.7(A)).

- Some operators also check for exit block by pacing at multiple sites within the PV or antrum (Fig. 20.7(B)).
- Ideally, electrical disconnection should be confirmed during isoprenaline or adenosine infusion.
- Differentiating residual PV potentials from far-field signals (arising from the LA, RA, LA appendage, or SVC) is often required (Fig. 20.8):
  - Distal CS pacing is commonly used to split the PV potentials from local atrial signals (Fig. 20.4), especially mapping within the left-sided veins.
  - Deflections >60 ms after a CS pacing spike are unlikely to arise from the LA body but could represent either PV potentials or far-field signals arising from the LA appendage.
  - Pacing within the LA appendage (via the ablation catheter) advances far-field LA appendage signals whereas true residual PV potentials remain delayed.
  - In the right-sided veins, post-ablation potentials that are low frequency and relatively early may represent far-field right atrial activity.
  - Rarely, delayed far-field signals arising from the SVC may be recorded within the right upper PV – pacing in the SVC with local capture should advance these far-field signals but not residual PV potentials.

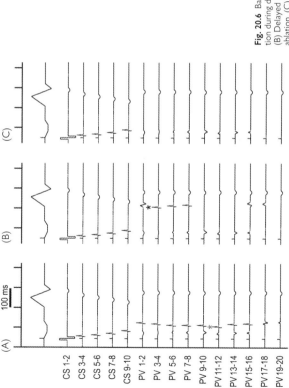

Fig. 20.6 Basic PV isolation technique. (A) Normal PV activation during distal CS pacing pre-ablation, with PV potential (*). (B) Delayed PV conduction (*) with altered activation during ablation. (C) PV isolation with loss of PV potentials.

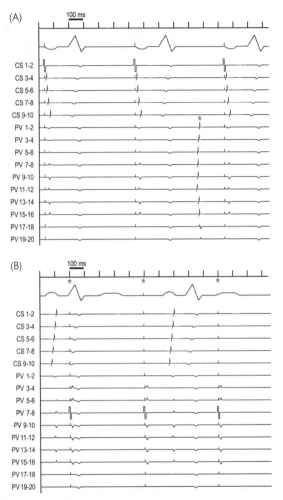

Fig. 20.7 PV dissociation. (A) During ablation, normal PV activation gives way to entry block with dissociation of PV potential (*). Isoprenaline infusion at 10 mcg/min restored 1:1 LA-PV conduction, confirming residual PV connection. Following application of further lesions at the site of earliest activation, PV dissociation was restored even during catecholamine infusion. (B) Pacing inside the vein results in local capture of the PV potential (*) but with exit block to the LA.

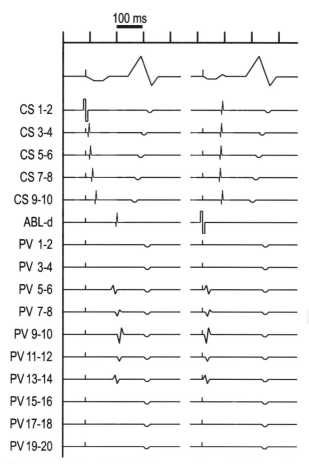

Fig. 20.8 Differentiation of far-field LAA electrograms from residual PV potentials within the left-sided veins. Following LACA, PV potential activity has diminished markedly but a circumferential PV mapping catheter in LSPV and the ablation catheter still show a sharp, delayed electrogram during CS pacing, consistent with residual PV connection (left). However, following placement of the ablation catheter within the LA appendage the timing of the electrogram in the PV mapping catheter is identical to LAA activation and is advanced by LAA pacing via the ablation catheter, confirming that this is an LAA far-field signal with complete isolation of LSPV (right).

Wide area/left atrial circumferential ablation (WACA or LACA)

This technique was originally pioneered by Pappone *et al.* and involves wide encirclement of the pulmonary veins (outside the antra) by sequential RF lesions, either of the ipsilateral veins in pairs or of each individual vein (Fig. 20.9).

- Usually guided by 3-D-mapping to ensure confluence/overlapping of RF lesions and complete encirclement.
- Most operators aim to achieve PV isolation as an explicit endpoint guided by a circumferential PV mapping catheter (□ p. 428). Some use an ablation catheter alone to assess residual PV conduction.
- A few operators undertake LACA using a purely anatomical approach without PV isolation as an explicit endpoint.
- PV isolation may require additional ablation at antral or ostial level, with breakthrough most often via sites within the intervenous ridges.
- In addition to PV isolation, LACA results in significant atrial substrate modification via debulking and possibly by isolating antral arrhythmogenic foci and ganglionated plexi.
- LACA is technically more challenging and may increase the tendency to LA macroreentry but improves outcomes compared to ostial segmental PV isolation, probably due to the exclusion of more arrhythmogenic tissue at the LA-PV junction.
- LACA reduces risk of PV stenosis and phrenic nerve injury.

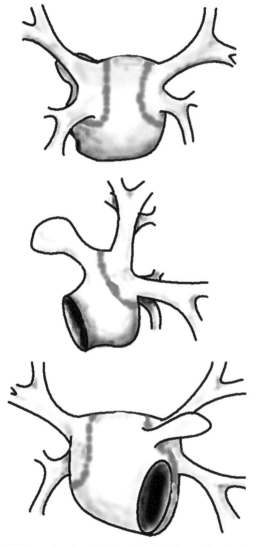

Fig. 20.9 Wide area circumferential ablation lesion set (without additional roof or mitral isthmus lines). Ipsilateral veins are encircled as a pair. It is sometimes necessary to perform additional ablation at the intervenous carina between the upper and lower veins to achieve isolation. Top panel = PA; middle panel = LLAT; bottom panel = AP.

Electrogram-guided ablation

Also known as 'rotor ablation' or 'defragmentation'. This approach was pioneered by Nadamanee and aims for atrial substrate modification to make AF less sustainable. It may be deployed either as a stand-alone treatment or as part of a 'stepwise approach' in conjunction with LACA ± linear ablation (📖 p. 448).

- Ablation guided by '**rotor mapping**', i.e. lesions delivered at sites exhibiting **CFAEs** characterized by short CL (<120 ms), fractionation, or continuous electrical activity **during AF** (induced for paroxysmal AF cases) (Fig. 20.10):
  - Such signals may indicate sites of delayed conduction, pivot/anchor points for re-entrant circuits, wavefront collision, and conduction block that facilitate fibrillation.
  - Potentially arrhythmogenic shortening of atrial refractoriness at sites of autonomic innervation ('**parasympathetic ganglia**', '**ganglionated plexi**') may also manifest as CFAEs.
- Ablation of a putative rotor site should continue until the local and immediately adjacent electrograms have attenuated.
- Ablation at the site of a ganglionated plexus may elicit severe bradycardia or even prolonged asystole. Treatment should be completed (if necessary with temporary pacing) as these 'vagal reactions' are associated with more favourable procedure outcomes.
- Most CFAE sites are located within the LA/PV antra and these are always targeted initially. If ablation of all identified LA rotor sites fails to achieve the endpoints (see below) of non-inducibility (paroxysmal AF) or termination of AF (persistent AF), further mapping/ablation of CFAE sites within the coronary sinus and RA/SVC may be undertaken.
- Ablation Frontiers offer customized catheters (MAC™ and MASC™) for mapping and ablation of CFAEs but at significantly increased cost.

Endpoints for electrogram-guided approach

Paroxysmal AF: Non-inducibility of sustained AF (>5–10 minutes) or other atrial tachyarrhythmias assessed by:
- Programmed stimulation (e.g. atrial pacing at 20 mA in 5–10 second bursts down to atrial refractoriness ± multiple sites); **OR**
- Isoprenaline infusion (up to 20 mcg/min) – probably has superior sensitivity and specificity to assessment by programmed stimulation.

Non-inducibility predicts improved long-term outcome (but continuing inducibility does not preclude a successful outcome).

Persistent AF: Ideally slowing and termination of AF to:
- Sinus rhythm **OR**
- An organized atrial tachyarrhythmia requiring further mapping/ablation to restore sinus rhythm (📖 p. 466).

Termination of AF predicts improved long-term outcome but is achieved in <40% of cases in most series. Failure to terminate AF by ablation does not preclude a successful outcome (sinus rhythm restored by DC cardioversion). Inducibility appears to be of limited predictive value in persistent AF cases (unlike paroxysmal AF).

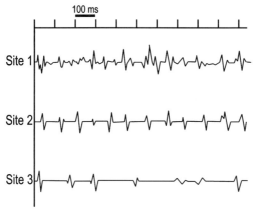

Fig. 20.10 Electrogram-guided ablation. Site 1: Example of typical CFAE signal exhibiting very short cycle length, fractionation, and continuous electrical activity, suitable for 'rotor' ablation or 'defragmentation'. Site 2: The local electrogram is relatively organized. Site 3: The local electrogram is even more organized and slower, therefore unsuitable for ablation.

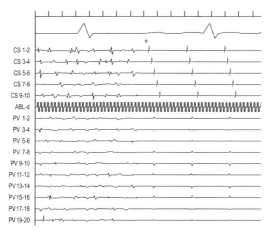

Fig. 20.11 Conversion of AF to an organized atrial tachyarrhythmia during ablation (*) with DCS-PCS activation during electrogram-guided ablation. Subsequent activation mapping and entrainment showed this to be peri-mitral flutter and sinus rhythm was restored by mitral isthmus ablation (p. 438).

Linear ablation techniques

Linear left atrial ablation for substrate modification is seldom undertaken as a stand-alone procedure but is used for patients with ongoing AF/atrial tachyarrhythmias despite LACA or other PV isolation techniques, the rationale being to prevent left atrial macroreentry. This applies to almost all persistent/permanent AF cases and 30–40% of paroxysmal AF cases, the latter usually identified on the basis of clinical recurrence of arrhythmias following an initial ablation procedure. Linear ablation techniques include:
• Mitral isthmus ablation by joining LIPV to the mitral annulus.
• LA roof line, joining LSPV to RSPV.
• Cavotricuspid isthmus ablation.

These are by far the most commonly performed 'lines'. Other linear lesions include:
• LA floor line plus CS roof – to disrupt CS-LA connections.
• Anterior left atrial transection – anterior connection of roof line to mitral annulus.
• Mitral isthmus ablation by joining RIPV to the mitral annulus.
• Infero-posterior wall of LA.
• Septal border of LA.

Mitral isthmus ablation

Peri-mitral flutter is a common form of macroreentry post-LACA and is prevented by linear ablation from lateral mitral annulus to LIPV. Achieving transmural conduction block is challenging due to the depth of the myocardium and possibly the cooling effect of the coronary sinus, which passes over the epicardial aspect of the isthmus region – adjunctive ablation within the CS is required in most patients.

- Usually performed with 3-D mapping, enabling:
  - Delineation of key landmarks – LIPV, MV annulus, LAA, and CS.
  - Correct placement of lesions.
  - Monitoring of catheter tip position during ablation in case of inadvertent dislodgement into inferior PV or LA appendage.
- Catheter setup:
  - Support sheath for ablation catheter, preferably steerable.
  - CS multi-polar catheter, ideally advanced so as to straddle/bracket the proposed linear lesion (i.e. distal poles just anterior to line).
  - If ablation is performed during sinus rhythm, circumferential PV mapping catheter is placed in the LA appendage for continuous pacing to assess isthmus conduction on a beat-to-beat basis.
- Technique – endocardial approach (Fig. 20.12(A) and (B)):
  - Catheter placed at lateral mitral annulus (approx. 4 o'clock in LAO), with A and V deflections in local electrogram (A < V).
  - Catheter/sheath assembly is rotated clockwise to extend the line posteriorly towards inferior PV (approx. 2 o'clock in LAO).
  - Lesions applied at 40–50 W near annulus and 35–40 W near inferior PV, for 30–60 seconds at each site or until local electrograms attenuate.
  - Recheck entire line for residual breakthrough electrograms if isthmus conduction intact after initial linear lesion completed. Occasionally a more anterior line close to the LA appendage is needed.
  - Only switch to epicardial approach if there is definite evidence of residual isthmus conduction (therefore if ablation is performed during AF, sinus rhythm should be restored and isthmus conduction checked by LAA pacing etc.).
- Technique – epicardial approach (Fig. 20.12(C)):
  - Required in 60–70% of cases to achieve isthmus block.
  - Should only be performed after complete endocardial ablation.
  - Should be performed during either: (i) peri-mitral flutter; or (ii) sinus rhythm with LAA pacing.
  - Ablation catheter advanced into CS until positioned opposite to the endocardial lesions.
  - Identify electrogram with early and/or fractionated atrial potentials (during LAA pacing) suggestive of an epicardial gap.
  - Lesions applied at 20–30 W for 30–60 seconds or until local electrograms attenuated before repositioning.
  - Some operators perform coronary angiography prior to ablation to check proximity of the circumflex artery.
  - Occasionally it may be necessary to switch back to the endocardial approach to deliver lesions *en face* to the epicardial sites in order to achieve isthmus block.

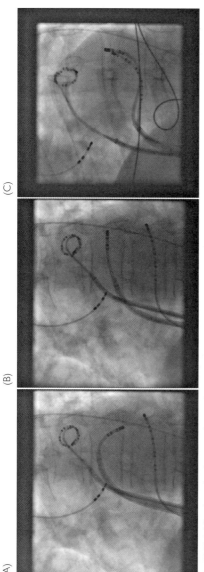

(A)

(B)

(C)

Fig. 20.12 LAO radiographs showing techniques for mitral isthmus ablation. (A) Endocardial approach with ablation catheter at lateral end of mitral valve annulus (4 o'clock) supported by steerable trans-septal sheath in deflected position. (B) Endocardial approach with ablation catheter just outside LIPV (2 o'clock). (C) Epicardial approach with ablation catheter introduced via CS and positioned beyond the distal poles of the CS multi-polar catheter, *en face* to the line of endocardial lesions; the circumferential PV mapping catheter is positioned within the LA appendage for continuous LAA pacing to assess mitral isthmus conduction on a beat-to-beat basis during ablation.

Determining mitral isthmus block

- Endocardial activation mapping during pacing from either side of the line, ideally as close as possible to the line. Usually done via 3-D system (📖 Chapter 6, p. 97).
- Analysis of CS activation pattern during LA appendage pacing (i.e. anterior to the line) with CS multi-polar catheter positioned just posterior to the line (Fig. 22.12):
  - Enables beat-to-beat monitoring of isthmus conduction during ablation (unlike endocardial activation mapping).
  - With intact isthmus conduction, activation will be DCS-PCS (Fig. 20.13 (A)).
  - Conduction delay during ablation may produce a 'chevron' pattern (Fig. 20.13(B)).
  - Onset of conduction block is usually signalled by an abrupt switch to PCS-DCS activation as paced impulses from the LAA are detoured and reach exclusively via the CS ostium (Fig. 20.13(C)).
  - CS-LA electrical disconnection may result in pseudo-block, therefore isthmus block should always be confirmed by endocardial activation mapping.
- Recording widely-split double potentials (>90 ms) along the ablation line during CS pacing or LA appendage pacing (Fig. 20.13(C)).
- Differential pacing should always be performed to exclude marked conduction delay as opposed to complete isthmus block (Fig. 20.14(B) to (C)):
  - Pacing from most distal CS poles results in longest S1-LAA interval.
  - With complete isthmus block, pacing from progressively more proximal CS poles should result in progressively shorter S1-LAA interval (using identical CS catheter position and recording poles in the LAA) (Fig. 20.14(C)).
  - Prolongation of S1-LAA intervals from more proximal poles implies isthmus conduction delay rather than block.
  - If the distal CS poles lie anterior to the line of block, pacing activation will be detoured and enter via the CS ostium, producing PCS-DSC activation in the more proximal poles.

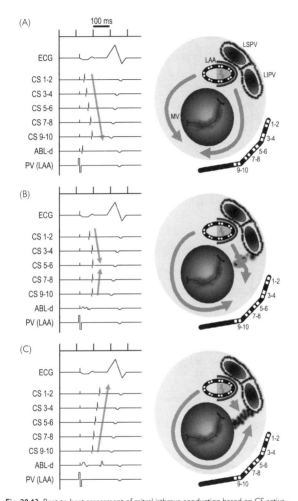

Fig. 20.13 Beat-to-beat assessment of mitral isthmus conduction based on CS activation during LAA pacing (NB requires restoration of sinus rhythm, either spontaneously or by DC cardioversion). Circumferential PV mapping catheter positioned within LAA for continuous pacing. CS multi-polar catheter positioned with distal poles just posterior to (i.e. just before) the ablation line. (A) At baseline, isthmus conduction is intact and LAA pacing results in DCS-PCS activation. (B) Following extensive endocardial ablation, isthmus conduction is delayed but still present as indicated by a 'chevron' CS activation pattern, but switching to an epicardial approach, mapping with the ablation catheter more distally identifies an 'epicardial gap' with early fractionated atrial electrograms. (C) Ablation at this site results in abrupt change in CS activation to PCS-DCS with a sudden increase in S1-DCS interval. There are widely split double potentials in ABL-d which is positioned on the line.

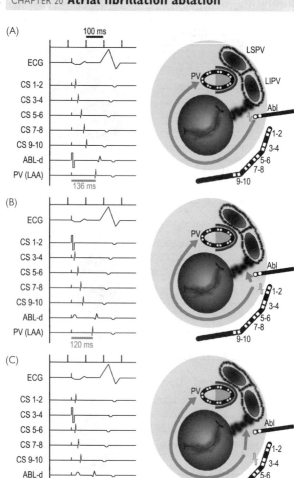

Fig. 20.14 Differential CS pacing is performed. (A) Initially pacing from the ablation catheter just posterior to the line of ablation with S1-LAA 136 ms. (B) Pacing most distal poles of CS and the S1-LAA interval shortens to 120 ms. (C) Pacing more proximally, S1-LAA interval shortens further to 108 ms, in keeping with complete isthmus block.

LA 'roof' line

Another commonly observed form of post-LACA left atrial macroreentry is peri-venous, i.e. macroreentry around the ipsilateral veins (📖 p. 294). This is prevented by creating a roof line connecting the two superior pulmonary veins, effectively connecting the encircling line of lesions generated around each vein during LACA.

- Usually performed using 3-D-mapping to:
  - Enable delineation of the key anatomical landmarks (right upper PV, left upper PV, and LA appendage).
  - Ensure accurate placement of lesions in a confluent line.
  - Monitor catheter tip position during ablation in case of dislodgement into one of the PVs.
- Catheter setup:
  - Support sheath for ablation catheter, preferably steerable.
  - Circumferential PV mapping catheter placed in the LA appendage for continuous pacing to assess conduction block.
- Technique:
  - Catheter tip positioned and ablation commenced near the LSPV, at or within the encircling linear lesion created during LACA.
  - Catheter/sheath assembly is dragged with clockwise torque, causing the tip to brush along the roof inferiorly and septally until the RSPV is reached.
  - RF lesions applied at 30 W for 30–60 seconds or until local electrograms attenuate before repositioning catheter tip.
  - Ablation of the roof near the RSPV junction may be challenging due to poor catheter stability. Occasionally this problem can be solved by using the steerable trans-septal sheath to fashion a large reverse loop with the ablation catheter.

Determining roof line conduction block

- Recording widely-split double potentials from the vicinity of the line during LAA pacing, with no 'breakthrough' electrograms (Fig. 20.15).
- Endocardial activation mapping during LAA pacing, i.e. pacing anterior to the line. In the presence of conduction block, activation is detoured resulting in infero-superior activation of the posterior wall, with the latest activation just below the roof line.
- Differential pacing from the posterior wall to distinguish marked conduction delay. Thus, the longest S1-LAA interval should be obtained by pacing near the line, with progressively shorter S1-LAA intervals pacing from more inferior sites (Fig. 20.15).

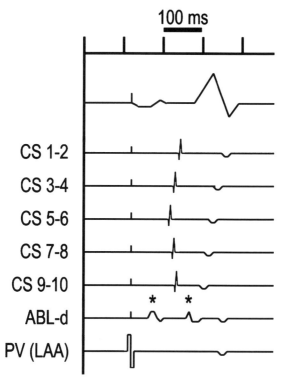

Fig. 20.15 Roof line block. During LAA pacing, mapping with the ablation catheter along a complete roof line identifies a widely-split double potential (* *), with the far-field component delayed by >100 ms compared to the near-field component due to the onset of roof line block.

Other ablation techniques

Linear ablation
- Cavotricuspid isthmus ablation – should only be performed if there is a prior history of typical flutter or isthmus-dependent develops during the ablation procedure.
- LA floor line plus CS roof – to disrupt CS-LA connections. Often performed as part of stepwise approach in persistent AF.
- Other ablation lines (see above).

Isolation procedures
- SVC encirclement.
- LA appendage encirclement.
- Isolation of ligament of Marshall.

Generic strategies for ablation of paroxysmal AF

The ablation techniques described in the previous sections are deployed in various combinations and permutations, with currently no universal agreement about the optimal approach. The commonest strategies are summarized below.

PV isolation only

- LACA.
- Ablation Frontiers (PVAC™ only).
- Ostial segmental/antral techniques.
- Endpoint = PV isolation.

Simplest, most widely used approach for paroxysmal AF. Offers shortest procedure times and minimizes radiation exposure/procedural risk, but recurrence rates may be higher. Nowadays empirical isolation of all four veins is the norm, apart from in a few younger patients with 'PV tachycardia' mapped to a single vein.

PV isolation + defragmentation (rotor ablation)

- LACA + CFAE mapping/ablation.
- Ablation Frontiers (PVAC™, MAC™, and MASC™).
- Endpoint = PV isolation plus non-inducibility.

Some evidence of superior efficacy and reduced re-do rates but at the expense of longer procedure times, increased radiation, and possibly higher risk of complications. Also some concern about pro-arrhythmic potential of defragmentation (by creating a substrate for microreentrant focal tachycardias).

Defragmentation only (Nadanamee)

- No LACA, just electrogram-guided ablation.
- Endpoint = non-inducibility.

Limited published data/experience apart from original authors.

PV isolation ± mitral isthmus line ± roof line

- LACA + roof line and/or mitral isthmus line.
- Ablation Frontiers (PVAC™ + TVAC™) but difficult to achieve isthmus block without irrigated-tip catheters.
- Endpoint = PV isolation plus conduction block across the lines.

Some evidence for improved outcome but involves a significantly more complex operation with increased procedure time/radiation and increased risk. Also concerns about pro-arrhythmic macroreentrant tachycardias if only conduction delay (rather than block) is achieved.

Generic strategies for ablation of persistent AF

In general, persistent AF requires more extensive ablation/substrate modification (compared to paroxysmal AF) to achieve rhythm-control, with a higher chance of repeat procedures.

PV isolation only
- LACA preferable to ostial/antral isolation procedures (more substrate modification).
- Endpoint = PV isolation.

Low efficacy. Now less used as a stand-alone treatment.

PV isolation + defragmentation (rotor ablation)
- LACA + CFAE mapping/ablation.
- Endpoint = PV isolation ± termination of AF.

More effective than stand-alone LACA but risk of left atrial macroreentry and possibly pro-arrhythmic effects of defragmentation (by creating a substrate for microreentrant focal tachycardias).

Defragmentation only (Nadenamee)
- No LACA just electrogram-guided ablation.
- Endpoint = conversion to sinus rhythm.

Limited published data/experience apart from original authors.

PV isolation + defragmentation + linear lesions 'stepwise approach' (Haissaguerre)
- Restores sinus rhythm in >80% of cases.
- LACA performed initially plus isolation of SVC and CS.
- Defragmentation.
- Linear ablation – mitral isthmus, roof line ± cavotricuspid isthmus:
  - Termination to sinus rhythm may occur directly at any stage; **OR**
  - Conversion to organized atrial tachyarrhythmia requiring further mapping/ablation to restore sinus rhythm.
- Endpoint = PV isolation plus conduction block across the lines plus ideally restoration of sinus rhythm *without* DC cardioversion.

More complex, longer procedure and still high (≥50%) re-do rates but significantly improved chance of long-term rhythm-control.

PV isolation + linear lesions
- LACA performed initially.
- DC cardioversion (unless cardiovert during LACA).
- Linear ablation – mitral isthmus, roof line ± cavotricuspid isthmus.
- Defragmentation ± CS isolation etc. only if immediate relapse to AF or AF refractory to DC cardioversion.
- Endpoint = PV isolation plus conduction block across the lines.

Less complex, shorter procedure than stepwise approach but limited data on comparative outcomes and need for redo procedures.

Ablation frontiers

Ablation frontiers can also be used in persistent AF (PVAC™ for LACA, MAC™ and MASC™ for defragmentation, and TVAC™ for linear ablation) but multiple catheters increase costs and it can be difficult to achieve linear block (especially mitral isthmus) without irrigated-tip catheters.

Repeat ablation procedures

A feature of current AF ablation techniques is the frequent requirement for repeat ablation procedures. Both published series and anecdotal experience indicate that 20–40% of paroxysmal AF patients and 50–75% of persistent AF patients will require more than one session of ablative therapy to achieve rhythm-control.

Time course of recurrences

- The early period after left atrial ablation procedures is often characterized by arrhythmia exacerbation, which may be self-limiting as post-operative inflammatory changes resolve and there is atrial healing/remodelling.
- This so-called 'blanking period' lasts for at least four weeks and possibly up to 3–6 months.
- Early post-op recurrent atrial tachyarrhythmias should be managed conservatively with anti-arrhythmic drugs and/or DC cardioversion if necessary, in the hope that they will settle without re-intervention.
- Repeat ablation is increasingly likely to be needed the longer the arrhythmias are ongoing – certainly beyond 4–6 weeks.

Types of recurrent atrial tachyarrhythmias

- ECG documentation of recurrent arrhythmias is essential.
- All 12-lead ECGs, rhythm strips, and ambulatory ECG recordings should be retrieved prior to repeat ablation.
- Although AF is the commonest recurrent arrhythmia, organized atrial tachyarrhythmias (focal and macroreentrant tachycardias) occur frequently post-LACA and may require specific evaluation, mapping, and ablation (📕 p. 466).
- Post-LACA tachyarrhythmias may be paroxysmal or persistent irrespective of the pre-op arrhythmia. For example, persistent atrial tachyarrhythmia may develop after ablation for paroxysmal AF and is often poorly tolerated.

Strategies for redo ablation

There is no universal approach but potentially there are three components to any redo ablation procedure:

- 'Re-touching' lesion sets delivered at the previous ablation:
  - Any PVs exhibiting reconnection should be isolated again, ideally by lesions applied at antral breakthrough sites.
  - Gaps in linear lesions should be mapped and ablated to restore bidirectional conduction block.
- Mapping/ablation of *de novo* organized atrial tachycardias manifesting since the first ablation, as described elsewhere (📕 p. 466):
  - Definitely any that occurred clinically.
  - Probably any that develop during redo ablation, either spontaneously or during programmed stimulation (however, it is uncertain that these induced atrial tachycardias predict recurrence).

- Additional ablation therapy:
  - Empirical, for example adding defragmentation and/or linear lesions if patient only underwent LACA at first session, or additional defragmentation for recurrent AF despite stepwise approach (LACA → defragmentation → linear lesions).
  - Targeted, for example SVC isolation if restudy suggests arrhythmogenic focus in that location.

Major complications

Tamponade

- Diagnose promptly by arterial pressure monitoring.
- Reduce risk by minimizing powers and gentle catheter handling.
- Pericardiocentesis/drain.
- May need reversal of anticoagulation to control.
- Awkward dilemma about how soon to restart post-operative anticoagulation:
  - Increased risk of re-bleed if continued.
  - Increased risk of stroke if anticoagulation stopped.

Stroke

- Avoid by careful peri-procedural anticoagulation.
- Further reduce risk by routine irrigation of trans-septal sheaths.
- Acute management of peri-operative strokes requires urgent CNS imaging plus specialist advice.

Pulmonary vein stenosis

- Presents with dyspnoea and haemoptysis.
- Diagnosed by cross-sectional imaging and lung perfusion.
- Avoid by ablating outside the pulmonary vein ostium.
- Treatment is difficult – nowadays usually managed by stenting.

Post-LACA arrhythmias (📖 p. 294)

- Manage medically by rate-control, anti-arrhythmics ± cardioversion in first six weeks post-op (📖 p. 450), as often they settle spontaneously with conservative approach.
- ECG documentation is essential as post-ablation atrial tachycardias are often mistaken for sinus tachycardia or AF.

Atrio-oesophageal fistula

- Rare but serious complication (fatal in >50%).
- Reduce risk by avoiding high power ablation settings when applying lesions on posterior wall, and by adjusting catheter position frequently.
- Typical symptoms are chest pain/dyspepsia and TIAs (due to air embolism).
- CT barium studies for diagnosis.

Ablation of other atrial tachyarrhythmias

Introduction

This section examines ablation techniques for atrial tachyarrhythmias other than common atrial flutter and atrial fibrillation:

- Focal atrial tachycardia (📖 p. 290), including sinus node re-entrant tachycardia (SNRT) and pulmonary vein (PV) tachycardia.
- Atypical right atrial flutter (📖 p. 294).
- Organized post-LACA atrial tachyarrhythmias, i.e. macro-, micro- and small loop re-entry tachycardias within the left atrium (📖 p. 294), including peri-mitral flutter, peri-venous (especially roof-dependent) flutter, and coronary sinus re-entry tachycardia. Such arrhythmias are commonly observed:
  - During LACA procedures, either through organization of AF or by induction testing.
  - Following LACA procedures.
  - Following Cox Maze operations.
  - In other patients with previous left atriotomy.

Successful ablation of these arrhythmias depends on a clear understanding of underlying mechanisms/pathophysiology, and of activation mapping and entrainment techniques.

Also included in this section is a brief consideration of sinus node modification for inappropriate sinus tachycardia.

Ablation of focal atrial tachycardia

In children and adolescents, FAT is a relatively common cause of SVT without underlying heart disease, although incessant cases may lead to rate-related cardiomyopathy. SNRT is a rare cause of paroxysmal SVT in adults but is frequently found incidentally at EPS and may sometimes be sufficiently troublesome to warrant ablation so that the main arrhythmia (e.g. AVNRT) can be induced and treated without interference. FAT in adults is usually seen with structural heart disease (may be multifocal) and increasingly in the post-LACA population due to microreentry.

The keys to successful ablation of FAT are:
• Inducibility of arrhythmia.
• Ensure correct diagnosis.
• Activation mapping.

Arrhythmia induction

Not required with persistent FAT. In paroxysmal cases, induction of the tachycardia by catecholamine infusion and/or programmed stimulation (📖 p. 154) is a pre-requisite for confirmation of the diagnosis and mapping/ablation but is often problematic:
• Non-inducibility or unreliable inducibility.
• Induction of non-clinical arrhythmias (requires careful comparison of ECGs of induced arrhythmia and clinical tachycardia).
• Commonest reason for failure to ablate FAT.
• Use of multi-electrode array (📖 p. 108) may occasionally be useful in cases of unreliable inducibility by enabling activation mapping on the basis of a few beats of tachycardia.

Confirmation of diagnosis of FAT

Usually straightforward based on standard ECG and EPS criteria (📖 p. 290).
• Commonest pitfall is misclassification of a macroreentrant atrial tachycardia (MRAT) as FAT with marked intra-atrial conduction delay (📖 pp. 290, 300). Always reconsider the possibility of MRAT if intracardiac mapping identifies electrical activity exceeding 50% of tachycardia cycle length.
• Misclassification of AVNRT with AV block as atrial tachycardia (📖 p. 236).

Activation mapping

Identification of the site of earliest atrial activation during tachycardia is the key to localization and ablation of FAT. Entrainment techniques are not applicable to automatic FAT and are of limited value in microreentrant FAT (📖 p. 298).

Left or right atrium?
• Review P wave morphology on surface ECG (Fig. 14.2).
• DCS-PCS activation always indicates left atrial origin.
• PCS-DCS suggests right atrial origin, certainly if HRA or LRA precedes PCS activation.

- PCS-DCS activation may be seen with PV tachycardias arising from right-sided pulmonary veins, FAT from left side of interatrial septum, or any left atrial FAT in patients that have previously undergone mitral isthmus ablation with complete block (📖 p. 440).
- Thus, in some cases detailed activation mapping of both the RA and LA may be required to identify the location of FAT.

Conventional mapping

- Display the surface ECG leads that most clearly show the P waves.
- In some cases, local atrial activation in the exploring electrodes (mapping/ablation catheter) can be timed from P wave onset but more often this is unreliable and it is necessary to time against a fixed intracardiac signal.
- If the multi-polar CS catheter is reasonably stable, timing can be referenced to any electrode pair exhibiting a sharp atrial electrogram (Fig. 21.1). Other standard electrode positions are usually too unstable for reliable referencing and so the alternative is to use an active-fixation bipolar or quadripolar electrode (can be positioned at any RA site but the interatrial septum is preferred if the patient is to be anticoagulated for left atrial mapping to avoid the chance of perforation).
- Ablation is performed at the site of earliest activation (Fig. 21.1A):
  - Will usually precede the P wave onset by >30 ms.
  - Unipolar recording shows negative QS deflection.
  - May exhibit fractionation if FAT is microreentrant.
- Following application of RF current at a successful site:
  - FAT may accelerate transiently before terminating, especially if the mechanism is automatic (Fig. 21.2).
  - Transient acceleration without termination suggests proximity to the focus but the catheter needs to be repositioned.
  - FAT may slow and terminate, especially if the mechanism is microreentrant (Fig. 21.1B).

3-D electroanatomical mapping

- Not required in all cases but may be preferred technique with complex anatomy or uncertainty about mechanism (FAT vs. MRAT).
- Requires intracardiac reference as above.
- Window of interest typically set to 50–80 ms ahead of P wave onset.
- Essential to obtain high density of points around site of early activation and ensure centrifugal spread of activation **in all directions** from 'hotspot'.
- Misclassification of MRAT as FAT may happen if activation is recorded at insufficient points. This error is more likely with a paucity of endocardial electrograms, for example post-LACA.

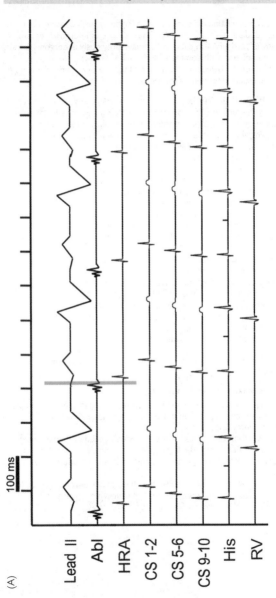

(A)

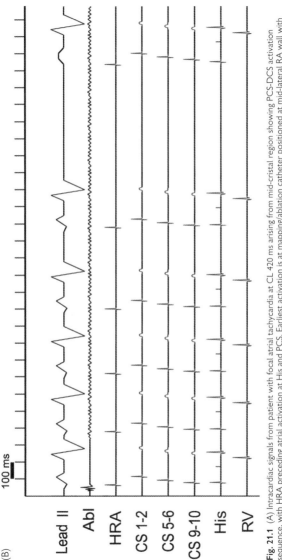

Fig. 21.1 (A) Intracardiac signals from patient with focal atrial tachycardia at CL 420 ms arising from mid-cristal region showing PCS-DCS activation sequence, with HRA preceding atrial activation at His and PCS. Earliest activation is at mapping/ablation catheter positioned at mid-lateral RA wall with complex fractionated electrogram preceding P wave onset by 40 ms. (B) Following application of RF lesion, tachycardia slows and terminates.

(B)

Lead II

Abl

HRA

CS 1-2

CS 5-6

CS 9-10

His

RV

100 ms

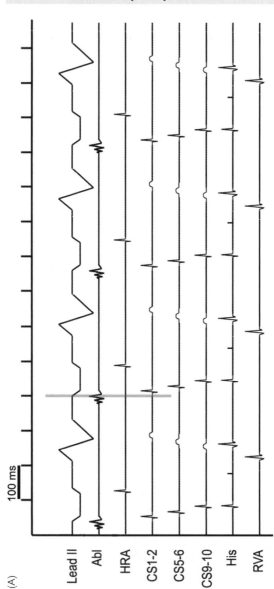

(A)

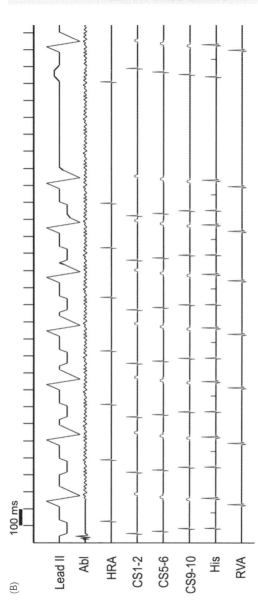

Fig. 21.2 Focal atrial tachycardia (automatic) at CL 350 ms. (A) CS activation is DCS-PCS with PCS earlier than HRA but similar to His. Earliest atrial activation is via mapping/ablation catheter positioned trans-septally close to but outside left lower pulmonary vein, preceding activation at DCS by 50 ms. Unipolar electrogram from distal mapping/ablation catheter confirms early activation with a QS pattern (not shown). (B) Application of an RF lesion at this site results in transient acceleration of tachycardia to CL 260 ms followed by termination.

Specific conditions

- **Sinus node re-entrant tachycardia (Fig. 21.3)**:
  - Common incidental finding at EPS.
  - Activation mapping and ablation is usually straightforward with conventional electrodes, exploring superiorly along the crista terminalis for the site of earliest activation.
  - Advisable to check for phrenic nerve stimulation prior to ablation by pacing at high output (e.g. 20 mA and pulse width 2 ms). Diaphragmatic twitching may be assessed by palpation and/or fluoroscopy. If present, the catheter should be repositioned and checks repeated. SNRT can often be successfully treated with lesions slightly away from site of earliest activation.
  - Successful ablation may be heralded by acceleration or slowing of the atrial rate prior to termination.

- **Pulmonary vein tachycardia**:
  - May occur as an isolated tachyarrhythmia in younger patients with structurally normal hearts and only involving a single vein.
  - Usually repetitive rather than sustained atrial tachycardia.
  - Activation mapping usually localizes earliest electrical activity to well inside PV ostium.
  - Unlike other forms of FAT, ablation at the site of earliest activation should be avoided due to the risk of PV stenosis. Ostial segmental or even circumferential PV isolation usually guided by a circumferential mapping catheter (📖 p. 424) will address the problem.
  - PV isolation will usually abolish the tachyarrhythmia and produce complete electrical silence within the vein but rarely the PV tachycardia persists with exit block and PVP dissociation from the atria.
  - Especially in younger patients, only isolation of the affected PV is usually required and empirical isolation of the other veins could be avoided to reduce the chance of complications (esp. PV stenosis).

- **Peri-nodal atrial tachycardia**:
  - Requires careful differentiation from typical and atypical forms of AVNRT (📖 p. 300).
  - Consider use of 3-D electroanatomical mapping to delineate geometry, including creation of a 'His cloud' to better define the extent of the AV junction region.
  - Cryoablation reduces the risk of iatrogenic AV junction injury compared to standard RF by enabling reversible lesions to be delivered at −20 to −30°C ('cryomapping').
  - If cryoablation is not available, consider RF application in power-mode with stepwise up-titration (e.g. 10 W → 15 W → 20 W etc.) until tachycardia is suppressed. If accelerated junctional rhythm is provoked, suggesting risk of AV block, RF application should be terminated immediately.

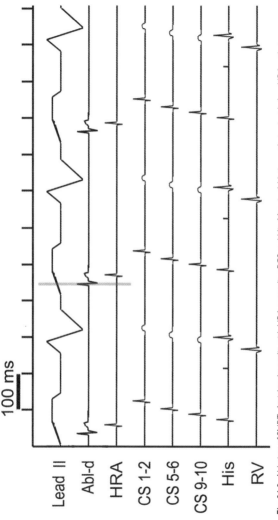

Fig. 21.3 Ablation of SNRT. Atrial tachycardia with HRA preceding PCS and His. Mapping/ablation catheter just below HRA catheter on crista terminalis exhibits earliest activation.

Ablation of atypical right atrial flutter

Atypical right atrial flutters, i.e. MRATs within the RA that are *not* isthmus-dependent, most commonly develop in the context of prior surgical atriotomy, for example for ASD closure. Typical and atypical right atrial flutter often occur in the same patient and may transition from one to the other, e.g. during cavotricuspid isthmus ablation. Because of the complex anatomy/landmarks, 3-D electroanatomical mapping is preferred:

- To delineate circuit/lines of block prior to delivery of ablative therapy.
- To exclude FAT with intra-atrial conduction delay (also relatively common in post-surgical patients).

Checklist for atypical right atrial MRAT includes:

- CS activation is PCS-DCS (DCS-PCS implies left atrial FAT or MRAT).
- Entrainment from DCS results in longer PPIs than PCS and RA sites.
- Consistent PPIs pacing from the same RA site (highly variable PPIs from one site suggests FAT).
- Entrainment from RA isthmus results in PPI – TCL >30 ms.
- Cavotricuspid isthmus ablation fails to terminate flutter despite achieving isthmus block.

Lesion-related or incisional MRAT (Fig. 21.4)

- Detailed 3-D electroanatomical mapping of RA:
  - Delineate SVC, IVC, and tricuspid annulus.
  - Voltage mapping to identify atriotomy scar.
  - Activation mapping to identify MRAT circuit around scar and confirm 'head-meets-tail'.
  - Adequate density of mapping points must be taken to avoid misdiagnosis of FAT with centrifugal activation spread.
- Circuit's rotation point is usually at the lower end of the scar near the IVC (occasionally via a gap in the atriotomy on the lateral RA wall).
- May detect double potentials along the scar with continuous fractionated electrograms at the lower rotation point (Fig. 21.4).
- Entrainment from isthmus or septal RA produces PPI > TCL by more than 20 ms, whereas entrainment at the lateral RA wall will produce PPI close to TCL. Entrainment within the lower rotation zone is often precluded by poor electrical capture.
- Linear ablation is performed through the lower turnaround, connecting the atriotomy scar to the IVC, and should result in slowing and termination of flutter.
- In view of the proximity of the phrenic nerve, it is advisable to check for phrenic nerve stimulation by pacing at high output prior to ablation.
- If not previously performed, consider undertaking cavotricuspid isthmus ablation in view of the frequent co-existence of typical flutter.

Atypical right atrial MRAT without prior atriotomy

- Various forms, for example rotation around the SVC with an area of functional block along the lateral RA wall (upper loop re-entry).
- 3-D mapping enables identification of activation circuit and scope for creating curative lesions.

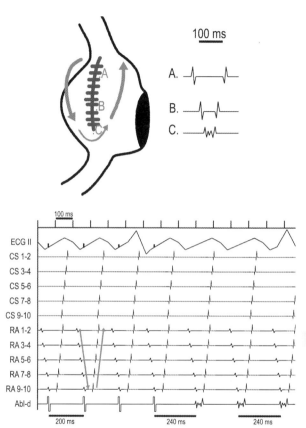

Fig. 21.4 Ablation of lesion-related MRAT. Patient underwent surgical secundum ASD closure 20 years ago and subsequently cavotricuspid isthmus ablation for typical atrial flutter but now presents in persistent flutter of different morphology at CL 240 ms. Top panel: 3-D-mapping suggests macroreentry around atriotomy scar. (A) Mapping/ablation catheter is positioned at top of scar and widely spaced double potentials are recorded. (B) With the mapping/ablation catheter at mid-lateral RA wall the double potentials are less widely spaced. (C) Mapping/ablation catheter just below atriotomy near the IVC exhibits long, fractionated electrogram consistent with rotation point. Bottom panel: CS multi-polar catheter shows PCS-DCS activation. Entrainment with the mapping/ablation catheter at C results in PPI 240 ms, i.e. within MRAT circuit with turnaround in activation. After checking for phrenic nerve stimulation, an RF lesion at this site slows and terminates flutter (NB subsequently bidirectional conduction block of the cavotricuspid isthmus was demonstrable from the earlier ablation procedure).

Ablation of post-LACA atrial arrhythmias

(See Table 14.2)

Because post-LACA tachyarrhythmias are self-limiting in 30–50% of cases, many groups attempt conservative management with pharmacological rate-control ± DC cardioversion/anti-arrhythmic drugs until at least 2–3 months post-ablation to allow time for atrial healing and remodelling. If re-intervention is required, the pre-operative work-up is identical to that used for first-time LACA procedures (📖 p. 419).

- Any 12-lead ECGs of the post-LACA atrial tachyarrhythmias should be available for comparison during the redo procedure, particularly if the condition is paroxysmal and PES is needed, as non-clinical arrhythmias may be induced.
- The possibility of right atrial arrhythmias (especially typical flutter or FAT) should always be considered.

Setup

- 3-D mapping is highly preferable because of the complex anatomical basis of the potential arrhythmia mechanisms.
- Mapping/ablation catheter (irrigated-tip) plus multi-polar CS catheter essential. Circumferential PV mapping catheter is desirable:
  - To facilitate geometric mapping.
  - To check PV status (connected or disconnected).
  - For LA appendage pacing to assess block in the mitral isthmus and/or roof lines.
- Geometric mapping of LA should ideally include delineation of mitral annulus as well as PVs and LA appendage.
- Arrhythmia induction if patient is in sinus rhythm initially.

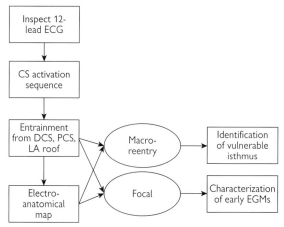

Fig. 21.5 Generic approach for post-LACA atrial tachycardias.

Approaches for identifying arrhythmia mechanism (see Table 14.2)

- **CS activation pattern**:
  - If PCS-DCS, may need to exclude RA mechanism (see above) but also consistent with counter-clockwise peri-mitral flutter, FAT arising near right-sided PVs or septum, 'CS flutter', or any left atrial mechanism with mitral isthmus block.
  - DCS-PCS most likely to represent clockwise peri-mitral flutter or FAT from around left-sided veins or LA appendage. Also peri-venous roof-dependent flutter with outer loop passing below left inferior PV.
  - Flat or 'chevron' CS activation may indicate peri-venous flutter via roof or FAT near LA roof or posterior wall.

- **Response to entrainment**:
  - Inconstant PPI suggestive of FAT. CS pacing at 10, 20, and 30 ms shorter than tachycardia cycle length differentiates MRAT vs. FAT on the basis of variability in PPI, viz. <10 ms for MRAT vs. >30 ms for FAT.
  - Concealed entrainment (PPI = TCL) at CS sites and mitral isthmus, with longer PPI pacing near LA roof and at RA sites, suggests peri-mitral flutter (Fig. 21.6).
  - Concealed entrainment from LA roof and either DCS or PCS but late PPI at RA sites suggest peri-venous flutter.
  - BUT entrainment may be precluded by poor endocardial electrograms resulting in failure of capture.

- **3-D activation mapping** (isochronal and propagation):
  - Centrifugal spread from a fixed point ('hot spot') indicates FAT (or RA tachyarrhythmia breaking through septum).
  - Full range of cycle length with 'early meets late' indicates MRAT.
  - Often hampered by paucity of endocardial electrograms.
  - Commonest pitfall is misdiagnosis of FAT (or small loop re-entry) as MRAT because of insufficient density of local electrograms combined with marked intra-atrial conduction delay due to prior LA ablation (especially linear ablation).

- **Trial of ablation**:
  - Often there remains a degree of uncertainty about the arrhythmia mechanism after activation mapping and entrainment.
  - Trial of ablation may be appropriate in these circumstances, targeting the best-guess diagnosis.
  - Linear ablation of roof or mitral isthmus if suspected MRAT.
  - Application of test lesions at sites of early fractionated atrial electrograms if suspected FAT or SLRAT.
  - Slowing/termination of tachycardia confirms the putative diagnosis.

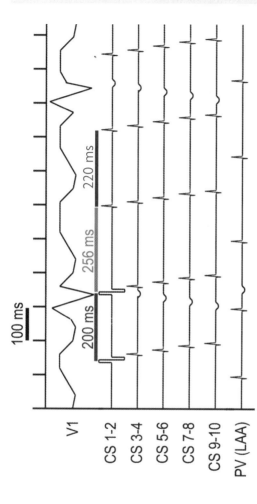

Fig. 21.6 Example of entrainment of clockwise peri-mitral flutter. Pacing at 200 ms from distal coronary sinus entrains the arrhythmia, which has a distal to proximal activation sequence in the coronary sinus. The post-pacing interval (grey) of 256 ms is 36 ms longer than the tachycardia cycle length (220 ms, red) because the distal coronary sinus is just outside the peri-mitral flutter circuit.

Ablation of specific targets

- MRAT:
  - Linear ablation of the roof and/or mitral isthmus as described for AF ablation (📖 pp. 438, 444).
  - Ablation guided primarily by anatomical landmarks but target sites should exhibit appropriately timed electrograms, with fractionation at breakthrough sites (Fig 21.7).
  - End-point is slowing/termination of MRAT **plus** confirmation of bidirectional conduction block across linear lesion as previously described (📖 pp. 440, 444).
  - Interrupting peri-mitral MRAT will require epicardial ablation (at 20–30 W) in 60–70% of cases.
- FAT or small loop re-entrant atrial tachycardia (SLRAT):
  - Ablation delivered at or around earliest atrial activation ('hot spot' on 3-D map), ideally with a long, fractionated local electrogram (Fig. 21.8A).
  - Endpoint is slowing/termination of tachycardia **plus** non-inducibility.
  - Both FAT and SLRAT often occur at conduction gaps in the original wide area encirclement lines, so may be associated with reconnection of the adjacent PV. Thus, ablation of FAT/SLRAT may simultaneously re-isolate the PV (Fig. 21.8B).
- CS re-entrant tachycardia:
  - Lesion delivered at site exhibiting fractionated electrograms, usually just outside ostium, will often terminate tachycardia.
  - Further lesions may be empirically delivered around CS ostium before confirming non-inducibility.

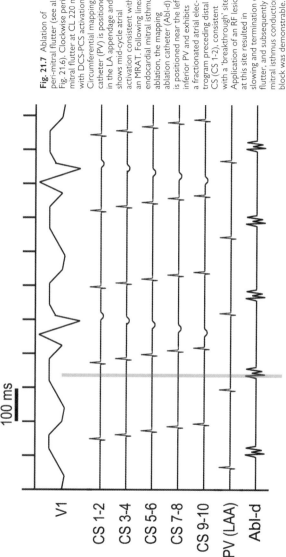

Fig. 21.7 Ablation of peri-mitral flutter (see also Fig. 21.6). Clockwise peri-mitral flutter at CL 220 ms, with DCS-PCS activation. Circumferential mapping catheter (PV) is positioned in the LA appendage and shows mid-cycle atrial activation consistent with an MRAT. Following linear endocardial mitral isthmus ablation, the mapping ablation catheter (Abl-d) is positioned near the left inferior PV and exhibits a fractionated atrial electrogram preceding distal CS (CS 1-2), consistent with a 'breakthrough' site. Application of an RF lesion at this site resulted in slowing and termination of flutter, and subsequently mitral isthmus conduction block was demonstrable.

100 ms

V1

CS 1-2

CS 3-4

CS 5-6

CS 7-8

CS 9-10

PV (LAA)

Abl-d

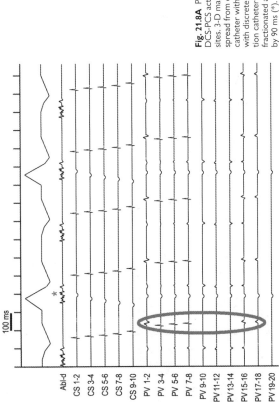

Fig. 21.8A Post-LACA atrial tachycardia, CL 330 ms, DCS-PCS activation and inconstant PPIs entraining from CS sites. 3-D map suggested early activation with centrifugal spread from outside LUPV. PV circumferential mapping catheter within ostium of LUPV shows residual connection with discrete PV potentials (grey circle). Mapping/ablation catheter just posterior to LUPV antrum shows long fractionated atrial electrogram preceding DCS activation by 90 ms (*).

100 ms

Abl-d
CS 1-2
CS 3-4
CS 5-6
CS 7-8
CS 9-10
PV 1-2
PV 3-4
PV 5-6
PV 7-8
PV 9-10
PV 11-12
PV 13-14
PV 15-16
PV 17-18
PV 19-20

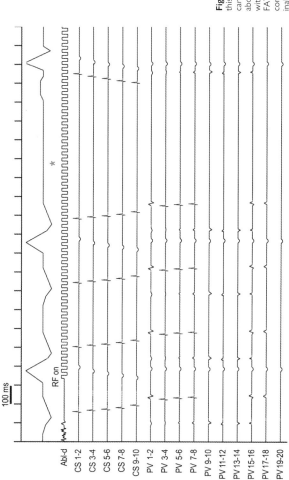

Fig. 21.8B RF ablation at this site terminates tachycardia (*) with simultaneous abolition of PV potentials within LUPV, suggesting FAT or SLRAT utilizing a conduction gap in the original PV encircling lesion.

Generic approach to paroxysmal post-LACA tachycardia

- Trans-septal puncture and geometric LA mapping.
- Check if PVs disconnected and if not re-isolate (📖 p. 450). This may concomitantly interrupt an FAT or SLRAT using the breakthrough site of the original encircling lesion.
- If linear ablation of the roof or mitral isthmus was performed at the first LACA procedure, conduction block in these lines should be checked during LAA pacing (📖 pp. 440, 444) and any breakthrough sites treated to eliminate residual conduction.
- Induce tachycardia (extrastimuli/burst pacing from DCS, PCS, and via roving catheter).
- If inducible proceed as for persistent tachycardia.
- If non-inducible perform empirical mitral isthmus and LA roof lines and consider cavotricuspid isthmus ablation.

Generic approach to persistent atrial tachycardia ablation

- Trans-septal puncture and geometric mapping of LA.
- Analysis of tachycardia mechanism based on CS activation, entrainment, and 3-D activation map as described above (see Table 14.2).
- Ablation of putative mechanism to restore sinus rhythm.
- If mitral isthmus and/or roof line ablation performed (including at first LACA procedure), conduction block should be confirmed during LAA pacing.
- Check for PV disconnection and re-isolate if necessary.
- Confirm non-inducibility of atrial tachycardia.
- Ordinarily if a second post-LACA atrial tachycardia is induced, this should be analysed and treated along the lines described above.
- Cavotricuspid isthmus ablation is only performed if typical flutter has been observed pre-operatively or during the ablation procedure.

Ablation strategies for inappropriate sinus tachycardia

There are three strategies considered for these patients, although none is common or entirely successful:
- Sinus node modification.
- Sinus node ablation and pacemaker implantation.
- AV node ablation and pacemaker implantation.

Sinus node modification

- This is not widely performed for this condition, although some groups have reported acute success up to 80% (defined as a resting heart rate reduced by 20–30 bpm, and a blunted response to adrenergic stimulation, normally isoprenaline infusion).
- Longer term it is quite common for recurrence to occur.
- The aim is to ablate the earliest activation recorded during sinus rhythm.
- This should result in atrial activation originating more inferiorly in the right atrium.
- This manifests as a flattened or inverted P wave in the inferior leads on the 12-lead ECG.
- 3-D mapping systems and non-contact mapping have been used for this type of ablation to assist in identifying the earliest site of activation and the subsequent change (Fig. 21.9).
- The phrenic nerve is often close to the SA node and ablation here may cause phrenic nerve damage – pacing at high outputs at any site before ablation is essential in this situation.
- Cryoablation has been used to try to prevent phrenic nerve injury. Balloons have also been inflated in the pericardium to lift the phrenic nerve away from the epicardial surface.
- Sometimes an idioventricular rhythm occurs with a faster rate than the new sinus rate. This can cause symptoms similar to pacemaker syndrome with dissociated atrial and ventricular contraction.

Sinus node ablation and pacemaker implantation

- Ablation of the entire sinus node is not as straightforward as ablation of the AV node usually is. The fibres can be extensive and the same issues as sinus node modification with phrenic nerve injury are a problem.
- Once ablated a dual chamber pacemaker is implanted.

AV node ablation and pacemaker implantation

- Performed in the same way as described in Chapter 16 with pacing of the ventricle alone.
- Loss of AV synchrony can result in symptoms of pacemaker syndrome.

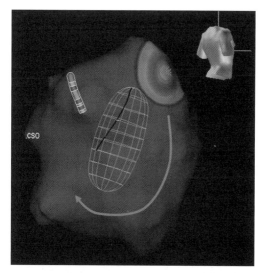

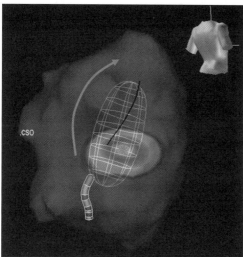

Fig. 21.9 Non-contact mapping during sinus node modification. Top panel: Sinus node activation initially shows earliest activation from high lateral RA, above crista terminalis, down around atrium. Bottom panel: After ablation the activation originates lower in the RA, around the lower end of the crista terminalis. (□ Plate 18 for colour version.)

Ventricular tachycardia ablation

Approach to the patient with VT

Once the diagnosis of VT has been made, the following investigations may be performed to guide further management.

Transthoracic echocardiography

The main question is whether the patient has a structurally normal heart. Apart from the implications this has for the type of VT (📖 p. 308), if a patient has severely impaired ventricular function they may warrant implantable cardioverter defibrillator implantation.

Cardiovascular magnetic resonance imaging (cardiac MRI)

Like transthoracic echocardiography this will primarily assess the cardiac structure and function, but the additional advantage is that with gadolinium contrast it is possible to assess changes in myocardial composition, i.e. to identify areas of scar/fibrosis/fatty infiltration (Fig. 22.1). This may demonstrate that there is substrate for re-entrant VT or indicate underlying pathology, e.g. ARVC (📖 p. 312).

Assessment of cardiac ischaemia

It is important to identify underlying cardiac ischaemia as this may need to be treated primarily. Coronary angiography is often performed in patients with VT, particularly if features of the history or other investigations suggest its presence, e.g. regional wall motion abnormality at echocardiography. It is essential to consider the clinical relevance of any coronary artery disease identified before proceeding to revascularization. Myocardial perfusion scanning, dobutamine stress echocardiography, and stress cardiovascular magnetic resonance may help in this regard.

Further management of the patient can be broadly divided into medical therapy, catheter ablation, and device implantation:

- Medical therapy not only includes anti-arrhythmic medication but also medication for treating any underlying condition, e.g. ischaemic heart disease and/or impaired ventricular function.
- Catheter ablation is reserved for those patients who either have VT despite medical therapy or for whom long-term medical therapy is undesirable, e.g. the young patient with idiopathic VT. It is also important to give consideration to the haemodynamic stability of the VT when deciding on the type of therapy used, and if ablation is being considered, how this should be performed, e.g. non-contact mapping (📖 p. 504).
- Device implantation may be appropriate irrespective of medical therapy/catheter ablation. Implantable cardioverter defibrillator (ICD) implantation is indicated on prognostic grounds in many patients with VT despite any other treatment given and in some of these cardiac resynchronization therapy (CRT) is also appropriate.

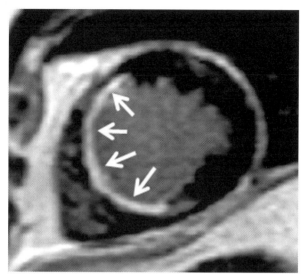

Fig. 22.1 Cardiovascular magnetic resonance scan of a septal infarct with gadolinium late enhancement. Mid-ventricular short axis image demonstrating the confluent area of infarction covering most of the wall thickness of the septum (white, arrowed), compared to the normal myocardium (black); the blood pool appears grey.

Intracardiac electrograms during VT

The intracardiac electrograms recorded at diagnostic EP study during a broad complex tachycardia may immediately make the diagnosis of VT clear. An almost pathognomonic feature of ventricular tachycardia is that ventricular and atrial activity is dissociated (Fig. 22.2). This is confirmed by findings when recording from atrial and ventricular catheters with absence of any consistent relationship between the atrial and ventricular electrograms.

However, it is possible to have 1:1 VA conduction during VT, with retrograde activation of the atrium from the ventricle. In order to distinguish this from an SVT with aberrant conduction, pacing manoeuvres are required (p. 206).

Atrial extrastimuli/pacing

Where retrograde AV nodal conduction is rapid enough, it is possible to see a one-to-one relationship between the atrial and ventricular electrograms with VT. To distinguish VT from the other causes of a broad complex tachycardia, pacing manoeuvres are performed to demonstrate that VA dissociation is possible. The introduction of atrial extrastimuli/atrial pacing at a cycle length shorter than that of the VT cycle length may transiently produce VA dissociation (p. 207).

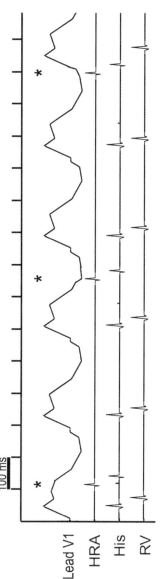

Fig. 22.2 Intracardiac electrograms from a three-wire EP study during VT. The surface ECG lead V1 is shown and demonstrates a broad complex tachycardia with evidence of dissociated P-wave activity (denoted by the *). The three diagnostic EP catheters are in the high right atrium (HRA), the His bundle position (His), and in the right ventricular apex (RV). The cycle length of the electrograms on the HRA (which coincide with the surface P-waves) is clearly slower than the electrogram on the RV catheter, and dissociated. The His catheter confirms the lack of a relationship between the atrial and ventricular components.

484 CHAPTER 22 **Ventricular tachycardia ablation**

Common aspects of VT ablation

Some aspects of ablation are common for all types of VT.

Success

Acute procedural success rates depend upon the type of VT:
- RVOT VT and fascicular VT: 90+%.
- Infarct-related VT (in patients with coronary artery disease): 70–85%.
- DCM-associated VT: 60–80%.
- ARVC VT: 70–90%.
- Bundle branch re-entrant VT: 80–90%.

NB These figures demonstrate the variation in reported success rates. Furthermore, in patients with scar-related VT (either ischaemic or non-ischaemic) these figures represent success for the *ablated* VT but not for freedom from *any* VT – subsequently a different VT may occur in many of these patients.

Complications

- Vascular access: haematoma; DVT; AV fistula; arterial pseudoaneurysm.
- Catheter manipulation: vascular damage; microemboli (particularly in the left ventricle) and risk of stroke; coronary artery dissection if retrograde aortic approach used; cardiac perforation and tamponade.
- RF application: cardiac tamponade; coronary artery damage if epicardial approach used. AV block is rarely reported but may occur in some patients with RVOT VT and fascicular VT. Also occurs after bundle branch re-entrant VT ablation, as intrinsic conduction disease is invariably present (📖 p. 316).
- Mortality is uncommon in 'normal heart' VT ablation (<0.1%) but may be up to 2% in some forms of infarct-related VT ablation.

Patient preparation

- Stop all anti-arrhythmic drugs at least five half-lives before procedure for patients with RVOT VT, fascicular VT, and where practical for other forms of VT ablation. In patients with incessant VT this may not be necessary.
- Conscious sedation can be used for all VT ablation but is preferred for the triggered/automatic VT types, e.g. RVOT VT and fascicular VT, as general anaesthesia (GA) may be more likely to render VT non-inducible in these patients:
  - Midazolam (up to 0.2 mg/kg/hr), and
  - Fentanyl (up to 2 mcg/kg/hr) IV.
- GA is more frequently used for VT ablation in patients with significant structural heart disease or in those undergoing epicardial ablation.

Choice of access (📖 p. 46)

- Femoral venous access is invariably required, at least for a catheter for programmed stimulation – more venous sheaths may be used, e.g. for His catheter in bundle branch re-entrant VT or for trans-septal access when required.
- Femoral arterial access may simply be used for haemodynamic monitoring or be required for catheter access.

General principles of VT ablation

Automatic vs. re-entrant mechanisms

Ablation of automatic/triggered VT such as RVOT VT is intrinsically dependent on inducing at least ventricular ectopy and if possible sustained tachycardia (📖 p. 510). Re-entrant VT is ideally mapped and ablated during tachycardia but it is possible to perform ablation even if no tachycardia is induced, e.g. ablation of Purkinje potentials in sinus rhythm in patients with fascicular VT or substrate ablation in infarct-related VT (📖 p. 526).

Activation mapping vs. pace-mapping

In simple terms activation mapping describes mapping of an arrhythmia whilst the arrhythmia is occurring. For automatic/triggered arrhythmias the aim during activation mapping is to find electrograms within the chamber of interest that are substantially earlier than the earliest surface activation, e.g. with RVOT VT the identification of an electrogram within the right ventricle that is earlier than the onset of the QRS complex on the surface ECG by 30–50 ms (📖 p. 513). For a re-entrant arrhythmia activation mapping aims to identify a series of electrograms that determine activation of as much of the entire circuit as possible (Fig. 22.3) and, in the example of scar-related VT, to try to identify the critical components of the circuit where ablation will lead to termination of the tachycardia and render it non-inducible (📖 p. 498). Pace mapping is performed when the patient is in sinus rhythm but the morphology of the clinical tachycardia is known. For VT, this mapping technique may be used where the VT is inducible but non-sustained or even for mapping ectopics alone. The theory underpinning this technique is that if pacing is performed at the same cycle length as tachycardia from the site of origin of an automatic/triggered VT, or at the exit site of a re-entrant VT, then the paced QRS morphology will match that of the clinical tachycardia. Pace mapping is generally described in relation to the number of leads of the standard 12-lead ECG that match the clinical arrhythmia, i.e. if all 12 leads during pacing from a given site match the clinical arrhythmia then it is said to be a '12/12 pace map' (Fig. 22.4).

Practical note

12/12 pace maps may be achieved over a relatively large area (in the ventricles in the case of VT up to 1 cm²) and so may not localize the most precise point for effective ablation. Activation mapping is much more specific and when early sites are found with automatic/triggered VT, or diastolic activity is identified in re-entrant VT, this is a much more precise indicator of the critical areas for ablation of the arrhythmia. In practice, e.g. where a patient has been very troubled by arrhythmia clinically but in the lab it is non-sustained, the operator has no option but to pursue pace mapping in the hope of achieving curative ablation rather than abandoning the procedure. Pace mapping in scarred tissue may also be misleading as the paced wavefront may activate normal myocardium (as the path of least resistance) rather than the critical tachycardia isthmus. Also block at the boundaries of the scar may be functional and so not reproduced exactly during pacing. Most operators will use a combination of techniques where possible to identify optimal sites for ablation.

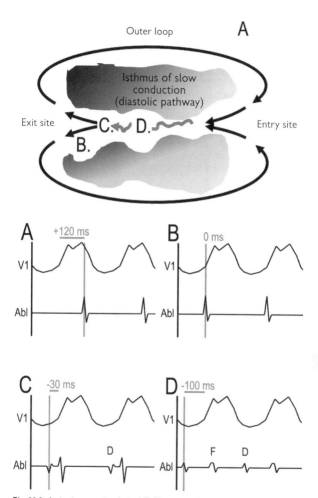

Fig. 22.3 Activation mapping during VT. The timing of the ablation catheter electrogram (Abl) in relation to the surface ECG QRS (V1) is shown for different positions in the VT circuit. The outer loop electrogram (A) is 120 ms later than the onset of the QRS. The exit site electrogram (B) coincides with QRS onset. Electrograms in the diastolic pathway often have more than one component. Nearer the exit (C) the electrogram has a pre-systolic component labelled D (−30 ms), and within the diastolic pathway (D) this component becomes earlier (−100 ms) with a far-field component within the QRS labelled F.

Mid-diastolic potentials

A potential occurring in the isoelectric segment may identify an area of slow conduction (the diastolic pathway – Fig. 22.3). These potentials occur 10–100 ms, or more, before the main ventricular deflection. Features of mid-diastolic potentials that support its importance as a critical part of the circuit include:

- Always precedes all tachycardia complexes during initiation and reset of tachycardia.
- Loss of potential with termination of arrhythmia.

If these potentials do not precede the QRS complex this area is a bystander. Continuous activity during the diastolic period represents slow/fractionated conduction in diseased myocardium but this may not be an essential area for the tachycardia circuit.

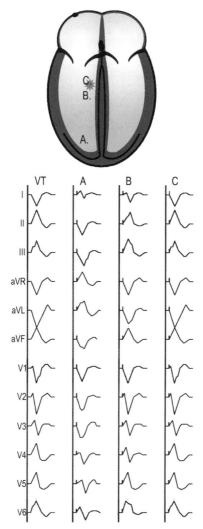

Fig. 22.4 12-lead ECG recordings are shown. When pacing at Site A, the 'pace map' (A) is very different to the clinical VT (VT). Site B has a better pace map but the precordial transition is not the same and the QRS morphology is not identical. Site C has a perfect (12/12) pace map suggesting that this is close to/at the exit site. (Note that ablation at perfect pace map sites may still not eliminate VT – 📖 p. 486.)

Pacing manoeuvres

Entrainment and post-pacing intervals

In order to understand the value of entrainment it is necessary to: (a) know how to perform the pacing manoeuvres required; and (b) to understand how to interpret the results obtained.

Performing entrainment pacing

This has to be performed whilst the patient is in tachycardia (assume VT for the purposes of this explanation). A catheter is placed in the ventricle of interest and pacing is performed from the distal portion (ideally this is unipolar for the purist signal, but routinely bipolar pacing is used in many labs). As an example, assume we have a clinical VT with a stable tachycardia cycle length (TCL) measured at 300 ms. To 'entrain' we need to pace slightly faster than the clinical TCL (between 10 and 50 ms faster) and capture the ventricle from the catheter at this faster rate. Once we are satisfied that the pacing stimulus is capturing at this faster rate, then the pacing is abruptly discontinued. The clinical tachycardia must then continue (at the same original TCL) and measurements can then be made.

Measurements to take when performing entrainment (Fig. 22.5)

First determine the nature of the fusion that is seen. 'QRS fusion' may be seen where the paced QRS is of a clearly different morphology to the clinical VT. In this case pacing is either being performed at a remote bystander site or in the outer loop. If the paced QRS complex is of the same morphology as the clinical VT then entrainment is said to be 'concealed' (Fig. 22.5). The post-pacing interval (PPI) must then be measured (Fig. 22.5). Where it is difficult to see the local electrogram on the pacing catheter immediately after pacing is terminated, an alternative in the same chamber may be used, but measurement must then be from the electrogram on that catheter at the last paced beat to the next non-paced electrogram on that catheter during tachycardia. The time from stimulus (S) to onset of QRS during pacing (S-QRS) and the electrogram (EG) on the same catheter to the onset of the QRS during VT (EG-QRS) are also measured.

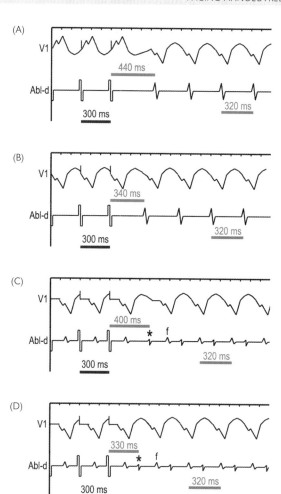

Fig. 22.5 Tachycardia cycle length (TCL) is 320 ms. Pacing at 300 ms CL entrains the tachycardia at each of the sites shown in Fig. 22.6. (A) At site A, a different QRS morphology to the tachycardia is seen and the post-pacing interval (PPI) is long (440 ms). (B) At site B the QRS morphology is similar to tachycardia and the PPI is close to the TCL, but the stimulus-QRS (S-QRS) time during pacing is short, confirming an exit site location. (C) At site C the PPI is longer but the S-QRS is longer and there is evidence of diastolic activity (*) and far-field ventricular activation subsequently (f). (D) At site D the QRS morphology during pacing is identical to tachycardia, PPI is less than 30 ms different to TCL, a longer S-QRS is seen, and mid-diastolic activity is seen during tachycardia (*) – an optimal ablation site!

Response to entrainment

Entrainment has several electrophysiological purposes:
- Confirms re-entry as mechanism for arrhythmia.
- Localizes re-entrant circuit to a particular cardiac chamber.
- Localizes critical components of the re-entrant circuit that sustain tachycardia, e.g. diastolic pathway (📖 p. 310).

Fused and concealed entrainment can be seen not only on the ECG (Fig. 22.5) but also on the intracardiac electrograms. Activation patterns can give an important indication of whether entrainment is genuinely concealed (i.e. the activation patterns are exactly the same) or fused (Fig. 22.5).

Determining location of pacing site in tachycardia circuit (Fig. 22.6)

The nature of entrainment (fused or concealed) and the post-pacing interval (PPI) can indicate where the pacing site lies within the circuit. This is shown diagrammatically in Fig. 22.6. First the nature of the entrainment is determined. When fusion is identified, this suggests the pacing site is in either a bystander, adjacent, or remote site (tissue that plays no part in sustaining the tachycardia) or in the outer loop. If the PPI equals the tachycardia cycle length (or is at least within 20–30 ms different) then it is in the outer loop, whilst if greater than 20–30 ms different it is in a bystander/ remote/adjacent site. Neither of these sites represents suitable targets for ablation. When entrainment is concealed, this could still represent a bystander or remote site (the PPI does not equal the CL). If concealed entrainment is accompanied by a PPI closely matching the tachycardia CL, the pacing site is within the more critical part of the circuit. It is possible to further define where the pacing site is within the circuit by using the formula (S-QRS/CL) × 100 (📖 Fig. 22.6). S-QRS is measured as described on 📖 p. 490. Ablation at any of these sites may successfully terminate a tachycardia and render it non-inducible, but central and proximal sites in the diastolic pathway are most successful.

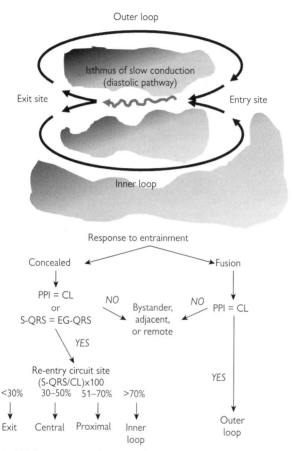

Fig. 22.6 Determining site of pacing in tachycardia circuit. See text for details on page opposite.

Ablation of VT in patients with coronary artery disease

Ablation of VT associated with ischaemic heart disease is important because it is relatively frequent, and can have a profound effect on both quality and quantity of life. It is common for these patients to already have an ICD *in situ* and this may have resulted in multiple therapies from the device prior to any ablation.

Useful information prior to ablation

Ideally before any ablation is performed:

- Underlying coronary artery disease and the presence of associated reversible ischaemia should be investigated. This may require coronary angiography.
- Non-invasive imaging should be performed to identify areas of scar that may act as potential substrate for VT and to assess ventricular function.
- A 12-lead ECG of the clinical VT may be available and identification of the exit site can be extrapolated (Table 22.1). A 12-lead ECG may not always be available, particularly where the VT is fast and haemodynamically poorly tolerated. In some cases the only recordings of VT are through an ICD *in situ*. This can still provide valuable information regarding the tachycardia cycle length of the clinical VT.

Also see 📖 p. 484.

Mapping and ablation with conventional electrodes

A single quadripolar catheter is used to induce VT, commonly from the right ventricle, but multiple different pacing sites may be used.

Ablation catheter access is most commonly needed to the left ventricle. This may be either via a trans-septal puncture (better for access to the lateral wall) or via the transaortic approach (better for access to the septum). In some cases both access routes may be used to improve mapping and to help with stability during ablation.

Activation mapping is used where the VT is haemodynamically stable (📖 p. 486). Pace mapping is used where either the VT is non-sustained, which prevents effective activation mapping, or where the VT is haemodynamically unstable (📖 p. 486). Where possible the diastolic pathway is identified using activation mapping and entrainment manoeuvres (📖 p. 490).

3-D mapping, non-contact mapping, and substrate mapping

There are several other techniques used to guide VT ablation that make use of more recent technologies. These are described in more detail both generally (📖 Chapter 6) and specifically related to VT (📖 pp. 500–504).

Table 22.1 Simplified approach to ischaemic VT localization from ECG

ECG finding	Area of localization
Bundle branch morphology	
Left	LV septum or right ventricle
Right	Other parts of the LV
Axis	
Superior (negative in II, III, AVF)	LV inferior wall or inferior septum
Inferior (positive in II, III, AVF)	LV anterior wall or anterior septum
Rightward	LV lateral wall or apex
Precordial transition (R > S)	
≤V3	Basal
≥V4	Apical LV
Positive concordance	Mitral valve annulus
Negative concordance	Apical
QRS upstroke	
Slurred (pseudo delta)	Epicardial (📖 p. 534)

Ablation targets

Diastolic pathway

This represents the critical isthmus of tissue required to maintain the re-entrant VT circuit and if it can be identified and ablation is performed here then success rates are highest (see below).

Features of the diastolic pathway:
- Typically lies within the infarct zone.
- Bipolar electrogram ≤0.5 mV and other characteristic features of the electrogram as shown in Table 22.2.
- Mid-diastolic potentials (📖 p. 488).
- Concealed entrainment during pacing (📖 p. 490).
- Post-pacing interval = TCL during VT (📖 p. 492).
- 12/12 pace map (📖 p. 486).
- Time from stimulus during pacing in sinus rhythm to the onset of the QRS is >50–70 ms or 30–50% of the TCL – described as 'latency' in this setting (📖 p. 493).

Exit site

The exit site will be a larger area of tissue than the diastolic pathway:
- Typically lies at the edge of the infarct zone.
- Bipolar electrograms between 0.5 and 1.5 mV are common but may also be larger.
- Pre-systolic potentials (20–50 ms pre-QRS).
- Concealed entrainment during pacing may still occur (📖 p. 491).
- Post-pacing interval = TCL during VT (📖 p. 492).
- 12/12 pace map (📖 p. 486).
- Time from stimulus during pacing in sinus rhythm to the onset of the QRS is short and <30% of the TCL (📖 p. 493).
- Similar findings can be demonstrated over a 1 cm^2 area of tissue (📖 p. 486).

Practical note

Although ablation at certain sites provides better success than at others, it may not always be possible to identify the very best sites, e.g. because the diastolic pathway is epicardial and only endocardial mapping has been performed.

Table 22.2 Electrogram features

Morphology	Definition	Interpretations/causes
Low amplitude	<1.5 mV	Area of fibrosis, scar, or any other process that destroys normal cellular structure
		Poor contact of catheter
		Far-field signal
Fractionated	Prolonged, low amplitude potentials with multiple peaks/troughs around the isoelectric baseline (often >70 ms in duration)	Peri-infarct area
		Slow conduction area
		Catheter movement
		Arborized myocardial connection
Split	Two components of the potential separated by an isoelectric interval (often >60 ms)	Local conduction block (anatomical, e.g. scar, or functional)
		Slow conduction area
Late component	A potential occurring after the end of the surface QRS	Delayed activation
		Slow conduction area or conduction block
Continuous	A potential that runs throughout the cardiac cycle with no diastolic isoelectric interval	Slow conduction area
		Artefact
		Electromagnetic interference (e.g. 50 Hz noise from main electricity)
Mid-diastolic	A potential that occurs in mid-diastole with isoelectric segments on either side	📖 p. 488
Low frequency	Small amplitude potential with shallow slope shown by a low dV/dt	Far-field signal
		Artefact
Monophasic action potential	Pattern seen with injury current	Too much contact pressure
		Injury to tissue locally

Endpoints for VT ablation in patients with CAD

Ideally termination of the clinical VT occurs during ablation and no further VT can then be induced. This may be regarded as an absolute endpoint. However, it is quite common in these patients to be able to induce further VT that may not be clinically relevant, or the clinical VT itself is non-sustained/haemodynamically poorly tolerated, making ablation during VT itself difficult. A pragmatic approach, therefore, is to aim for the absolute endpoint but accept that this may need to be modified in some circumstances. Also, finish the procedure when only haemodynamically poorly tolerated VT can be induced after ablation if the original VT was well-tolerated and slower – further induction testing and ablation in this setting is only likely to lead to complication and carries a significant mortality risk.

Success rates

For abolition of the *clinical* VT:
If the diastolic pathway is identified – 70–90%.
If the exit site is identified – 70–80%.
Substrate mapping and pace mapping alone – 70–80%.

Complications

General complications are as listed on p. 484. These patients often have depressed ventricular function and concomitant illnesses, and ablation may be a late attempt to control refractory arrhythmias. Significant complications are therefore more common:
- Stroke, transient ischaemic attack, myocardial infarction, cardiac perforation requiring treatment, or heart block occur in 5–8%.
- Mortality is 1 to 3% depending upon the patient population.

Troubleshooting the difficult case

Non-inducible tachycardia or only able to induce fast, haemodynamically unstable VT:
- Substrate/scar mapping and ablation in sinus rhythm (📖 p. 502).
- Use of non-contact mapping (📖 p. 504).
- Support of blood pressure during VT with positive inotropes, intra-aortic balloon pump insertion.
- Slow rate of VT pharmacologically but may affect inducibility.
- Try high dose isoprenaline where induction is essential the procedure.

Ablation at favourable site unsuccessful:
- Most commonly because of inadequate energy delivery. Irrigated (or large-tip) ablation catheter may overcome this.
- If early in mapping then continue to map with more detail.
- Consider mapping with different catheter shapes/sizes or change approach, e.g. from transaortic to trans-septal.
- Consider another form of VT.
- Use of unipolar electrograms as well as bipolar signals.
- Consider an epicardial path (📖 p. 534).

3-D mapping in VT ablation

Mapping systems are commonly used for ablation of complex arrhythmias. There are a number of different mapping systems available commercially but they share many similar features.

Electroanatomical mapping (CARTO, 📖 p. 100 and Fig. 22.7)

Anatomical information

A 3-D computer-generated representation of the ventricle being mapped is created (often referred to as a 'geometry'). The catheter is navigated around the chamber of interest and endocardial points are serially acquired to create the geometry. At the same time points of interest may be marked or 'tagged', e.g. His bundle, valves.

Electrical information

Electrograms (EGMs) are recorded from the catheter tip. EGM timing is compared to a stable electrical reference (the surface ECG or another intracardiac EGM). A colour-coded activation map is then superimposed on the 3-D geometry.

> **Tips and tricks**
>
> - Position of catheter updates from cardiac cycle – can use pacing to ↑ refresh rate.
> - Set timing window appropriately:
>   - For re-entry aim to cover 90% TCL, e.g. for TCL 300 ms set −140 to +140 ms.
>   - For focal arrhythmia set window to appropriate time pre-surface ECG, e.g. 50–80 ms pre-QRS for RVOT VT.

Impedance-based catheter localization (NavX, 📖 p. 104 and Fig. 22.7)

Location information is used to construct a 3-D geometry of the ventricle. Activation maps are constructed by comparing the timing of an EGM (usually the ablation catheter) to a stable timing reference electrode and are superimposed upon the geometry (like CARTO above).

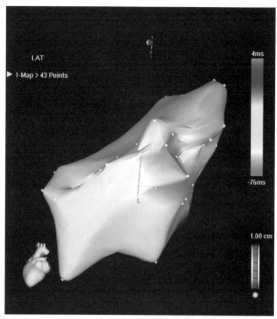

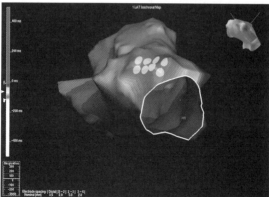

Fig. 22.7 Top panel shows CARTO map of focal VT in the left ventricle. Bottom panel shows a NavX map of a focal VT near the mitral valve annulus (MVA). Circles represent the ablation lesions that terminated VT. (See Plate 20 for colour version, which shows earliest activation during tachycardia in red on the CARTO map and white on the NavX map.)

Substrate/scar mapping

Up to 25% of patients considered for stable VT ablation cannot be ablated using conventional mapping techniques as described earlier (📖 p. 486). Those with haemodynamically unstable VT are even more difficult to ablate with conventional methods. Substrate/scar mapping was originally developed for surgical ablation. Mapping systems have been an essential development in this process for the transition to a percutaneous approach (Fig. 22.8).

Principles of substrate mapping

- That identification of the location of scar can be useful in targeting ablation of VT during sinus rhythm.
- Bipolar electrograms of <0.5 mV identify dense scar.
- Electrograms of 0.5 to 1.5 mV identify border zone scar.
- Electrograms >1.5 mV represent normal tissue.
- Linear lesions from scar to anatomical barriers, e.g. mitral valve annulus, or to normal tissue can approximate to surgical subendocardial resection.

How to do it

- A mapping system is used to generate an anatomical representation of the cardiac chamber (📖 p. 500).
- The chamber is systematically mapped and voltages recorded during sinus rhythm. Density of mapping, i.e. number of points collected, can be relatively low in normal tissue but should be higher in abnormal tissue.
- Once these are recorded the scar and border zone can be identified by setting the colour representation to a range of 0.5–1.5 mV, e.g. with a CARTO map the voltage window is red for any area below 0.5 mV and then there is progression through the colour scale to a light purple, which is normal myocardium (📖 p. 100).

Ablation can then be performed in a number of ways:

- The entire scar may be encircled with ablation but this is technically challenging, the area may be large, and it is almost impossible to create a complete continuous line.
- Mapping may be enhanced by pace mapping if the ECG morphology of the clinical VT is known and then ablation performed at the border zone of the scar that matches most closely (the presumed exit site).
- Areas where there is 'latency' with pacing (📖 p. 496) may be ablated.
- Areas of normal myocardium may be identified amongst the scar tissue (by pacing and showing it is excitable within the scar region) and then ablated as possible re-entrant circuit isthmuses. Also, abnormal electrograms (📖 p. 497) are targeted in the regions identified from the substrate map and ablated.
- Brief inductions may be performed with the mapping catheter at the 'best' sites as defined by the above techniques and then entrainment manoeuvres performed briefly.
- Normally several of these techniques are used in combination.

- Ablation is normally performed along a short section of the scar zone (1–2 cm) both tangentially and perpendicularly. Multiple lesions (no more than 5 mm apart) are delivered, and perpendicular lesions may be extended to another area of conduction block (either anatomical, e.g. valve annulus/other scar tissue, or functional, e.g. anatomical crista).

Endpoints for tissue ablation with substrate mapping
- Decrease in contact impedance at ablation site of >5 Ω.
- Decrease in electrogram voltage by >75%.
- Doubling of the pacing capture threshold.

Note

Substrate mapping is not used exclusively in patients with non-inducible/ haemodynamically poorly tolerated VT and may also be used in conjunction with more conventional mapping and ablation techniques in patients with stable VT where other strategies have proved unsuccessful (🔲 p. 498).

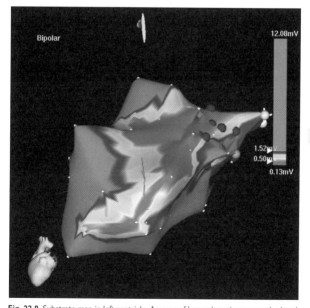

Fig. 22.8 Substrate map in left ventricle. An area of low voltage is seen on the basal lateral wall (red colour in Plate 14). The white balls mark the mitral valve annulus (MVA) and the blue ball an area of double potentials (DPs). The best pace maps for the clinical VT (which was fast and haemodynamically unstable) were in the region of the very basal scar and therefore a set of ablation lesions (red balls) were performed around the margin of the low voltage area, extending through the area of DPs and to the MVA. This rendered the VT non-inducible. (🔲 Plate 14 for colour version.)

Non-contact mapping in non-sustained or haemodynamically unstable VT

The concept of non-contact mapping

- An endocavity probe electrode is able to record endocardial signals without being in contact with the endocardium.
- The potentials recorded are low amplitude and a process of amplification and mathematical reconstruction is used to create an electrogram resembling the endocardial electrogram as it would appear with a contact mapping catheter.

The clinical non-contact mapping system

The non-contact mapping system used clinically consists of:

- *A catheter-mounted multi-electrode array (MEA)*: The MEA is a woven braid of 64 0.003-inch-diameter wires mounted on a 7.6 ml balloon on a 9 F catheter. Each wire has a 0.025 inch break in insulation, producing a non-contact unipolar electrode.
- *A custom-built amplifier system*: The raw far-field electrographic data from the MEA are acquired and fed into a multichannel recorder and amplifier system.
- *A workstation to run specially designed system software*: This makes it possible to reconstruct >3300 unipolar endocardial electrograms simultaneously.

A ring electrode located on the proximal shaft of the MEA catheter in the descending aorta is used as a reference for both non-contact and contact unipolar electrogram recordings.

Before deployment of the MEA, patients are given 10 000 IU heparin with later boluses to maintain activated clotting time at 300 to 400 seconds. The MEA catheter is deployed via the retrograde transaortic route over a 0.032-inch J-tipped guidewire advanced to the LV apex. With the pigtail of the MEA in the LV apex, the guidewire is withdrawn and the balloon inflated with a contrast-saline mixture.

The system is also able to locate any conventional catheter in space with respect to the MEA by passing a low-current 'locator' signal between the catheter being located and alternately between ring electrodes proximal and distal to the MEA on the non-contact catheter. This locator signal serves two purposes. First, it is used to provide measured samples for the geometry matrix of the inverse solution by constructing a 3-D computer model of the endocardium (a so-called 'virtual endocardium'). This is achieved by dragging a mapping catheter around the LV chamber, building up a series of coordinates for the endocardium (contour geometry – Fig. 22.9) and generating an anatomically accurate endocardial model. Secondly, the locator signal is used to display and log the position of the mapping catheter on the virtual endocardium during a study.

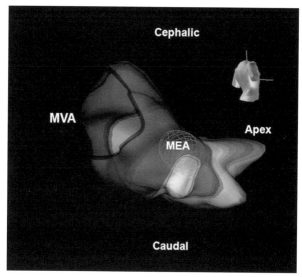

Fig. 22.9 Left ventricular geometry created using a multi-electrode array (MEA). The colours represent electrical activation (📖 Chapter 6). The torso in the top right corner depicts the orientation of the chamber. MVA – mitral valve annulus. (📖 Plate 17 for colour version.)

Practical use of a non-contact mapping system for VT ablation (see Table 22.3)

- Patients are studied in the post-absorptive state under local anaesthesia.
- A standard quadripolar catheter at the right ventricular apex is used for programmed stimulation (📖 p. 80).
- For mapping the LV, two mapping and ablation catheters (trans-septal and retrograde approach) may be used. This has the advantage of allowing access to areas of the endocardium that may be restricted by the MEA from either approach (in general the LV septum may be reached more easily from the transaortic approach, whilst the trans-septal route provides better access to the lateral wall).
- Continuous systemic (and sometimes pulmonary artery) pressures are monitored throughout the study.
- The MEA catheter is deployed as described on 📖 p. 504. It is important to carefully position the MEA in dilated LVs, as reconstruction of electrograms and catheter-location accuracy decreases at distances >34 mm from the MEA centre.
- The mapping catheter is dragged around the endocardial surface to collect a large series of points and construct a geometric model representative of the LV. Trabeculations may limit catheter manipulation, and it can be helpful to use a catheter inversion technique to access some parts of the LV to complete the reconstruction. This creates the 'virtual endocardium' (Fig. 22.9).
- The electrograms derived from the reconstruction process are then superimposed onto the endocardial model to produce dynamic high-resolution isopotential maps (Fig. 22.10). Isopotential maps are colour-coded to represent changes in potential difference on the endocardium. Maximum −dv/dt with endocardial activation is seen as a spectral change from resting purple to white colour on the isopotential map.
- Once the basic geometry is configured, VT is induced and mapping undertaken as follows: (1) Identification of diastolic pathways is started by identification of the VT exit site, which is defined as a rapidly spreading focus of activity coincident with onset of the QRS complex on the surface ECG, leading to systolic activation of the ventricle. Diastolic activity during VT is then defined as activity progressing in a continuous fashion to the VT exit site. In practice the exit site can be seen as a white spot of activation when an isopotential map is displayed at the onset of surface ECG QRS complex. Diastolic activity is then identified by moving the isopotential map display back in time. When a discrete spot of diastolic activity can no longer be seen on the map then the limit of the diastolic pathway identified by the system has been reached and all diastolic activity identified before this is ignored. (2) Ablation catheters are navigated to the targets of interest identified by non-contact mapping. (3) Complimentary conventional mapping techniques are then used to assess and reconfirm target sites before ablation. (4) Ablation is performed during VT if possible.

- The ability to visualize the catheter and mark ablation sites with mapping systems means that it is possible to create accurate linear lesions during ablation, in preference to single spot lesions. If VT is terminated then attempts are made to re-induce tachycardia.

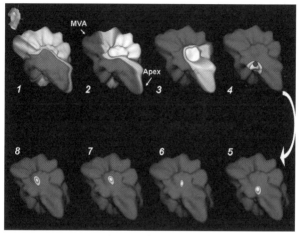

Fig. 22.10 A reverse-time sequence of eight isopotential maps during VT. In (1) the left ventricular virtual endocardium is translucent and the multi-electrode array position can be seen. The translucency has been removed in the rest of the maps. Systolic activation is shown during VT in (1) and (2). The VT is then mapped backwards in time. (3) and (4) show the probable exit site of the VT. (4) to (8) show slow conduction (inferred from the small distance covered by the activation on the isopotential maps during a time period of 150 ms). This presumably represents part of the diastolic pathway for the VT circuit. Ablation at the exit site (marked by a red circle on map 4) terminated VT and rendered it non-inducible. MVA – mitral valve annulus. (📖 Plate 19 for colour version.)

Pitfalls and limitations of non-contact mapping for VT ablation

Difficulties in demonstrating the diastolic pathway/diastolic potentials

Although the ability to map the entire tachycardia cycle length within a single cycle is clearly an inherent advantage when mapping unstable VT, it is not always possible to accurately demonstrate the diastolic pathway. Several factors contribute to this:

- It is possible that the re-entry circuit is not entirely confined to the endocardial surface, with intramural or subepicardial areas of slow conduction.
- The volume of the tissue forming the diastolic component of the circuit may be insufficient to produce electrograms that can be identified by the non-contact mapping system.
- Saturation of the isopotential maps occurring with repolarization of the LV leads to similarities between the lower frequency and amplitude diastolic potential electrograms detected by the system and those of repolarization.

Filter settings

Changing the filter settings used to display virtual electrograms can have a profound effect on the morphology of the electrogram (as it can with contact electrograms). When trying to identify and display the low amplitude unipolar signals associated with diastolic potentials, adjustment of filtering may be necessary to differentiate true electrical activity from noise. Local activation on a unipolar electrogram is associated with the first negative deflection from baseline. It can be difficult to distinguish the deflections of a unipolar virtual electrogram from baseline wander. Increasing the high pass filter can help to distinguish such noise from true electrical activation on the isopotential maps but it should be remembered that it may also filter out the virtual electrograms associated with true activation for this reason. A number of different filter settings may therefore need to be tried with the operator looking at the electrograms produced at the region of interest on the isopotential map, rather than relying on the isopotential map alone to guide ablation.

Dynamic substrate mapping

It may be possible to address some of the limitations of mapping the VT itself by using dynamic substrate mapping. This technique allows identification of low voltage areas that may be the substrate for the arrhythmia and can be performed in sinus rhythm. As with isopotential mapping, the array may be used to acquire surface voltage characteristics during a single cardiac cycle. It is then possible to identify potential voltage barriers, such as scar tissue, and the threshold for low-voltage detection may be manually adjusted. The same limitations as for isopotential mapping are seen with this technique, i.e. reduced accuracy with increasing distance from the MEA and alterations of the voltage map according to the filter settings. Ultimately, the technique has yet to be validated in ischaemic VT, but may give additional guidance when diastolic potentials cannot be identified.

Anatomical problems
- Very low amplitude signals may not be detected, particularly if the distance between the MEA and endocardial surface >34 mm.
- If the geometry of the LV is created during sinus rhythm, changes in the LV size and contraction pattern during VT may in theory adversely affect the accuracy of the location of the endocardial electrograms. In practice this does not seem to be a big issue.
- Movement of the MEA within the LV during the procedure inevitably leads to inaccuracies in mapping. This appears to only be a significant issue if the MEA has not been located in a stable position at the apex of the LV or in patients with normal LV function who have dynamic hearts that can push the MEA out of position.
- The MEA can result in difficulties with ablation catheter manipulation but the use of two mapping catheters (one via a trans-septal puncture and the other retrogradely across the aortic valve) will usually allow access to all regions of the LV.

Table 22.3 Clinical experience of non-contact mapping in post-MI VT

Total no. of patients studied (no. of patients with infarct related VT)	Total no. of VTs induced (clinical)	Total no. of VTs successfully ablated/ mapped (clinical)	Percentage of VTs where diastolic pathway component identified	Recurrence
52 (52)	132	74/124	—	33% of any VT over 18 months
24 (19)	97 (24)	38/81 (14)	80%	5.4% of ablated VT over 18 months
40 (40)	140 (36)	67/81 (27)	55%	7.5% of ablated VT over 36 months
68 (9)	9	8/9	—	12.5% had same symptoms after 20 months

Ablation of RVOT VT

Clinical features and the mechanistic aspects of RVOT ectopy and VT can be found on 📖 p. 318. Catheter ablation of RVOT VT is increasingly considered first-line therapy. When approaching ablation of these patients the following are important in the process.

Understanding the anatomy of the RVOT

The RVOT is defined by the following anatomical landmarks:
- The pulmonary valve superiorly.
- The superior margin of the tricuspid valve inferiorly.
- The interventricular septum posteriorly.
- The right ventricular free wall anteriorly.

Localization of the RVOT focus from the 12-lead ECG

Although the RVOT is a relatively small area, the ECG characteristics of the RVOT ectopy or VT can give useful clues regarding its specific location and guide the operator to within 1 cm of the site for successful ablation (Table 22.4).

Induction and catheter setup

- A quadripolar catheter is placed in the RV apex for programmed stimulation/burst pacing to induce the tachycardia (this is often used even if the VT/ectopy is almost incessant).
- Easiest to ablate when spontaneous VT/ectopy is present. Any anti-arrhythmics should be discontinued for at least five half-lives and sedation limited to minimize rendering the patient non-inducible. Induction may need to be augmented by the use of isoprenaline and is more commonly successful with burst pacing from the RVOT itself.
- A standard RF medium sweep or 'D' curve ablation catheter is often used.
- Commonly used ablation settings: temperature limited RF at 50–60°C, with powers of 40–60 W, for 60 seconds at a time (for lesions in the aortic cusp start with lower powers, 10–15 W, and up-titrate to achieve catheter tip temperature – 📖 p. 516).
- Where there is difficulty achieving adequate power, irrigated RF ablation may be used. This may be because the catheter is lodged under the pulmonary valve or in a trabeculated area with lower blood flow.
- Cryoablation has been used, particularly when the best ablation site is near the His bundle or maintaining stability through the time of an entire RF lesion is problematic, as the cryoablation catheter becomes adherent to the tissue once it reaches the appropriate 'freezing' point (📖 p. 44).

Table 22.4 ECG localization of an RVOT focus

ECG finding	Area of localization
Precordial transition (R > S)	
≤V3	Septum
≥V4	RV free wall
QRS duration	
≤140 ms	Septum
Lead morphology	
Lead I R or Rs	Right (posterior)
Lead I rs or qrs	Middle
Lead I qs or rS	Left (anterior)
Notching in II, III, aVF	RV free wall
QS amplitude aVR < aVL	Left (anterior)
Initial R wave in V1 and V2 > 0.2 mV	Below the pulmonary valve
V3 R:S ratio <1	RVOT (rather than LVOT)

Standard ablation technique

RVOT ectopy and VT ablation is normally guided by a combination of activation and pace mapping (📖 p. 486). The ablation catheter is advanced into the RVOT. If spontaneous ectopy or VT is present then activation mapping can be performed looking for local bipolar electrograms that precede the QRS during ectopy or VT by at least 30 ms (Fig. 22.11). If a unipolar recording is available this should have a QS pattern. Because of the size of the ablation tip, the first such signal recorded may still not represent the very best ablation site and pace mapping should also be performed. Pacing at an output high enough to capture the ventricle at a rate similar to the VT tachycardia CL (or at a rate of between 600 and 400 ms where only ectopy is present) should demonstrate a 12/12 pace map. It is important to carefully map and find the best site before performing any ablation as sometimes this site is not in the RVOT itself (📖 p. 516). During RF delivery, a positive sign is acceleration of the VT or a burst of VT with the same morphology as the ectopy, which disappears as the lesion is completed. It is common practice to deliver further consolidation ablation (2–4 lesions) in the successful area. Conventionally this procedure can be guided by fluoroscopy alone (often facilitated by biplane imaging), but 3-D mapping equipment may be very useful for labelling and returning to sites of interest once a complete map of the area has been made.

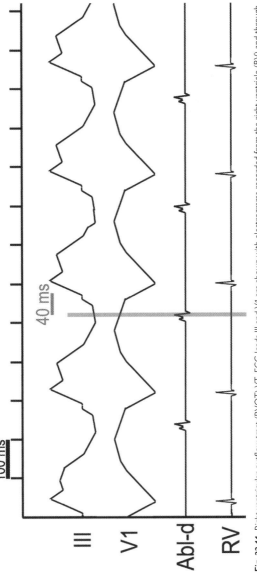

Fig. 22.11 Right ventricular outflow tract (RVOT) VT. ECG leads III and V1 are shown with electrograms recorded from the right ventricle (RV) and through the ablation catheter (Abl-d) at a site in the RVOT. The electrogram on Abl-d is 40 ms before the QRS onset, which suggests it may be at the exit site of the VT.

3-D mapping

3-D mapping may be particularly useful where a large area of the RVOT and surrounding structures needs to be mapped and areas of interest returned to later (Fig. 22.13). Where only non-sustained VT or ectopy are present, non-contact mapping may be used (📖 p. 504):

- The non-contact mapping array is inserted into the RVOT and used to map the non-sustained VT/ectopy.
- The array is positioned in the RVOT as shown in Fig. 22.12. NB It is important to remain below the pulmonary valve but not to be too low in the outflow tract either, as many of these will be high in the RVOT and accuracy diminishes further away from the array.
- An ablation catheter is inserted (📖 p. 510) and an anatomical representation of the RVOT generated by manipulating the catheter within this area. Once this is done a single ectopic can be mapped and targeted for ablation.
- Need to be aware that multiple exit sites may be present and catheter manipulation within the RVOT can be difficult with the array in position, as space may be physically limited.

Endpoints for RVOT ablation

- Where VT or ectopy was sustained prior to ablation, termination of VT during ablation with no further VT or ectopy is a very good sign of success.
- If it is only possible to get infrequent non-sustained VT or infrequent ectopy, despite provocation with pharmacological agents such as isoprenaline or pacing manoeuvres, then the ablation endpoint becomes more difficult. In this case, when good pace maps have been achieved, ablation characteristics have been good (i.e. early signals during the infrequent ectopy and accelerated rhythm during RF), and there has been an absence of further ectopics for 30–60 minutes after ablation, the case may be finished.

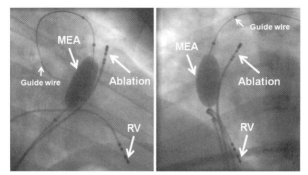

Fig. 22.12 Non-contact multi-electrode array (MEA) deployed in the right ventricular outflow tract (RVOT). The ablation catheter is also in the RVOT, a quadripolar catheter is in the RV, and the guidewire supporting the MEA is in the right pulmonary artery. RAO projection on the left and LAO on the right.

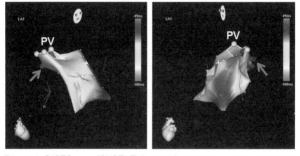

Fig. 22.13 CARTO map of RVOT VT. An area of early activation (area indicated by arrow) is seen just below the pulmonary valve (PV). RAO projection on the left and LAO on the right. (📖 Plate 8 for colour version.)

Related tachycardia sites

Basal left ventricular/left ventricular outflow tract VT

- Anatomy of the area: aortic valve superiorly and medially, and the myocardium bordering the mitral valve annulus septally, anteriorly, laterally, and inferiorly.
- As with RVOT, LVOT VT can initially be localized according to the 12-lead ECG morphology – generally right bundle branch block predominates but parahisian/septal LVOT VT will have a LBBB appearance (Table 22.5).
- Like RVOT, mapping and ablation may be performed conventionally and/or using 3-D mapping techniques. A transaortic approach is commonly used and as these patients mostly have normal-sized left ventricles, a small sweep or 'B' curve catheter is normally best.

Aortic cusp VT

- VT may originate from the left and right coronary cusps or the sinus of Valsalva (Table 22.6).
- The pulmonary valve and RVOT are anterior and superior to the aortic valve. The right coronary cusp is adjacent to the posterior septal aspect of RVOT whilst the left coronary cusp is adjacent to the more anterior septal aspect.
- Careful mapping of this region should be performed when a broad area of early activation is found in the RVOT adjacent to this region.
- Coronary angiography needs to be performed before and after ablation to demonstrate that the coronary ostia are at least 1 cm or more away and that no damage has occurred.

Epicardial focus

- Where no clear discrete area of early activation is identified during endocardial mapping, the epicardial approach may be considered (📖 p. 534). Again, caution needs to be exercised because of the proximity of the epicardial coronary arteries to possible ablation sites, and coronary angiography performed before any ablation.

Multiple foci

- Although multiple foci may suggest a more cardiomyopathic process such as ARVC (📖 p. 319), it is also possible for multiple foci to be seen in the normal heart. If ectopy of a different morphology is seen after ablation of the clinical VT, consider deferring any further ablation unless VT is inducible or occurs with the new morphology. Also, if there are other catheters in the RVOT or an array for non-contact mapping, these may be triggering the new ectopy.

Table 22.5 LVOT/basal VT localization from ECG

	Lead I morphology	Lead V1 morphology	Precordial transition
Septal/parahisian	R or Rs	QS or Qr	Early (≤V2)
Aortomitral continuity	Rs or rs	qR	None (positive concordance)
Superior mitral annulus	rs or rS	R or Rs	None (positive concordance)
Superolateral mitral annulus	rS or QS	R or Rs	None (positive concordance)
Lateral mitral annulus	rS or rs	R or Rs	None (positive concordance) or >V5

Table 22.6 Aortic cusp VT localization from ECG

	V1 morphology	Precordial transition
Right coronary cusp	QS or QR (predominantly a Q wave)	≥V3
Left coronary cusp	Multiphasic, i.e. 'M' or 'W' type pattern	≤V2

Success and complications

- Success rates are between 90 and 95%, with 5–10% requiring more than one procedure.
- Complications (□ p. 484): The RVOT is a thin-walled structure on the free wall side so there is an increased risk of cardiac perforation, particularly if higher powers and irrigated ablation are used.

Troubleshooting the difficult case

Non-inducible tachycardia or very infrequent spontaneous ectopy:

- Try high dose isoprenaline (>10 mcg/min sometimes needed), aminophylline (6 mg/kg intravenously over 20 minutes followed by an infusion 0.5 mg/kg/min), or epinephrine (25–50 mcg/kg/min). Sometimes the VT/ectopy will be more frequent in the 'cool down' phase so try turning off the infusions and wait for heart rate to normalize.

Large area of early activation:

- Consider mapping other related tachycardia sites as described earlier.
- Try using unipolar electrograms to help narrow the area.

Best site near the His bundle:

- Consider the use of cryoablation.

Ablation at favourable site unsuccessful:

- If early in mapping then continue to map with more detail.
- If powers are low, consider irrigated or large-tip ablation catheter.
- Consider mapping other related tachycardia sites.

Ablation of fascicular VT (idiopathic left ventricular VT)

Clinical features and the mechanistic aspects of fascicular VT can be found on □ p. 322). Catheter ablation of fascicular VT is increasingly considered first-line therapy. When approaching ablation of these patients the following are important in the process.

Induction and catheter setup (Fig. 22.14)

- A quadripolar catheter is placed in the RV apex for programmed stimulation/burst pacing to induce the tachycardia.
- A quadripolar catheter may also be placed in the His bundle position to help with distinguishing His electrograms from Purkinje potentials (□ p. 522).
- A multi-polar catheter may be placed along the left ventricular septum with the distal electrode nearer the apex to record left bundle/Purkinje potentials.
- Induction of fascicular VT can be achieved using programmed electrical stimulation from the ventricle (□ p. 80). A characteristic feature of this tachycardia is that it may also be induced from the atrium.

NB Whilst operating in the left ventricle it is important to anticoagulate to minimize the risk of thrombus formation and thromboembolism. Unfractionated heparin is given intravenously before the catheters are introduced into the arterial system – routinely 5000 IU is given as a bolus and if the procedure is longer than an hour then ACT may be checked and further heparin given to maintain an ACT of between 250 and 300.

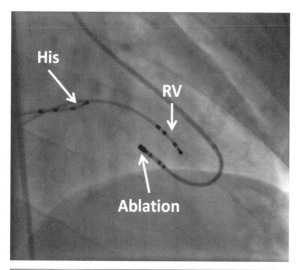

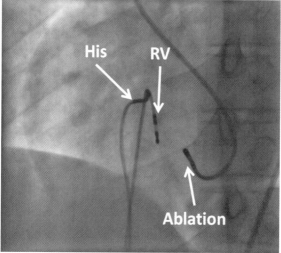

Fig. 22.14 Traditional catheter positions during ablation of fascicular tachycardia. The ablation, His, and right ventricular (RV) catheters are shown in the RAO (top) and LAO (bottom) fluoroscopic views.

Understanding the intracardiac electrograms of fascicular VT

- During sinus rhythm and during VT, discrete potentials (Purkinje potentials) can be recorded from the mid-septum. The relationship of Purkinje potentials to the ventricular electrogram and His differs during sinus rhythm and VT and this can be used to identify them (Figs. 22.15 and 22.16).
- Purkinje potentials can be divided into late diastolic (P1) and pre-systolic (P2). During sinus rhythm P2 is seen as a pre-systolic potential and represents activation through the posterior fascicle anterogradely. P1 represents slow conduction in a Purkinje fibre but is either buried in the ventricular electrogram or very late during sinus rhythm as it is activated slowly anterogradely and retrogradely. A critically-timed extrastimulus can initiate VT by allowing conduction anterogradely through the slow-conducting Purkinje fibre (activating P1) and then retrogradely activating the posterior fascicle (P2 may be delayed) (Figs. 22.15 and 22.16).
- To confirm the diagnosis/separate it from the differential diagnosis of SVT with aberrant conduction, particularly where there is retrograde 1:1 VA conduction:
  - Demonstrate His activation is retrograde.
  - HV interval is shorter during tachycardia than during sinus rhythm.
  - Compared to bundle branch re-entry where His activation precedes left bundle activation, the His activation comes after bundle activation.
  - Entrainment may be possible from either the atrium or the ventricle. PPIs at the site of P1 or P2 will reproducibly closely match the tachycardia cycle length.
  - With left posterior fascicular VT, earliest ventricular activation during VT is recorded at the apical septum and diastolic potentials in the mid-septum.
  - With left anterior fascicular VT, earliest ventricular activation during VT is recorded from the anterolateral LV and diastolic potentials in the mid-septum.
- A standard RF catheter is often effective as the Purkinje network is relatively superficial and easy to ablate.
- A small sweep or 'B' curve ablation catheter is often used via a retrograde approach as this gives good access and stability in the region of the LV of interest.
- Commonly used ablation settings: temperature limited RF at 50–60°C, with powers of 40–50 W, for 60 seconds at a time.
- Where there is difficulty achieving adequate power, irrigated RF ablation may be used but this is unusual. Occasionally a trans-septal approach is required.

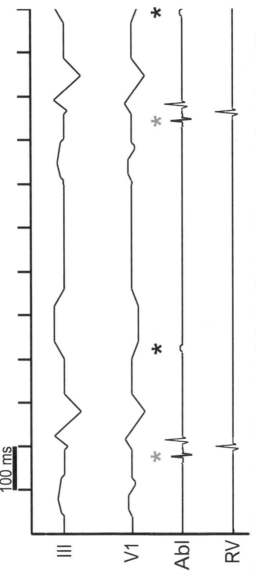

Fig. 22.15 Purkinje potentials recorded during sinus rhythm. ECG leads III and V1 are shown with electrograms recorded from the right ventricle (RV) and through the ablation catheter (Abl) at a site in the left ventricle such as that shown fluoroscopically in Fig. 22.14. A ventricular electrogram is seen on the ablation catheter with a pre-systolic Purkinje potential (P2) labelled by the grey asterisk and a late diastolic Purkinje potential (P1) labelled by the black asterisk.

Standard ablation technique

The ablation catheter is introduced into the LV via a transaortic approach. The catheter is fully inverted before crossing the aortic valve. Once in the left ventricle the catheter is turned clockwise, whilst still fully deflected and positioned in the region of the apical septum. VT is then induced and activation mapping is performed (📖 p. 486). The aim is to identify the Purkinje potentials (P1 and P2 electrograms) and ablate during VT if stable and well tolerated. For posterior VT, ablation is ideally performed at P1 but sometimes this cannot be identified as a separate electrogram to P2 and ablation can be equally successful at the fused P2 site in these circumstances. For left anterior fascicular VT, Purkinje potential mapping is also performed to identify the optimal ablation site. Conventionally this procedure can be guided by fluoroscopy alone (often facilitated by biplane imaging), but 3-D mapping equipment may be very useful for labelling and returning to sites of interest.

Features of optimal ablation site

- Diastolic potential (P1) in the antegrade limb of the VT circuit (mid-septum) – not necessarily the earliest, but the more apical the site, the less risk of creating LBBB (P1-QRS can be from 30 to 130 ms).
- Tachycardia slowing and termination within 15 seconds of RF onset.
- If this site is ineffective then move to a more proximal site.
- Pre-systolic potential (P2) at the VT exit site if P1 not found.
- With upper septal fascicular VT, identify PS and ablate in this instance during sinus rhythm to prevent missing inadvertent AV block (use lower powers, e.g. 10–20 W, and gradually increase whilst monitoring for junctional rhythm or AV block).

3-D mapping

3-D mapping may be particularly useful where the operator wishes to map the Purkinje potentials and document their relationship to the His but without using multiple catheters. Where only non-sustained VT is present, non-contact mapping may be used (📖 p. 504) but this is very rare and it is often easier to use other techniques (📖 p. 526).

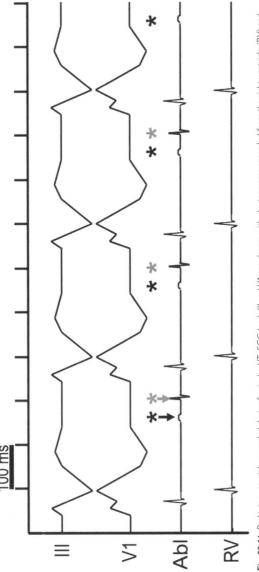

Fig. 22.16 Purkinje potentials recorded during fascicular VT. ECG leads III and V1 are shown with electrograms recorded from the right ventricle (RV) and through the ablation catheter (Abl) at a site in the left ventricle such as that shown fluoroscopically in Fig. 22.14. Compared to Fig. 22.15 the Purkinje potential timings seen on the ablation catheter have changed, with the Purkinje potential (P2) (grey asterisk) still pre-systolic but now the Purkinje potential P1 (black asterisk) is activated antegradely first and precedes P2.

Endpoints for fascicular VT ablation
- Non-inducibility of VT with programmed electrical stimulation after previously inducible VT.
- P1 moves from pre-QRS to post-QRS – indicates block in the direction from P2 to P1, i.e. unidirectional so **not** a reliable endpoint.
- Atrial pacing at different cycle lengths will induce premature ventricular ectopics with the same morphology as the VT ('ventricular echoes') if there is still unidirectional conduction, but these are not seen with bidirectional block between P1 and P2.
- Where pharmacological provocation, e.g. isoprenaline, was initially necessary for VT induction, testing should be performed with isoprenaline again after ablation.

Success and complications
- Success rates are between 90 and 95%, with 5–10% requiring more than one procedure.
- Complications (☐ p. 484): LBBB and AV block may occur. However, as long as the most distal ablation sites are targeted first and care is taken to avoid areas near to the His electrogram, this risk is very small and often only transient.

Troubleshooting the difficult case
Non-inducible tachycardia:
- Try high dose isoprenaline (>10 mcg/min sometimes needed) or epinephrine (25–50 ng/kg/min).
- The Purkinje fibre may have been 'bumped' during mapping – this is relatively easily done as the fibres are very superficial. Need to wait to see if VT inducible after a period of time (up to 30 minutes or more).
- Can map the ventricular echo beats during atrial pacing.
- Can map and ablate Purkinje potentials in sinus rhythm if identified. An anatomical approach is used in this instance (see below), aiming to transect the middle to distal third of the left fascicular tract where Purkinje potentials are recorded. This may be combined with pace mapping but this is often unreliable and the endpoint is difficult to define.

Unable to find good Purkinje potential electrograms:
- Try using a multi-polar catheter if not already being used.
- Change catheter for a different shape/curve, or change the approach, e.g. from transaortic to trans-septal.
- Can perform an anatomical ablation – linear lesion created at mid-septum, perpendicular to the long axis of the LV, 10 to 15 mm proximal to the site of best QRS by pace mapping.

Poor catheter stability:
- Fascicular VT may be very rapid and the excessive cardiac motion causes catheter instability. A different catheter or cryoablation can be used. Also, ablation may be performed during sinus rhythm. Where frequent ventricular ectopy occurs during ablation and displaces the catheter, overdrive pacing the ventricle may also help.

Ablation of bundle branch re-entrant VT

It is important to consider this form of VT in the differential diagnosis of a broad complex tachycardia (📖 p. 190), particularly in patients with structurally abnormal hearts as described on 📖 p. 316. When approaching ablation of these patients, the following are important in the process:

Initial electrophysiological testing, induction, and catheter setup (Fig. 22.17)

- In these patients with a broad complex tachycardia of uncertain origin, a three-wire setup may be used initially. A quadripolar catheter is placed in the high right atrium, in the His bundle position, and in the RV apex. A coronary sinus catheter may also be used, either in addition to or instead of the high right atrial catheter.
- At baseline virtually all patients have HV prolongation (60–110 ms).
- Programmed stimulation from the right ventricle, particularly using a short-long protocol, will normally induce VT (short-long means a standard drive train followed by a relatively early extrastimulus and then a later one by 100–200 ms longer, e.g. S1 600, S2 250, S3 400).
- Rarely left ventricular pacing is required to induce RBBB morphology bundle branch re-entrant VT. NB The induced VT BBB morphology may not match the clinical VT, particularly where the clinical VT was RBBB, but this does not mean the mechanism is different.
- Isoprenaline may be needed to induce VT.
- Diagnostic criteria for bundle branch re-entrant VT are described on 📖 p. 203.

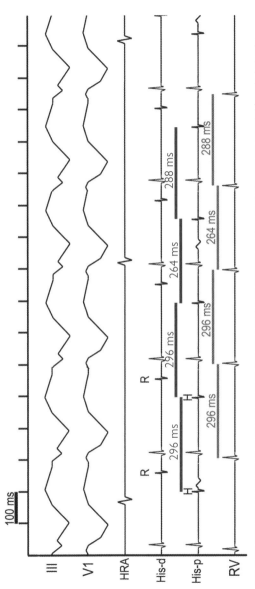

Fig. 22.17 Intracardiac recordings during bundle branch re-entrant VT. ECG leads III and V1 are shown with electrograms recorded from the high right atrium (HRA), His distal (His-d) and proximal (His-p), and the right ventricle (RV). The atrium is dissociated from the ventri-cle confirming VT (with a left bundle branch morphology). The His-d records a right bundle branch potential (R) before every ventricular electrogram. If recorded, a left bundle branch potential would be seen just after the ventricular electrogram followed by His bundle activa-tion eventually (H). Changes in the H-H interval (red) are fol-lowed by changes in the V-V interval (grey).

Standard ablation technique

Ablation of either the right or left main bundle branch will prevent VT. Although left bundle branch disease is more common, the target for ablation is generally the right bundle branch because:

- Ablation of the left bundle involves more extensive ablation of both the anterior and posterior fascicles.
- There is no need for arterial access.
- Even where there is a degree of left bundle conduction disease on the resting ECG, ablation of the RBBB will not necessarily mean a pacemaker is required.

> ### Practical note
>
> Whilst mapping the right bundle it is common to cause transient block by catheter trauma alone. If complete heart block then occurs it is clear that the patient will need a pacemaker if the right bundle is formally ablated. In this situation consider ablating the left bundle branch instead. Also, if mapping of the left bundle is performed and left bundle potentials are only recorded intermittently or after the ventricular electrogram in sinus rhythm, then it is likely that there is complete antegrade LBBB already.

Ablation of the right bundle branch

Commonly a large sweep/'F' curve standard 4 mm ablation catheter is introduced into the RV. The right bundle branch is identified along the basal RV septum (Fig 16.2). As the catheter enters the RV at the basal anterior septum a His electrogram is often recorded. The catheter is then advanced apically (often in the RAO projection) and a right bundle branch potential identified. Often the right bundle branch may be ablated with a single lesion with powers between 20 and 60 W at 60°C.

Features differentiating His from right bundle branch potential

- The absence of an atrial electrogram (occasionally a very small atrial signal) suggests a right bundle branch potential.
- If both electrograms are recorded the His-RBB interval >15 ms.
- If RBB delay is present during sinus rhythm it may be obscured by local ventricular activation and only be visible retrogradely during VT.

Ablation of the left bundle branch

Typically 1–3 cm long and 1 cm wide but there is large individual variation. To record an LBB potential, an ablation catheter (usually small/medium sweep, 'B'/'D' curve) is advanced via a transaortic approach directly towards the inferior apical septum. The catheter is then withdrawn towards the His bundle until an LBB potential is recorded. The LBB often needs more than a single lesion to ablate. Often a line of lesions from the anterior superior septum to the inferior basal septum is required. Care needs to be taken not to ablate the His, which is close. The anterior and posterior fascicles can be targeted (📖 p. 520) but ablation of one alone will not prevent VT.

Features of left bundle branch potential

- Usually 1–1.5 cm inferior to His recording site.
- Potential ventricular interval typically <20 ms.
- A:V ratio of <1:10.

Success and complications

- Success rates are reported to be close to 100% where this form of VT is identified. Recurrence is uncommon.
- Complications (📖 p. 484): High grade AV block occurs in 10–30% and many patients may have an indication for an ICD. Where an ICD is implanted further VT is common but not normally a recurrence of bundle branch re-entrant VT.

Troubleshooting the difficult case

Non-inducible tachycardia:

- Intermittent complete bidirectional BBB or insufficient conduction slowing may make inducibility difficult. Isoprenaline infusion may improve conduction whilst class Ia agents such as procainamide may slow conduction.
- Consider short-long pacing protocols.
- Try left ventricular pacing.

Unable to record/ablate right bundle branch potential:

- Anatomical ablation of the RBB can be performed by ablating perpendicularly to the axis of the RBB distal to where a His signal is recorded.
- Ablate the LBB instead.
- Map/ablate during VT.

VT remains inducible after successful bundle branch ablation:

- Consider other mechanisms for the residual VT, e.g. scar-related VT (inducible in 30–60% of BBB RVT patients after successful bundle branch ablation), an automatic focus, or the initial diagnosis was incorrect (📖 Chapter 8).

AV block risk is high with bundle branch ablation:

- It may be apparent that conduction tissue disease is extensive and the risk of complete AV block is high with ablation. In this case ablate the bundle with the worst intrinsic conduction (📖 p. 530). Also, the need for pacemaker/ICD after ablation is performed must be assessed.

Polymorphic VT/VF ablation

The techniques used for monomorphic VT ablation cannot be applied reliably to polymorphic VT (PMVT) or VF. Premature ventricular beats from relatively predictable anatomical locations have been shown to be the initiators of PMVT/VF in some patients and can therefore be targeted and ablated. Although some clinical success has been demonstrated with this strategy, the numbers of patients are small and the technique relies on the frequency of these PVCs being high enough to perform activation mapping for the best results, or at least to have a 12-lead morphology to perform pace mapping (which as always has inferior clinical efficacy).

PMVT/VF ablation in patients with a structurally normal heart

Survivors of PMVT/VF arrest without structural heart disease have been identified with isolated PVCs of identical morphology that trigger PMVT/VF. These PVCs can be mapped and commonly arise from the RV/LV Purkinje system or RVOT. Purkinje potentials are commonly seen at these sites. During sinus rhythm the potentials are approximately 10–15 ms pre-QRS at the site of the PVC, but between 10 and 150 ms pre-QRS with the initiating PVC. Ablation of these PVCs when identified has been very effective in rendering PMVT/VF non-inducible in these patients.

PMVT/VF ablation in patients with a structurally abnormal heart

Activation and mapping of these PVCs has shown that they arise from Purkinje-type fibres at the scar border zone in patients with structural heart disease and Purkinje-type potentials are again recorded at the sites of successful ablation, if they can be identified.

Epicardial approach

When endocardial mapping/ablation of VT fails, a critical epicardial component of the circuit should be considered. Features suggestive of epicardial VT are shown in Table 22.7.

Routes for epicardial catheter ablation

- Aortic root – for idiopathic outflow tract VT (📖 p. 516).
- Coronary sinus – access to epicardium limited by venous anatomy.
- Coronary arteries – access again limited by anatomy.
- Sub-xiphoid approach.

Sub-xiphoid approach

- Approach is similar to pericardiocentesis.
- Some operators use a special spinal needle (Tuohy needle) with a curved end, which may reduce the risk of cardiac perforation, but a normal pericardiocentesis needle may be used too.
- The puncture is made between the left border of the sub-xiphoid process and the lower left rib.
- The needle is advanced towards the left shoulder, initially at a steep angle to go under the rib and then flattened to aim for the cardiac margin.
- Needle position is then monitored under fluoroscopy.
- In LAO the needle is advanced towards the edge of the dome of the diaphragm where it meets the cardiac silhouette (Fig. 22.18).
- Injections of small amounts (0.5–1 ml of contrast) are used to demonstrate where the needle tip is. When in the sub-phrenic space contrast stains the tissue (Fig. 22.18). As the needle enters the pericardial space there is often slight resistance just before it enters, followed by a sensation of passing through the pericardium. Injected contrast now washes around the pericardium, and remains in the space.
- The guidewire is advanced through the needle and into the pericardial space. There should be no ectopy and the wire should stay within the cardiac silhouette.
- A standard 8 French sheath is inserted over the guidewire into the pericardial space.
- An ablation catheter can then be manipulated around the ventricle and mapping performed in the same way as endocardially.

Practical tip

Given that endocardial ablation in the LV may have been attempted prior to epicardial mapping, it is likely that the patient will have been formally anticoagulated. This may raise some concern about possible visceral perforation. Some operators will place a sheath in the pericardial space before endocardial mapping in patients with VT undergoing ablation, particularly where the VT ECG is suggestive of an epicardial circuit (Table 22.7).

Table 22.7 12-lead ECG criteria suggestive of an epicardial VT circuit

ECG finding	Definition
QRS duration >198 ms	
Pseudo delta wave >34 ms	Earliest ventricular activation to earliest fast deflection in any precordial lead
Intrinsicoid deflection time ≥85 ms	Interval from earliest ventricular activation to nadir of the first S wave in any precordial lead
RS complex duration ≥121 ms	Interval from earliest ventricular activation to peak of R wave in lead V2
Delayed maximal peak deflection index ≥0.54	Interval from earliest ventricular activation to peak of R or nadir of S wave divided by total QRS duration

Success and complications

- Success rates from epicardial VT ablation may be >80% depending on the underlying substrate (greater with ischaemic than non-ischaemic VT).
- Complications of epicardial VT ablation include damage to the epicardial coronary arteries, acute pericarditis, ventricular perforation or other visceral damage from a sub-xiphoid approach, and theoretically phrenic nerve damage.

Troubleshooting

Avoiding the epicardial coronary arteries:

It is essential to perform coronary angiography prior to ablating at a given epicardial site to ensure there are no branches that are big enough to be seen within 1 cm of the catheter tip.

- Some operators will perform angiography at the start of the case and use these initial images to delineate safe areas to ablate.
- Many operators will perform angiography once the ablation catheter is in a site for ablation and immediately identify the relationship of the epicardial coronary arteries.

Inadequate energy delivery:

- Epicardial fat may insulate tissue and prevent adequate energy delivery to the underlying myocardial tissue.
- With a lack of cooling from blood flow, standard RF catheter tip temperatures rise rapidly, limiting power delivery. Irrigated RF is helpful, but the irrigant accumulates in the pericardial space and must be drained through the side arm of the percutaneous sheath to prevent cardiac tamponade (continuous monitoring of arterial pressure is useful to identify this).

Post-cardiotomy ablation:

Access to the pericardial space and manipulation within the space may be more difficult where the pericardium has already been instrumented and/or adhesions are present (e.g. after previous open cardiac surgery). This does not prevent use of this approach but access may be more difficult – adhesions are generally less common at the inferior cardiac margin.

Pericarditis:

Pericarditic chest pain is common after this approach but is usually managed easily:

- Routine administration of non-steroidal anti-inflammatory drugs (e.g. ibuprofen 400 mg tds) is sufficient in most cases to limit pain.
- If the pericardial space is aspirated to dryness with no bleeding evident then the sheath should be removed at the end of the case. Leaving a sheath/pericardial drain *in situ* increases the likelihood of ongoing pericarditis.
- The use of other agents (e.g. steroids) injected into the pericardial space may limit the pericarditic reaction but no definite evidence is available to support this in routine practice.

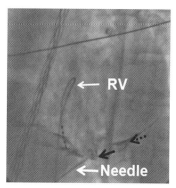

Fig. 22.18 Epicardial approach. **Top panel:** The needle (labelled) is seen to enter the pericardium with small volumes of contrast injected and initially staining the parietal pericardium (solid arrow) and then filling the pericardial space (dashed arrow). The quadripolar catheter is in the right ventricle (RV).

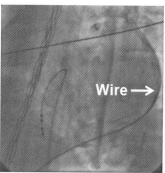

Middle panel: The guidewire (labelled) is passed through the needle into the pericardial space. The wire should move freely in the space and not outside the cardiac silhouette. No ventricular ectopy is seen if the wire is in the pericardial space.

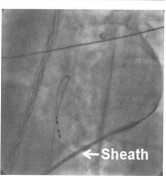

Lower panel: A dilator is used to dilate the tract into the pericardial space and then a standard sheath (labelled) is inserted over the guidewire. An ablation catheter can then be passed through the sheath into the pericardial space. NB If an open irrigated catheter is used then fluid will accumulate in the pericardial space and eventually cause tamponade. This is prevented by intermittently aspirating any accumulated fluid through the sheath side-arm.

Alcohol ablation

Alcohol ablation has been used successfully in cases of VT where endocardial mapping fails, particularly where the origin is felt to be in the deep septum. Its use is less common now that percutaneous epicardial VT ablation is more routinely performed.

Technique (Fig. 22.19)

- The coronary artery that supplies the territory of interest is catheterized using a standard percutaneous coronary intervention (PCI) guide catheter.
- A PCI guidewire is then used to select the specific branch of the coronary artery that is believed to supply the area of myocardium to be ablated.
- A selective balloon occlusion catheter is advanced over the wire and ice-cold saline is first infused, with the balloon inflated, to demonstrate termination of the VT (if the VT is not incessant then it is induced). If VT does not terminate another branch is selected and the saline infused again. This is repeated until the branch that terminates VT is identified.
- The balloon is deflated and the alcohol prepared. The VT is likely to resume if it was previously incessant. The balloon is then inflated again and 1 ml of 100% ethanol infused into the vessel. Care needs to be taken to ensure complete occlusion of the vessel before alcohol infusion, normally by injecting a small amount of contrast to demonstrate that there is no leak. The balloon is left inflated for 8–10 minutes after alcohol infusion.
- It may be necessary to ablate more than one branch to render the VT non-inducible (e.g. more than one septal branch of the left anterior descending artery for a septal VT). Once non-inducible, the coronary artery should be checked with a coronary angiogram to ensure no damage to the main vessel.
- If the VT is not incessant a small French diagnostic mapping catheter (e.g. the Cardima Pathfinder, Fremont, California) may be positioned in the branch of interest and pace mapping performed.

Complications

- A rise in CK/troponin is expected as is some degree of pain, which can be controlled with analgesia.
- AV nodal damage has been described, requiring permanent pacemaker insertion.
- Damage to a significant amount of viable myocardium may lead to worsening heart failure.

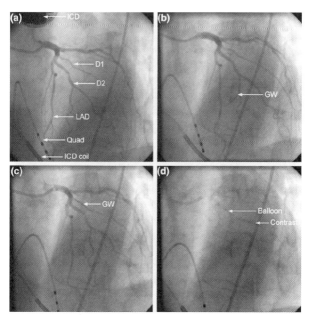

Fig. 22.19 Ethanol ablation of left ventricular VT. (a) Left coronary angiography (LCA) demonstrates the coronary artery anatomy. The left anterior descending artery (LAD) and its diagonal branches (D1 and D2) are labelled. An ICD, the right ventricular ICD coil, and a quadripolar EP catheter (Quad) can be seen. (b) A standard angioplasty guide wire is passed through the catheter and into the LAD. It is initially placed in a branch of D2. (c) This is not the desired branch so the wire is pulled back and positioned in D1. (d) A small balloon catheter is advanced over the wire, the wire removed, and cold saline infused (see text on opposite page). If this terminates VT then a small amount of contrast is injected to confirm there is no leak into the main vessel and then alcohol injected to ablate the myocardium (see text opposite). (Figure kindly provided by Dr Anthony Chow, The Heart Hospital, London, U.K.)

Index